Resources for People with Disabilities

A National Directory

Second Edition

Ferguson Publishing Company, Chicago, Illinois

Editor: Shawn Woodyard

Cover Design: Shelly Leonard Design

Ferguson Publishing Staff:
Andrew Morkes, *Managing Editor, Career Publications*
Carol Yehling, *Senior Editor*
Anne Paterson, *Editor*
Nora Walsh, *Editorial Assistant*

Library of Congress Cataloging-in-Publication Data

Resources for people with disabilities : a national directory / edited by Shawn Woodyard.—2nd ed.
p. cm.

Includes bibliographical references and index.

ISBN 0-89434-309-2
1. Handicapped—Services for—United States—Directories. 2. Handicapped—Services for—United States—Finance—Directories. 3. Self-help devices for the disabled—United States—Directories. I. Woodyard, Shawn.

HV 1553 .R48 2000
362.4'048'02573—dc21 00-039317

Published and Distributed by
Ferguson Publishing Company
200 West Jackson Boulevard, Suite 700
Chicago, Illinois 60606
800-306-9941
http://www.fergpubco.com

Printed in the United States of America

X-9

Table of Contents

Foreword

Approximately twenty-five years ago, I left the world of the able-bodied and entered the world of people with a disability. I was twenty-seven. I had undergone a series of tests that resulted in my being diagnosed with multiple sclerosis. At the time there was little help for people who did not fit the mold of the average able-bodied American. Welfare programs and rudimentary job training programs took care of us as long as we stayed segregated from the general population. But if we wanted to remain in the world of the able-bodied, we were pretty much on our own.

For years I had been experiencing some of the symptoms that were eventually defined as MS, but not until 1975, when I was working as a correctional officer at Montana State Prison, did I begin to develop a limp. Since I knew that my condition would only get worse, I applied for every desk job that came along. Time and time again, I was denied these jobs. There were jobs in the tower, jobs writing grants, and jobs sorting mail in the mail room, but these were always offered to someone else, even when I was the only candidate with a college degree. At the time such discrimination was not discussed, and there were no laws to back up complaints against employers. Out of ignorance, I accepted my employer's decision. I came to work on my crutches, handed in my uniform, and quit the job. I just didn't feel safe walking on crutches in a locked cell with sixty inmates. I applied for government programs and was accepted immediately, since that was the way different people were handled. I was expected to collect my check and stay out of the way.

Instead, I contacted the vocational rehabilitation office. The folks there were accustomed to finding mediocre jobs that were more of a hobby than a vocation. I wasn't interested in taking a position that was just time-consuming, so I began to explore the limits of the system. With the help of a counselor who was willing to take a chance, I became their first client to enter college at the postgraduate level. I started an M.B.A. program at the University of Montana.

All around the country people were challenging the establishment. Laws were passed that required any recipient of federal funds to make its programs accessible. Building modifications such as ramps were just beginning, but money was scarce and changes were slow. After three years of finding creative solutions to the accessibility problems at my university, I completed what should have been a two-year program and received an M.B.A. At that point I thought my search for meaningful employment would be easy, but I found that the struggle was just beginning.

I decided to pursue a job with the federal government, assuming that, since it had passed laws requiring accessibility, it would be a good place to start. To get a federal job, an evaluation test was needed. On the application, there was a space in which I was to request special accommodations. I asked that the test be given in a room with no stairs and easy access to a rest room. When I got to the testing site, there were two stairs into the room and the closest restroom (a ladies room) was four floors up. Though given the option of taking the test at another time, I decided to get it over with. Even after receiving a score of 98 percent on the test, however, I was offered only one interview for a job in a far away city.

After looking for work in other areas and being turned down, I took an extended trip that included Washington, DC. I was surprised by the building modifications that had been made. I could actually roll my wheelchair into the Lincoln Memorial, the Washington Monument, and the Smithsonian Institution. These experiences were so unlike my university days, but after all, this city was a showcase for the world and the center of funding. When I returned to Montana, I was determined to help my local area achieve standards that were equal or at least similar.

It was 1980, and the independent living movement was building momentum throughout the country. When a local center was established in my hometown, I started to work with them. At Summit Independent Living Center, I did not only peer counseling to help people adjust to their own disability but also advocacy work to bring about changes in accessibility and disability rights. At first these changes were slow to develop and usually involved much letter-writing as well as testimony before legislative committees. Finally, laws changed to make compliance mandatory rather than voluntary, and the rate of change accelerated. Assistive technology expanded along with advancements in computers, and the world became friendlier to people with disabilities. More and more people became involved, and accessible parking spaces, curb cuts, and ramps began to appear around the state in testament to our advocacy work.

Because of the Tech Act of 1988, funding was made available that allowed me to work with individuals in locating and purchasing equipment and technology to meet their specific needs. Although I would help people to meet specific goals, there was always the goal of people being independent and advocating for themselves. The emphasis was on self-reliance—provide a curb cut for someone and they get off of their block; teach someone how to get a curb cut for themselves and you have given them access to the world. This was the motto of the independent living movement.

Unfortunately, most programs for people with disabilities rely upon grants for funding. Patient services often have to be sacrificed, so that there is enough time and staff to write grants that justify the existence of the program. In addition there is an apathy among people who see parking spaces and ramps and feel that enough has been done for this minority group. On the other hand, tremendous strides have been made, especially with legislation that provides leverage in fighting job and housing discrimination and insuring access to assistive technology, public spaces, and public services. Even the university that I attended now has a full-time staff to help students with disabilities and to correct accessibility problems.

There are many areas where improvements can still be made. Looking back over the years, I do not regret the battles fought. If there had been access to the resources contained in this book, my experiences would have been easier. But I do not see my past as a hardship; I have found the challenges to be rewarding. With today's resources, a person can accomplish just about anything, including working and becoming (or continuing to be) a contributing member of society. The only challenge for which we still have no resource is that of changing people's attitudes toward disabilities. Only time and integration will break down the barriers brought about by stereotypes: Store clerks and waiters still ignore me and speak to my companion when asking about my needs; and even a doctor, trying to make polite small talk during a recent exam, asked innocently how long it had been since I had quit working. My answer, of course, was that I am still working and will continue as long as there are barriers to overcome.

John Bradford
January 6, 1998
Missoula, Montana

Introduction

Information—The First Step to Access

What Is a Handicap?

Over the last 25 years, a portion of our society has emerged after being invisible and forgotten—invisible because they could not access public spaces, forgotten because the adage "out of sight, out of mind" holds true for too many of us. Rather than being handicapped themselves, people with disabilities have found that their environment and the attitudes of the people around them have handicapped them. With the help of new technologies, changing attitudes, and better legislation, however, things have begun to improve. For example, people with disabilities are finding it easier to shop for their own groceries, attend universities, and remain active members of the workforce.

As this population speaks up, it reminds us again and again of the need to escape the old stereotype of being "taken care of" and move on toward the idea of independence and self-determination. Fulfilling this need requires access to information about assistive technologies, about funding to purchase those technologies, and about organizations that can help people with disabilities to take their places as active and productive members of society.

Resources for People with Disabilities: A National Directory provides easy access to this information. With more than 8,000 listings, it is the most comprehensive directory of its kind. Readers can explore and compare options for purchasing assistive computer devices, participating in vocational rehabilitation, joining an online support group, or seeking legal aid, for example. Librarians and teachers will find that this one-point reference work is an excellent resource for launching people on their individual quests to make personal decisions about their lives.

Who Are the People with Disabilities?

The Census of Americans with Disabilities: 1991\1992, published in January 1994, reports that nearly 50 million people with disabilities live outside institutions. This number translates to approximately 20 percent of the population. In other words, one out of every five people has trouble performing one or more daily-living tasks, and these are the people with permanent disabilities. Other people, perhaps as many as one out of every three, experience a temporary disability, such as a broken arm or leg. As the American population continues to grow, disability numbers will no doubt continue to increase as well. Whether these disabilities are permanent or temporary, people need some sort of assistance to make up for the losses they experience.

Introduction

The following numbers for people with physical disabilities come from the President's Council on Employment of People with Disabilities and were last updated in January 1997. See the Council's web site (http://www.pcepd.gov) for more information.

PEOPLE WITH DISABILITIES

Men	22,900,000
Women	26,000,000
Under Age 15	6 %
Ages 15-64	60 %
Ages 21-64	56 %
Ages 65 and older	34 %
African Americans	4,100,000
Asian and Pacific Islanders	515,000
Persons of Hispanic Origin	2,400,000
Whites not of Hispanic Origin	22,600,000
American Indian, Eskimo, or Aleut	285,000

PEOPLE WITH SEVERE DISABILITIES

Total	24,100,000
Men	9,900,000
Women	14,200,000

EMPLOYMENT STATUS

Total Employed Persons aged 21-64	108,700,000
Total Employed Persons with Disabilities	14,300,000
Men	7,900,000
Women	6,400,000
Total Employed Persons with Severe Disabilities	2,900,000
Men	1,300,000
Women	1,600,000

LEADING CAUSES AND RESULTS OF DISABILITY

More than 27 million individuals aged 15 and over reported having a limitation in physical or daily living activity, causing a disability. Following are the leading causes and results.

Arthritis/rheumatism	7,200,000
Back/spinal problems	5,700,000
Heart trouble	4,600,000
Lung/respiratory trouble	2,800,000
High blood pressure	2,200,000
Stiffness or deformity of the foot, leg, arm, or hand	2,000,000
Diabetes	1,600,000
Use a wheelchair	1,500,000
Use a cane, walker, or crutches for six months or longer	4,000,000
Even when wearing corrective lenses, have difficulty seeing words or letters in ordinary newsprint	8,100,000
Even when wearing corrective lenses, cannot see the words or letters in newsprint at all	1,600,000
Have difficulty hearing a normal conversation with another person	10,000,000
Can not hear what is said in a normal conversation	924,000

HEALTH CARE COVERAGE

Following is the status of health care insurance coverage for 29.5 million Americans with disabilities between the ages of 15 and 64.

People without a disability	135,600,000
Private insurance coverage	80 %
Government plan coverage	5.2 %
No coverage	14.8 %
People with a disability	16,300,000
Private insurance coverage	74.1 %
Government plan coverage	7.2 %
No coverage	18.7 %
People with a severe disability	13,200,000
Private insurance coverage	48.1 %
Government plan coverage	36.2 %
No coverage	15.7 %

Attitudes and Stereotypes

People with disabilities still depend heavily on the government for health care and general living expenses, a dependence that perpetuates negative stereotypes and attitudes toward disabilities.

One of the most common stereotypes about people with disabilities is that they are impoverished and, therefore, are not viable consumers. This misconception makes businesses less willing to spend the money necessary to make their buildings and products accessible. The more people with disabilities are seen in the workplace, however, the more this misconception is dispelled; but in order for most people with disabilities to be employed, some sort of resource modification to overcome a particular limitation is usually needed. Herein lies the importance of access to information about helpful resources. When people with disabilities have access to modern resources, they become more independent, which helps to dispel the negative stereotypes, which leads to greater accessibility.

Another common misconception is that a physical limitation prevents a person from making and communicating his or her own decisions. Many times, for example, store clerks or waiters will talk to a companion rather than speak directly to a person using a wheelchair. This mistake usually involves the method of payment, which is tied to the poverty stereotype. As individuals use modern technologies to become more independent, people will see that consumers with disabilities are able to handle their own business, even though the method may be unconventional.

Changing attitudes means responding to people as people first, without concentrating on their particular disability. It means understanding that the expressions "overcome a disability" or "in spite of a disability" inaccurately reflect the problems faced by people with disabilities, who succeed not in spite of their disabilities but in spite of an inaccessible and discriminatory society.

History of the Independent Living and Disability Rights Movements

As it did with the civil rights movement and affirmative action programs, government has stepped in with laws and mandates to level the playing field and eliminate stereotypes for people with disabilities. It all began back in 1962, when Ed Roberts rolled onto the campus at the University of California, Berkeley, to begin classes. Nobody knew how to handle the "helpless cripple" who wouldn't take no for an answer. Buildings were inaccessible, alternate formats of learning materials were inconceivable, and there were no appropriate living quarters.

As he chipped away at the barriers, Roberts saw the need for laws to help with enforcement. Ed Roberts completed his education and, in 1975, was made director of California's Department of Rehabilitation. He is known as "the father of the independent living movement." Because of the efforts of Ed Roberts, the government provided funds to set up regional independent living centers. Their philosophy is simple: "Provide a curb cut and a person gets off their block; teach them how to get their own curb cut, and they gain access to the whole world." These centers teach people to advocate for themselves and change deficiencies in laws as well as in structures. The following list shows the major pieces of legislation that have resulted from such advocacy.

1964 Civil Rights Act prohibits discrimination against various minority groups in America, most notably women and minorities categorized by race, religion, and national origin.

1968 Architectural Barriers Act prohibits architectural barriers in all federally owned or leased buildings.

1970 Urban Mass Transit Act requires that all newly purchased mass-transit vehicles be equipped with lifts. The American Public Transit Association (APTA) sought and won a court injunction barring implementation of the proposed regulations, virtually holding this law hostage until the ADA passed.

1973 Rehabilitation Act Title V (particularly Sections 503 and 504) forbids discrimination on the basis of disability in programs receiving federal funds. The language used is parallel to that of the Civil Rights Act of 1964.

1975 Individuals with Disabilities Education Act (formerly called the Education of All Handicapped Children Act) requires a free, appropriate public education in an integrated setting for children with disabilities. This law has been the least effective of all those passed to support the integration of people with disabilities into our society because it has created, essentially, a separate, segregated system of "special education." This law is commonly referred to by its acronym, IDEA.

1988 Air Carrier Access Act provides for equal access on private airlines and air carriers; forbids discrimination on the basis of disability in air travel.

1988 Civil Rights Restoration Act clarifies that any organization or corporation receiving federal funds may not discriminate in any of its programs on the basis of race, ethnicity, religion, national origin, gender, age, or disability. For the first time, people with disabilities were included as a protected class with other classes protected by the Civil Rights Act of 1964.

1988 Fair Housing Amendments Act prohibits discrimination against people with disabilities (along with families that have children) in housing and provides for universal design (architectural accessibility) in new construction of housing units of various types and sizes beginning in March 1991.

1988 Technology-Related Assistance for Individuals with Disabilities Act (Tech Act) established money to form state agencies that help people with disabilities to obtain assistive devices by evaluating their needs and finding sources for equipment and funding.

1990 Americans with Disabilities Act creates broad civil rights protections for people with disabilities; modeled after the Civil Rights Act of 1964 and Section 504 of the Rehabilitation Act of 1973.

1992 Civil Rights Act permits women and individuals with disabilities to sue for punitive damages when employment discrimination has been proven in court (up to a maximum of $250,000).

1996 The Telecommunications Act of 1996 requires manufacturers of telecommunications equipment or customer-premises equipment to ensure that the equipment is designed, developed, and fabricated to be accessible to and usable by people with disabilities.

1996 The Small Business Job Protection Act of 1996 creates the Work Opportunity Tax Credit to encourage employers to hire certain groups of individuals, including people with disabilities.

We will examine four of these more carefully in order to understand better the rights of people with disabilities and the opportunities that they can pursue when the proper connections and resources are available.

Individuals with Disabilities Education Act (IDEA). This law guarantees people with disabilities, especially children and young adults, educational opportunities. These are some of its basic principles:

1. All children with disabilities are entitled to a free public education appropriate to their needs.
2. As much as possible, children with disabilities should be educated with students without disabilities, as close to home as possible, and in the least restrictive environment.
3. Children with disabilities must be provided with supplemental services, such as physical therapy and assistive technologies.
4. A fair assessment, with parental agreement, must be completed to determine the student's educational needs.

The Individual Education Program (IEP) for each child must be reviewed annually to incorporate products and services that maximize educational goals. Assistive technologies cannot be denied a student, if they are part of the IEP. Assistive technology devices are not restricted to those used in school; the law applies to devices used in an individual's home as well. See page 9 of this book for a list of vendors of assistive technology.

Americans with Disabilities Act (ADA). This law expands upon earlier accessibility mandates and other civil rights legislation that made discrimination illegal, since disabilities were not included in those previous laws. The act covers more than 900 separate disabilities. In specific sections, it covers accessibility and accommodation requirements for all public places, state and local government services, transportation, employment, and communications. This law strives to ensure equal opportunities for people with disabilities in all these areas.

Employers must make reasonable accommodations for qualified workers with disabilities, so that job requirements and structure do not become barriers to employment. These accommodations must be made unless the employer shows that it would cause undue hardship. Accommodations usually include assistive technologies or technology access. If you have had trouble with an employer, potential employer, or public facility, see *Legal Assistance Organizations* on page 427 of this book.

Technology-Related Assistance for Individuals with Disabilities Act (Tech Act). This act mandates that federal funds be provided to assist states in developing programs that allow easy access to assistive technologies, technology services, and information. A landmark phrase in this legislation is "consumer responsive," which means that states must evaluate and respond to the concerns of people with disabilities.

The act set standard definitions for assistive technologies that have been used in subsequent legislation. Assistive technology is defined as "any tool that increases, maintains, or improves functional capabilities of individuals with disabilities" in such areas as seating, mobility, daily living, and environmental control. These devices are not necessarily computerized. They can be as simple as a hand-held magnifier.

For a list of agencies funded by the Tech Act, see *State Tech Act Programs & Organizations* on page 555. Funds are generally used to provide information and referral in order to eliminate barriers that prevent access to assistive technologies by consumers. A list of funding sources for purchasing assistive technology begins on page 353.

Rehabilitation Act Amendments of 1992. People with significant disabilities have benefited the most from these amendments in gaining access to rehabilitative services. Earlier laws evaluated people on their "employability," "feasibility of employment," and "rehabilitation potential." The amendments are based on the presumption that a person with a severe disability can achieve employment and other rehabilitation goals. The older laws did not provide for rehabilitative support except in cases of "full" employment potential.

Vocational rehabilitation agencies are now required to look for employment solutions rather than evaluate needs. Support to gain employment must now be given unless there is absolutely no possibility that an individual is employable, even with the aid of assistive devices. This way of regarding disabilities is a significant turnaround from previous attitudes. The burden of finding the proper technology is placed upon government agencies that are, in most cases, unaware of the most recent technologies. By using this book, people can match their needs to the proper equipment and receive support from state vocational agencies in order to purchase the equipment. See the sections in this book on *Vocational Assistance & Employment Organizations* (page 617) and *Rehabilitation Centers* (page 472).

Assistive Technology

Understanding the Basics

When he's on a baseball diamond coaching his team of Little Leaguers, Bill Chatterton doesn't think much about technology. He's more concerned about whether the eleven-year-old outfielder will be able to catch a pop fly.

Ask Chatterton about the assistive technology that allows him to use a computer, though, and he'll say without hesitation that it has "opened up a new life" for him. In 1991, Chatterton was in a motorcycle accident that resulted in a severe spinal injury causing paralysis from the neck down. After five years on a ventilator, Chatterton discovered that he could function without it, and he began attending a state university. At first, he didn't have a computer and was reliant on other people for a number of tasks, including carrying books and papers back and forth from school and turning pages as he read from textbooks. "It was very time consuming," he recalls. After one semester, he purchased a computer, which he operates via an infrared dot placed with adhesive on his nose. Now, his textbooks are scanned and put on disk by the college's disability services, and notes and assignments are sent directly to his computer so that he can view them without assistance. "I have an incredible amount of freedom," he says. In fact, despite his studies and his part-time research work at the university, Chatterton has time left over to coach not just the Little League team but also a YMCA basketball team.

For an increasing number of people with disabilities, computers and assistive technology are making it possible to tackle everyday tasks and activities more independently than ever before. This equipment has also drawn people with disabilities into the workplace, public libraries, and classrooms, where they can be recognized as peers and given equal opportunities.

In its simplest definition, assistive technology is anything that provides alternatives to the standard way of using a computer's keyboard, monitor, or printer. What paved the way for the explosion of new assistive equipment was the Technology-Related Assistance for Individuals with Disabilities Act. Better known as the Tech Act, it focused on developing state-by-state programs that have a lasting impact on the way people with disabilities access and obtain technology devices. In every state, Tech Act projects offer such services as referral centers, assistance in obtaining devices, equipment exchange and recycling, financial loans, and training.

In spite of the advancements of the past decade, the science of making computer hardware and programs accessible to everyone with a disability is still evolving. "Universal access is, and will continue to be, a tough nut to crack, until there are widely accepted protocols [for input and output] that can be put into a modality each computer user can access," points out Denis Anson, author of *Alternative Computer Access: Making Appropriate Selections.* "A software package that is perfectly accessible to a blind user might still be completely inaccessible to a person with a spinal injury or a person with spastic cerebral palsy."

As Anson indicates, it's not a one-size-fits-all selection process, and it's important to find assistive equipment that accommodates your individual needs. The following sections will get you started exploring the assistive technologies available to specific disability populations. For more personalized guidance, contact the Tech Act project in your state, a vocational rehabilitation counselor, or one of the other resources listed in this section.

Mobility Impairments

For people with mobility impairments, the key word is adjustability. Components such as the desk, chair, armrests, monitor, and keyboard all need to be positioned according to an individual's needs. An adjustable-height desk, for example, allows someone in a wheelchair to get close enough to the monitor, even when the computer is shared by several users. This is more than an issue of comfort. "The height of a computer in relation to the wheelchair is critical for someone with a severe spinal cord injury. You don't want to do something that causes secondary strain," emphasizes Jude Monson, education coordinator for an independent living center.

A person who cannot use a standard keyboard because of limited use of his or her hands can use a headpointer, mouthstick, or other mechanical pointing device to press keys on the keyboard. There also are lightweight head-tracking devices that require only a small, dot-sized item placed on a person's face. These devices utilize an infrared beam to access an on-screen keyboard on the computer. In addition, there are a number of keyboard adaptations. Expanded keyboards have keys that are spaced farther apart to help people with limited fine motor control. Conversely, smaller-than-standard keyboards are useful for those who use one hand to type or who lack the range of motion to use a larger keyboard.

Other assistive solutions are the result of new software utilities. Someone who types using one of the devices mentioned above, for instance, cannot easily use programs that require a person to simultaneously press two or more keys (such as "Shift" and "D"). Sticky keys have solved that problem; they stay pressed down so that sequential, rather than simultaneous, keystrokes will work. Repeat keys eliminate the problem of unwanted key repetitions, caused when a person with limited motor control can't release a key before it starts to repeat. Slow keys are helpful for people who often strike unwanted keys before hitting the one they want. These keys have to be pressed longer in order to be decisively selected, thus eliminating excessive corrections. Another item that can help with making a precise selection on the keyboard is a keyboard guard, a simple template with holes over each key. Similarly, plastic disk guides make it easier to insert and remove diskettes from a computer's disk drive.

Word-prediction software is useful for people with limited mobility and for people who tire easily from typing. It reduces input strokes by "guessing" the rest of a word or phrase after several keystrokes are made. Word abbreviation software (in which you could type "imdy" or "imy" for the word "immediately") is also effective.

As an alternative to typing, speech-input systems (also called voice-recognition systems) respond to voice commands. These systems require "discrete" speech; that is, the person has to pause between words to indicate that sounds should be interpreted as words. Speech input can enable a person to compose an essay on word processing software, surf the Internet, or search for files on the hard drive, among other functions. Bill Chatterton says that it took some time to "train" his system to recognize his speech patterns. "But now, I've got the computer set up to respond to voice commands to open doors in my house and turn the stereo on and off," he says.

Visual Impairments

Low Vision. Two of the most common assistive technologies for people with low vision are screen-enlargement software and a large (ideally, at least seventeen-inch) monitor. The screen-enlargement software allows everything on the computer screen to appear in a larger-than-standard font. Some people also find that adjusting the foreground and background colors on the monitor can be helpful. For instance, people with light sensitivity can usually read white text on a black background best.

A scanner allows a person to input text from any source (such as a magazine article or class syllabus), then use screen enlargement software to enlarge it.

Inputting on a standard keyboard is usually not problematic for people with low vision, but those just learning to type might find large-print key labels helpful.

Blindness. While most people who are blind are comfortable using standard keyboards, Braille keyboards are another option. Other available Braille devices include Braille printers and refreshable displays that provide detailed, line-by-line Braille translation of the text on the computer screen.

Paul Peterson works full time, running both a community disability advocacy program and a peer-support program. His disabilities stem from diabetes; he has no vision, is hearing impaired in one ear, and uses a wheelchair because of nerve damage. To do his job, he makes extensive use of screen-reading software and a speech synthesizer that speaks the text out loud. Since he types on a standard keyboard, he finds it particularly useful to have the computer read aloud as he types. He also uses a scanner to scan printed material into his computer in order to store or read it easily. "I wouldn't be able to do my work without [my computer]," he acknowledges. "It would be monumentally expensive for my office to hire a full-time person to read everything to me." For taking notes and keeping track of his schedule, Paul also uses a small portable device that has a seven-key Braille keyboard and a "voice."

Hearing Impairments

Generally, hearing impairments do not affect a person's ability to use a computer. Most computer operating systems now have built-in visual cues—such as a flashing screen or musical note in one corner of the screen—as alternatives to computer sound cues.

Speech Impairments

A person with a serious speech impairment who wants to communicate verbally in class, at work, or in other settings can use a portable communication device (also called a speech synthesizer) as his or her voice. The user can input frequently used sentences or can type out an original sentence, then press a button to make the device "speak."

Learning Disabilities

Many computer users with learning disabilities are utilizing adaptive tools designed originally for visually impaired users. Scanners and voice-output systems, for instance, can help people who have trouble comprehending what they read directly from books. Screen-enlargement software can assist people who have certain reading difficulties.

Other helpful software features are real-time spell checking, vocalized text (which talks as you type), word highlighting, and word prediction.

What's on the Horizon?

Typically, when a new computer technology sweeps the nation, there's a lag before computer users with disabilities are provided with adaptive solutions. However, more technology manufacturers are recognizing the potential in this large group of consumers. Sun Microsystems and IBM recently announced that they are making special "tool kits" for developers so that new applications can be made accessible when they are first released. Changes like this will make it possible for people with disabilities to work and study on a level playing field with their nondisabled peers.

Another obstacle for people with disabilities is the technology that exists outside the home and workplace. Going out into the "real world" and trying to use an ATM, for instance, presents a barrier. To use the touchscreen, a person has to be able to both reach and visually read the screen. Not being able to use an ATM isn't the end of the world, but now that similar electronic information systems are being used in education and employment, their accessibility to people with disabilities is becoming crucial. The Trace Center at the University of Wisconsin-Madison works with designers to integrate disability access features into these technologies. When you stop by your bank's ATM next year, don't be surprised if it talks back to you. Also in the works is a "talking fingertip" design that will allow people who are blind or have low vision to hear the screen instead of reading it.

Sources

Action Without Borders

350 Fifth Avenue, Suite 6614
New York, NY 10118
212-843-3973
info@idealist.org
http://www.idealist.org

A network of individuals and organizations that share ideas, information, and resources in order to help people live free, dignified, and productive lives.

Alliance for Technology Access

2175 E. Francisco Boulevard, Suite L
San Rafael, CA 94901
415-455-4575
atainfo@ataccess.org
http://www.ataccess.org/

ATA is a nationwide network of resource centers that are dedicated to providing information and support services to children and adults with disabilities and to increasing their use of standard, assistive, and informative technologies.

DO-IT

University of Washington
PO Box 354842
Seattle, WA 98195-4842
206-685-DOIT
doit@u.washington.edu
http://www.washington.edu/doit

DO-IT (Disabilities, Opportunities, Internetworking, and Technology) works to increase the participation of individuals with disabilities in academic programs and careers.

Rehabilitation Engineering and Assistive Technology Society of North America (RESNA)

700 N. Moore Street, Suite 1540
Arlington, VA 22209-1903
703-524-6686
TTY: 703-524-6639
http://www.resna.org/reshome.htm

Contact RESNA or visit its web site to find information about Tech Act projects in your home state.

Trace Research and Development Center

University of Wisconsin-Madision
5901 Research Park Boulevard
Madison, WI 53719-1252
608-262-6966
TTY: 608-263-5408
info@trace.wisc.edu
http://www.trace.wisc.edu

This is an interdisciplinary research, development, and resource center on technology and disability located at the University of Wisconsin at Madison.

Computers & Technology

These companies develop, sell, or distribute items related to technology and computers. The items may include computer hardware and software, communication aids, or controls such as switches.

2JT Incorporated
PO Box 55287
Washington, DC 20040
202-829-7577
Disability Served: all

This company manufactures a telephone holder for standard and cordless telephones.

A4 Tech (USA) Corporation
20256 Paseo Robles
Walnut, CA 91789
909-468-0071
Disability Served: all

This company manufactures a cordless mouse, trackballs and joysticks that emulate mouse controls, flatbed scanners, modified keyboards, and other specialty mouses.

Abacus
5370 52nd Street
Grand Rapids, MI 49512
616-698-0330, 800-451-4319
Disability Served: all

This company designs a mouse emulator software program.

Abaton Technology Corp.
5020 Brandin Court
Fremont, CA 94538-3140
510-683-2226, 800-444-5321
Disability Served: all

This company manufactures a trackball that emulates mouse control and an optical character recognition scanner.

Ability Center of Greater Toledo
Rehabilitation Technology Department
Sylvania, OH 43560
419-885-5733
Disability Served: all

The Center makes a keyboard wrist support to alleviate repetitive motion disorders.

Ability Research, Inc.
PO Box 1721
Minnetonka, MN 55345-1721
612-939-0121
http://www.skypoint.com/~ability/
Disability Served: all

This company manufactures and markets assistive technology devices for persons with physical and/or cognitive disabilities. One product is the Action Voice, a digital voice recorder and communicator.

Able Ergonomics Corporation
11305 Rancho Bernardo Road, Suite 116
San Diego, CA 92127
619-675-0040
Disability Served: all

This company manufactures keyboard wrist supports, rotating desk organizers, and computer monitor stands.

Able-Phone
7061 Claremont Mesa Boulevard, Suite 201
San Diego, CA 92111
619-296-9705, 619-537-2918
Disability Served: all

This company manufactures a variety of telephones to accommodate persons with disabilities, including speaker phones and cordless phones with headset receivers. The company also manufactures wireless remote controls.

AbleNet, Inc.
1081 Tenth Avenue, SE
Minneapolis, MN 55414-1312
612-379-0956, 800-322-0956
Disability Served: all

This company manufactures a wide variety of switches, including pull switches, touch switches, button switches, and switch adapters.

AbleNet also makes direct selection communicators, mounting hardware, and adaptive devices designed to convert appliances and toys to switch-activated units.

Abracadata Ltd.

PO Box 2440
Eugene, OR 97402
541-342-3030
Disability Served: all

This company develops software programs for drawing and creating graphics.

Academic Software, Inc.

331 West Second Street
Lexington, KY 40507
606-233-2332, 800-842-2357
http://www.acsw.com
Disability Served: physically disabled

This company develops academic software programs as well as switches.

Access Systems International Ltd.

415 English Avenue
Monterey, CA 93940
408-375-5313
Disability Served: vision

This company develops Braille printers.

Acrontech International, Inc.

5500 Main Street
Williamsville, NY 14221
800-245-2020
http://www.acrontech.com
Disability Served: vision

This company supplies software, audio mixers, and closed-caption televisions.

ADAMLAB

33500 Van Born Road
Wayne, MI 48184-2497
313-467-1415
http://www.wcresa.k12.mi.us/adlab/index.htm
Disability Served: communication

ADAMLAB sells voice output communication aids to students.

AdapTek Interface

4832 East Mercer Way
Mercer Island, WA 98040
425-230-0076
Disability Served: physically disabled

This company manufactures a keyboard emulating program, a mouthstick cursor control interface, and a mouse emulating program.

Adaptek Systems

2320 Brighton-Henrietta Town Line Road
Rochester, NY 14623
716-475-9770, 800-685-4566
Disability Served: vision

This company develops a voice output module designed to work with the Kurzweil voice-recognition system. The device provides voice output of what the computer hears for persons with visual impairments.

Adaptivation, Inc.

224 SE 16th Street, Suite 2
Ames, IA 50010
515-233-9086, 800-723-2783
Disability Served: all

This company manufactures environmental control switches, auditory paging systems, a mouse emulator program, and communication devices.

Adaptive Computer Systems

1835 Hafor Street
Iowa City, IA 52246
319-338-1449
Disability Served: all

This company designs web page creation software and on-screen keyboard programs.

Adaptive Computers

11 Fullerton Street, Suite 204
Albany, NY 12209
518-434-8860
Disability Served: all

This company makes a drawing software program designed for single-switch users.

Adaptive Innovations

66 Hale Road
East Walpole, MA 02032
508-660-2635
Disability Served: all

This company manufactures a portable computer that can be plugged into a wheelchair battery, a word prediction software program, and a bidet.

Adhoc Reading Systems Inc.

228 East 85th Street, #12B
New York, NY 10028-3058
212-717-4835
Disability Served: vision

This company manufactures an optical character recognition scanner and Braille personal note-taking devices.

Advanced Gravis Computer Technology

1602 Carolina Stree, D12
Bellingham, WA 98226
360-434-7274
Disability Served: physically disabled

This company designs joysticks to replace the mouse or keyboard for persons with physical disabilities.

Advanced Input Devices

West 250 AID Drive
Coeur d'Alene, ID 83814
208-765-8000
Disability Served: physically disabled

This company makes modified keyboards.

Advanced Peripheral Technologies

14416 Erin Court
Lockport, IL 60441
708-301-4508
Disability Served: physically disabled

This company manufactures a hands-free telephone system.

Advanced Videotech Corp.

1840 Count Line Road
Hunting Valley, PA 19006
215-322-4600, 800-233-0013
Disability Served: all

This company manufactures a hands-free, two-way radio system that is voice activated.

Affinity Micro Systems Ltd.

1900 Folsom Street, Suite 205
Boulder, CO 80302-5723
303-442-4840, 800-367-6771
Disability Served: all

This company designs macro creation software programs.

Ai Squared

PO Box 669
Manchester Center, VT 05255-0669
802-362-3612
http://www.aisquared.com
Disability Served: vision

This company develops software for the visually impaired.

Aicom Corporation

2318 Zanker Road, Suite 160
San Jose, CA 95131
408-577-0370
Disability Served: vision

This company develops speech synthesizers for computers to accommodate persons with limited vision.

AIMS Media

9710 Desodo Avenue
Chatsworth, CA 91311-4409
818-773-4300, 800-367-2467
Disability Served: vision

This company manufactures a voice output math tutorial software program for children with visual impairments.

Akron Resources, Inc.
11627 Clark Street, Suite 101
Arcadia, CA 91006
818-358-1133
Disability Served: hearing

This company manufactures infrared amplification systems for televisions or stereos.

Al Kalashian
3234 South Villa Circle
West Allis, WI 53227
414-327-4051
Disability Served: all

This manufacturer designs battery-operated communication devices and voice input control switches designed to operate battery-operated products and toys.

Alco Electronic Products Inc.
PO Box 2510
Attleboro Falls, MA 02763-0893
508-699-9800
Disability Served: all

This company manufactures button switches.

ALDS Inc. (Assistive Listening Device Systems)
2-11220 Voyageur Way
Richmond, BC V6X 3E1 Canada
604-244-0269, 800-665-2537
http://www.alds.com
Disability Served: hearing

This company manufactures products for the hearing impaired. The products include a computerized note-taking system and communication devices for one-on-one group meetings or large gatherings.

Alice Lee
29 Maple Drive
Swoyersville, PA 18704
717-283-2091
Disability Served: vision

This company manufactures a voice output check-writing software program and a voice output program for storing and printing mailing and telephone lists.

All Packaging Machinery and Supplies
90 13th Avenue
Ronkonkoma, NY 11779
516-588-7310
Disability Served: all

This company manufactures packaging machines and plastic-bag sealers.

Alpha Software Corporation
168 Middlesex Turnpike
Burlington, MA 01803
617-272-3680, 800-451-1018
Disability Served: all

This company develops a keyboard expansion program that makes use of macros.

Alton Technical Services
9492 Township Hall Road
Rapid River, MI 49878
906-474-9477
Disability Served: all

This company manufactures environmental control units, switches, keyboard covers, and direct selection communication aids.

ALTRA
520 West Cedar Street
Rawlins, WY 82301-5639
800-726-6153
http://www.altra.com
Disability Served: physically disabled

This company manufactures and sells a pointing device for computers to assist computer users with carpal tunnel syndrome.

ALVA Access Group, Inc.
5801 Christie Avenue, Suite 475
Emeryville, CA 94608
510-923-6280
TTY/TDD: 510-923-6286
http://www.aagi.com
Disability Served: vision

This company develops and manufactures computer-screen readers and computer-screen magnifying software programs to assist those with low vision.

American Occupational Therapy Association

4720 Montgomery Lane
Bethesda, MD 20814-3425
301-652-2682
http://www.aota.org/
Disability Served: all

The Association develops a software program designed to interpret tests and produce reports in occupational therapy.

American Thermoform Corporation

2311 Travers Avenue
City of Commerce, CA 90040
213-723-9021
http://www.atcbrleqp.com
Disability Served: vision

This company markets equipment and supplies for the blind population. Products include Braille embossers, thermoform and graphic machines, Braille paper, labeling material, and Braille displays.

Ameriphone, Inc.

12082 Western Avenue
Garden Grove, CA 92841-2913
714-897-0808, 800-874-3005
Disability Served: hearing

This company manufactures aids for the hearing impaired, including amplification systems, telephone accessories, text telephones, and wireless signal transmitters.

Amidon Publications

1966 Benson Avenue
St Paul, MN 55116
612-690-2401, 800-328-6052
Disability Served: all

This company designs prereading tutorial software programs for persons with cognitive disabilities.

Amtel Systems Corporation

8701 100th Street
Kenosha, WI 53142-7718
414-947-0600, 800-999-8903
Disability Served: hearing

This company manufactures paging systems for interoffice communication and for personal use.

Andersen Corporation

100 4th North
Bayport, MN 55003
612-439-5150
Disability Served: all

This company manufactures a remote control window operator.

Andy Schoenberg Rehabilitation Engineering Lab

University of Utah
Salt Lake City, UT 84112
801-581-2548
Disability Served: physically disabled

This lab designs a trackball or joystick mounting system for computer users who manipulate trackballs or joysticks with head movement.

Animated Voice Corp.

PO Box 819
San Marcos, CA 92079
619-744-8190, 800-942-3699
Disability Served: communication

This company designs software programs designed to enhance speech communication skills.

Anthro Technology Institute

10450 SW Manhasset Drive
Tualatin, OR 97062
503-691-2409
Disability Served: physically disabled

This company manufactures and develops height-adjustable desks and computer work stations as well as rolling carts.

Apple Computer, Inc.

Worldwide Disability Solutions Group
Cupertino, CA 95014
408-974-7910, 800-600-7808
TTY/TDD: 800-755-0601
Disability Served: all

This company develops large-print programs and keyboard modification programs.

Applications Express Inc.

179 Avenue at the Common
Shrewsbury, NJ 07702
908-389-3366
Disability Served: vision

This company develops a voice input terminal control interface.

Applied Science & Engineering Laboratories

University of Delaware/duPont Hospital for Children
Wilmington, DE 19899
302-651-6830
TDD: 302-651-6834
http://www.asel.udel.edu
Disability Served: all

ASEL is a program jointly operated by the duPont Hospital for Children and the A.I. duPont Institute of the Nemours Foundation and the University of Delaware. ASEL focuses on research and development, as well as public policy and systems change, relating to the use of advanced rehabilitation and assistive technology by people with disabilities.

APT Technology, Inc.

236A North Main Street
Shreve, OH 44676-9421
330-567-2001, 888-549-2001
http://www.apt-technology.com
Disability Served: physically disabled

This company provides assistive devices to people with severe physical disabilities, including computer access, environmental controls, and adaptive switches.

Ariel Corporation

433 River Road
Highland Park, NJ 08904
908-249-2900
Disability Served: communication

This company develops a speech analysis software program.

Arkenstone Inc.

555 Oakmead Parkway
Sunnyvale, CA 94086-4023
408-752-2200, 800-444-4443
TDD: 800-833-2753
Disability Served: vision

This company develops optical character recognition devices, reading tutorial software programs for the visually impaired, voice output computers, and a voice output map that analyzes the user's surroundings.

Arthur J. Cloran

309 Little Building
East Liverpool, OH 43920
216-385-0352
Disability Served: physically disabled

This company offers a telescoping mouthstick.

Artic Technologies International, Inc.

55 Park Street, Suite 2
Troy, MI 48083
810-588-7370
Disability Served: vision

This company manufactures speech synthesizers, voice output screen review programs, large-print programs, and low-vision reading systems.

Artificial Language Laboratory

Michigan State University
East Lansing, MI 48824
517-353-5399
Disability Served: physically disabled

The Laboratory develops switches, including eye switches and touch switches.

Artificial Speech Aids

2027 Read Street, #53
Omaha, NE 68112
402-453-6320
Disability Served: communication

This company manufactures a speech aid for persons who have had laryngectomies.

Asaflex Manufacturing
Southeast 525 Water Street
Pullman, WA 99163
509-332-2205
Disability Served: all

This company develops switches that can be operated by sound or muscle movement.

Asher Engineering Corp.
15115 Ramona Boulevard
Baldwin Park, CA 91706
818-962-4063
Disability Served: all

This company manufactures trackballs that emulate mouse control.

Assistive Device Center
California State University—Sacramento
Sacramento, CA 95819-6027
916-278-6679
Disability Served: all

The Center develops software programs, including skills training and assessment programs and control switch assessment programs.

Assistive Industries Marketing
PO Box 1663
Paradise, CA 95967-1663
530-877-7191
Disability Served: all

This company markets assistive products for people with disabilities.

Assistive Technology, Inc.
850 Boylston Street, Suite 317
Chestnut Hill, MA 02167
617-731-4900, 800-793-9227
http://www.assistivetech.com/
Disability Served: learning disabled

This company offers solutions for communication and learning disabilities through therapeutic hardware and software tools.

AT&T CPU Leasing
5 Woodhollow Road, #2A21
Parsippany, NJ 07054-2821
800-233-1222
TTY/TDD: 800-833-3232
Disability Served: all

This company manufactures telephones and accessories, including text telephones, telecommunication devices for the deaf, speech amplifiers, speakerphones, big button telephones, auxiliary bell ringers, and more.

AT&T Information Products and Systems
650 Liberty Avenue, Room 2-202
Union, NJ 07083-8107
908-851-3084, 800-327-7440
Disability Served: all

AT&T manufactures accessible telephones for persons who are visually or hearing impaired.

Attainment Company Inc.
PO Box 930160
504 Commerce Parkway
Verona, WI 53593
608-845-7880, 800-327-4269
http://www.attainmentcompany.com
Disability Served: all

This company develops and distributes a wide variety of educational materials, including augmentative communication devices, printed materials, software, and videos.

Audex/Audiometrics Inc.
710 Standard Street
Longview, TX 75604
903-295-8244, 800-237-0716
http://www.audex.com
Disability Served: hearing

This company manufactures infrared amplification systems for televisions and wide-area applications, personal amplification systems for persons with hearing disabilities, and hearing-aid compatible cellular and cordless telephones.

Audio Computer Information, Inc.
PO Box 216
Spring Grove, MN 55974
507-498-3279

Disability Served: vision

This company manufactures computer training audiocassettes for persons with visual impairments.

Audio Enhancement

12613 South Redwood Road
Riverton, UT 84057
800-383-9362
http://www.audioenhancement.com
Disability Served: hearing

This company provides personal and classroom amplification systems for the hearing impaired.

Audiological Engineering Corp.

35 Medford Street
Somerville, MA 02143
617-623-5562, 800-283-4601
TTY/TDD: 800-955-7204
http://www.tactaid.com
Disability Served: hearing

This company manufactures personal amplification systems and vibrotactile amplification systems which turn sounds into vibrations.

Auditory Display Inc.

162 Schoolhouse Lane
Mount Laurel, NJ 08054
609-234-4446
Disability Served: hearing

This company manufactures a portable telecommunication device for the deaf that can be used on any telephone.

Augmentative Communication Consultants Inc.

280-B Moon Clinton Road
Moon Township, PA 15108
412-264-6121
http://www.ACCIinc.com
Disability Served: communication

This company distributes communication devices, educational software, switches, resource books, environmental controls, and wheelchair mounting systems.

Augmentative Communication Service

2430 11th Avenue North
Birmingham, AL 35234
205-251-0165
Disability Served: communication

This service provides evaluations and other services relating to augmentative communication.

Aurora Systems, Inc.

2647 Kingsway
Vancouver, BC V5R 5H4 Canada
604-436-2694, 800-361-8255
http://www.djtech.com/aurora
Disability Served: all

This company provides software solutions for individuals with speech impairments, motor control disabilities, learning disabilities, and physical disabilities. Aurora 2.0 for Windows provides Windows users with learning disabilities assistance with their writing through spoken feedback and spelling help.

Automated Functions Inc.

6424 North 28th Street
Arlington, VA 22207-1114
703-536-7741
Disability Served: vision

This company designs voice output computers and speech synthesizers.

AVSI

17059 El Cajon Avenue
Yorba Linda, CA 92886
714-524-4488, 800-628-5837
http://www.mastervoice.com
Disability Served: all

This company supplies an environmental control system that gives complete control over appliances, lighting, and heating by time, touch, situation, and voice.

Axis Corporation
555 Sparkman Drive, Suite 1618 G
Huntsville, AL 35816
205-722-0922
Disability Served: communication

This company designs a communication computer program that allows persons to synthesize speech and compose text by operating a switch.

Baktec Inc.
7614-301 Boulevard
Sarasota, FL 34243
941-359-1647, 800-332-1647
http://www.tenasu.com
Disability Served: all

This company manufactures orthotics for the lower back.

Balloons Software
5201 Chevy Chase Parkway NW
Washington, DC 20015-1747
202-244-2223
Disability Served: vision

Base Resource, Inc.
181 South Riverside Avenue, Suite 126
Croton-on-Hudson, NY 10520
914-739-5602
http://www.shakeawake.com
Disability Served: hearing

This company distributes assistive technology devices for the deaf, hearing impaired, and senior citizens.

Baudville Inc.
5380 52nd Street SE
Grand Rapids, MI 49512
616-698-0888, 800-728-0888
http://www.baudville.com
Disability Served: all

This company manufactures desktop publishing solutions.

Baylor Biomedical Services Inc.
2625 Elm Street, Suite 102
Dallas, TX 75226
800-365-1890
Disability Served: all

This company manufactures speakerphones, remote control switches, communication devices, and cursor control interface programs for computers.

Bear Medical Systems Inc.
2085 Rustin Avenue
Riverside, CA 92507
800-232-7633
Disability Served: communication

This company makes a speech amplifier for people who use ventilators.

Behavioral Controls
Division of Alps Inc.
Milwaukee, WI 53215
414-671-3332
Disability Served: communication

This company manufactures a speech-teaching device.

Benjamin Bayman
3611 Abbott Avenue South
Minneapolis, MN 55410
612-920-1358
Disability Served: vision

This company develops large-print word processing programs for persons with low vision.

Berkeley Systems Inc.
2095 Rose Street
Berkeley, CA 94709
510-540-5535
Disability Served: vision

This company develops software programs, including large-print programs and voice output programs.

Beyond Sight
26 East Arapahoe Road
Littleton, CO 80122
303-795-6455
http://www.beyondsight.com
Disability Served: vision, learning disabled

This is a retail store with more than 800 products for the blind and visually impaired that also provides adaptive technology services.

BILBO Innovations, Inc.

1290 Oakmead Parkway, Suite 118
Sunnyvale, CA 94086
408-736-6086
http://www.bilbo.com
Disability Served: all

This company manufactures Step On It! keyboard control pedals for repetitive strain injury.

BioControl Systems, Inc.

2555 Park Boulevard
Palo Alto, CA 94306
650-329-8496
http://www.biocontrol.com
Disability Served: all

This company manufactures and sells the hands free mouse for computer users.

Biolink Computer R & D Ltd.

4770 Glenwood Avenue
North Vancouver, BC V7R 4G8 Canada
604-984-4099
Disability Served: all

This company designs battery accessories for wheelchair batteries and voice output screen review software programs.

Blazie Engineering

105 East Jarrettsville Road
Forest Hill, MD 21050
410-893-9333
Disability Served: vision

This company designs Braille equipment and accessories, including Braille printers, word processors, keyboard expansion programs, and voice output software programs.

Blissymbolics Communication International

1630 Lawrence Avenue West, Suite 104
Toronto, ON M6L 1C5 Canada
416-421-8377
http://home.istar.ca/~bci
Disability Served: communication

This company develops Blissymbol tutorial programs and Blissymbol reference aids, including flash-cards, stamps, dictionaries, and software.

Borland International

1800 Green Hills Road
Scotts Valley, CA 95066
408-439-1604
Disability Served: all

Borland produces a keyboard enhancement software program that allows the user to define macros.

Boston Educational Systems & Technology, Inc.

63 Forest Street
Chestnut Hill, MA 02167
617-277-0179
Disability Served: all

This company develops educational software programs designed to teach cognitive skills, as well as modified keyboard programs.

Boys Town Press

14100 Crawford Street
Boys Town, NE 68010
800-282-6657
http://www.ffbh.boystown.org/btpress
Disability Served: hearing

This company produces sign language tutorial videos.

BP Manufacturing

311 South Anthony
Anthony, KS 87005
316-842-3176
Disability Served: all

This company develops software programs designed to teach independent living skills to children.

Bradley Enterprises

1204 Beech Street
Wilmington, DE 19805-4325
302-658-0203
Disability Served: communication

This company sells the Bradley Board, a communication board. It is a write and wipe board with fifty-six items pictured, a word list, and a writing area.

Brainchild Corporation
425 8th Street South
Naples, FL 33940
941-263-0100, 800-522-8171
Disability Served: all

This company manufactures the Brainchild, an electronic educational device with software cartridges.

BrightEye Technology
2 Westwood Place
Asheville, NC 28806
704-253-6658
http://www.brighteye.com
Disability Served: all

This company provides technology products for the learning disabled, ESL students, sight and hearing impaired, and adults with reading deficits. One of its products is Scan-A-Word, which allows users to hear out loud what they are attempting to read.

Broderbund
PO Box 6121
Novato, CA 94948
415-382-4400
Disability Served: all

This company develops educational software programs for children.

BRYTECH Inc.
600 Peter Morand Crescent
Ottawa, ON K1G 5Z3 Canada
613-721-5800, 800-263-4095
http://www.brytech.com
Disability Served: vision

This company manufactures reading systems for the blind, deaf-blind, and visually impaired that provide voice-output identification of U.S. and Canadian paper currency.

C-CAD Center for Computer Assistance to the Disabled
1950 Stemmons Freeway, Suite 4041
Dallas, TX 75207
214-746-4217
TTY/TDD: 214-746-5303
Disability Served: all

This company develops a keyboard modification program that enables one-finger and mouthstick computer users to perform commands that require simultaneous key pressing.

Cadkey Inc.
4 Griffin Road North
Windsor, CT 06095-1527
203-298-8888
Disability Served: all

Cadkey develops a computer-aided design program that allows alternative input, such as voice input, eye gaze input, or pneumatic switch input.

Cafet Inc.
4208 Evergreen Lane, Suite 213
Annandale, VA 22003
703-941-8903
Disability Served: communication

This company develops software programs designed to treat stuttering.

Canon USA Inc.
One Canon Plaza
Lake Success, NY 11042
516-488-6700
Disability Served: all

Canon manufactures communication boards with printing capabilities, voice output calculators, large-print calculators, large-print typewriters, and optical character recognition scanners.

Capability Corporation
5805 East Sharp Avenue, Suite 103
Spokane, WA 99212
800-541-5006
Disability Served: all

This company develops a software program that assesses job interests and skills.

Cape Software

PO Box 800
Harwich, MA 02645
508-432-2435
Disability Served: all

This software company produces single-switch text processing programs that allow users to input text and perform word processing functions without the use of a standard keyboard.

Carlon

Division of Lamson & Sessions
Beachwood, OH 44122
216-831-4000, 800-321-1970
Disability Served: physically disabled

This company offers an oversized light switch and a sound-activated light switch.

Castle Special Computer Services, Inc.

9801 San Gabriel Street NE
Albuquerque, NM 87111-3530
505-293-8379
Disability Served: all

This company develops a software program designed to teach coin recognition and counting as well as a spelling tutorial program.

CBAT, Inc.

140 South Arthur, Suite 420
Spokane, WA 99202
509-533-1409, 800-500-1453
Disability Served: all

This company offers evaluation, equipment set-up and configuration, equipment training, and follow-up.

CE Software Inc.

1801 Industrial Circle
West Des Moines, IA 50265
515-224-1995
Disability Served: all

This company produces a keyboard expansion software program that allows the user to customize keys and create macros.

Celadon

610 22nd Street, Suite 303
San Francisco, CA 94107
415-252-7199
Disability Served: all

This company manufactures a programmable remote control device.

Centigram

91 East Tasmond Drive
San Jose, CA 95134
408-428-3500
Disability Served: vision

Centigram makes a speech synthesizer for personal computers.

CH Products

970 Park Center Drive
Vista, CA 92038
619-598-2518, 800-624-5804
Disability Served: physically disabled

This company manufactures a trackball for use with computers.

Chinon America Inc.

615 Hawaii Avenue
Torrance, CA 90503
310-533-0274
Disability Served: vision

This company manufactures scanners used to input text into computers.

Cirque

433 West Lawndale Drive
Salt Lake City, UT 84115
801-467-1100
Disability Served: all

This company manufactures touch pads and modified keyboards.

Clever Computers

1205 East Hintz Road, Suite 303
Arlington Heights, IL 60004
847-392-6451
Disability Served: all

This company designs an expanded keyboard.

Clever Devices Ltd.
133 Glenwood Road
Glenwood Landing, NY 11547
516-674-8000, 800-872-6129
Disability Served: vision

This company develops voice output computers as well as voice output calipers.

Cognetics Corporation
PO Box 3029
Princeton, NJ 08543-3029
609-799-5005, 800-229-8437
Disability Served: all

This company produces a word processor program called Hyperties.

Comm-Tel
1208 Kahului Street
Honolulu, HI 96825
808-396-5941
Disability Served: hearing

This company offers Software Interface for the Deaf and Disabled (SIDD) which is a TDD automated messaging system designed to work with IBM PCs.

Command Corp, Inc.
3761 Venture Drive
Duluth, GA 30096-5598
770-813-8030
http://www.commandcorp.com
Disability Served: all

This company manufactures speech recognition software.

Common Cents Systems
PO Box 110514
Nashville, TN 37222
800-805-9278
http://www.box-talk.com/
Disability Served: communication

This company develops communication devices to assist nonspeaking individuals.

Communication Devices, Inc.
421 Coeur d'Alene Avenue, Suite 5
Coeur d' Alene, ID 83814
800-604-6559
http://www.comdevices.com
Disability Served: communication

This company manufactures portable communication devices for nonspeaking persons.

Communication Intelligence Corporation
333 Ravenwood Avenue, PS 357
Menlo Park, CA 94025
650-328-1311
Disability Served: all

This company develops a form processor software program.

Communication Skill Builders
3830 East Bellevue
Tucson, AZ 85733
520-323-7500
Disability Served: communication

This company develops language training systems, communication boards, and other alternative and augmentative communication tools.

Communications Applied Technology
11250-14 Roger Bacon Drive
Reston, VA 22090
703-481-0068
Disability Served: vision

This company develops a wireless link system that transmits speech from a remote location to the voice input module of a computer.

CompTech Systems Design
PO Box 107
Waconia, MN 55387
612-442-9776, 800-343-2406
Disability Served: all

This company develops a screen print program that allows the immediate printing of the contents of the computer screen.

Compu TTY Incorporated
3315 Lackland Road
Ft Worth, TX 76116
817-738-2485, 800-366-9950
TTY/TDD: 817-738-8993
Disability Served: hearing

This company is the manufacturer of telephone accessories for the hearing impaired.

Compu-Tations Inc.
PO Box 487
Southfield, MI 48037
248-557-9280, 800-345-2964
Disability Served: all

This company develops prereading tutorial software programs.

ComputAbility Corporation
40000 Grand River, Suite 109
Novi, MI 48375
248-477-6720, 800-433-8872
Disability Served: all

This company manufactures computer accessories and software programs primarily for those with visual and/or hearing impairments.

Computer Counsellors!
2008 North Via Establo
Santa Maria, CA 93454-8201
805-925-5780
Disability Served: all

This company provides computer voice technology and other adaptive devices for the disabled. They offer set-up, installation, and on-site training.

Computer Support Corporation
15296 Midway Road
Dallas, TX 75244
214-661-8960
Disability Served: all

This company manufactures a remote keyboard that allows the user to control a computer from a distance of up to forty feet.

Computerade Products
2346 Wales Drive
Cardiff, CA 92007
760-942-3343
http://www.computerade.com
Disability Served: communication

This company is a consulting and software development firm. Its products include Catch the Cow and Board Builder.

Computers to Help People, Inc.
825 East Johnson Street
Madison, WI 53703
608-257-5917
http://www.globaldialog.com/index.shtml
Disability Served: all

This company provides computer consulting, assistive technology, and special software to help people with disabilities.

Conover Company
PO Box 155
Omro, WI 54963
920-231-4667, 800-933-1933
Disability Served: all

This company develops software programs, including training and assessment programs.

Consultants for Communication Technology
508 Bellevue Terrace
Pittsburgh, PA 15202
412-761-6062
Disability Served: all

This company manufactures and distributes software and hardware products for persons with disabilities that affect speech.

Conveyant Systems
2332 McGaw Avenue
Irvine, CA 92714
714-756-7100
Disability Served: vision

This company manufactures an attendant-operated work station that provides voice output and magnified screen text for telephone operators who are blind or have visual impairments.

Corning Inc.
Corning Medical Optics, MP 21-2
Corning, NY 14831
800-742-5273
Disability Served: all

This company manufactures optical lenses designed to reduce glare.

Cornucopia Software Inc.
PO Box 6111
Albany, CA 94706
415-528-7000
Disability Served: vision

This company produces a Braille text translation program as well as a spelling checker.

CoStar Corporation
100 Field Point Road
Greenwich, CT 06830-6406
203-661-9700, 800-426-7827
Disability Served: all

This company manufactures a trackball that emulates a mouse.

Creative Switch Industries
PO Box 5256
Des Moines, IA 50306
515-287-5748
Disability Served: all

This company manufactures assorted switches, including contact switches, electro-mechanical switches, body position switches, switch interfaces, and switch accessories.

Crestwood Company
6625 North Sidney Place
Milwaukee, WI 53209-3259
414-352-5678
http://www.communicationaids.com/
Disability Served: communication

This company is a manufacturer and distributor of communication aids for children and adults. The company offers more than 275 products through a mail order catalog.

Crofter Publishing
4546 South Semoran, #690
Orlando, FL 32822
407-273-8975
Disability Served: vision

This company develops software programs for persons with low vision, including a large-font electronic mail reader program, modified game programs, and large-print file reader programs.

Curriculum Associates Inc.
5 Esquire Road
North Billerica, MA 01862-0901
508-667-8000, 800-225-0248
http://www.curriculumassociates.com
Disability Served: all

This company develops software programs designed to create individual education plan (IEP) reports for use by instructors.

Curtis Manufacturing Company Inc.
30 Fitzgerald Drive
Jaffrey, NH 03452
603-532-4123, 800-955-5544
Disability Served: physically disabled

This company manufactures the MVP Mouse, a trackball with three buttons that emulate the functions of a mouse.

Custom Grids
24460 Sandy Creek Road
Minerva, OH 44657
330-894-2300
Disability Served: communication

This company manufactures accessories for communication devices.

Data Collection & Dispersal Inc.
42 Skinner Road
East Windsor, CT 06016
860-623-7364
http://www.dcdinc.com
Disability Served: hearing

This company manufactures portable communication aids and custom systems.

David Favin
221 Queens Drive South
Little Silver, NJ 07739
201-949-7602
Disability Served: communication

This company develops software programs, including communicator programs, keyboard tutorial programs, spelling tutorial programs, and prereading tutorial programs.

David Hauck
PO Box 901
Jacksonville, IL 62651
217-243-1020, 217-245-4101
Disability Served: vision

This company develops a voice output game program to accommodate basic math skills.

Dawn Sign Press
9080-A Activity Road
San Diego, CA 92126-4421
619-549-5330
TTY/TDD: 619-549-5333
Disability Served: hearing

This company develops sign language training books, finger spelling cards, and finger spelling posters designed to teach American Sign Language to students who are hearing impaired.

Dazor Manufacturing Corp.
4483 Duncan Avenue
St Louis, MO 63110
314-652-2400, 800-345-9103
http://www.dazor.com
Disability Served: vision

This company manufactures fluorescent, incandescent, and halogen task lights to include illuminated magnifiers.

Deaf Communications of Cinncincinnati
550 Palmerston Drive
Cincinnati, OH 45231
513-451-3722
Disability Served: hearing

This company manufactures the Answerall, an answering machine modified to accept both voice and TDD phone calls for persons with hearing impairments.

Deafworks Co.
PO Box 1265
Provo, UT 84603-1265
801-465-1957, 800-877-8973
TTY/TDD: 801-465-1957
http://www.deafworks.com
Disability Served: hearing

This company manufactures, sells, and repairs adaptive and assistive devices and products for the deaf and hard of hearing.

DEKRO Inc.
2758 Margaret Mitchell Drive, NW
Atlanta, GA 30327-1857
Disability Served: all

This company designs cognitive rehabilitation software programs called VISPA. VISPA is available in a variety of languages and is offered in adult and child versions.

Designing Aids for Disabled Adults
249 Concord Avenue, #2
Toronto, ON M6H 2P4 Canada
416-530-0038
Disability Served: physically disabled

This company designs keyboard interfaces and keyboard modification devices.

Development Systems Inc.
402 The Highland Building, Suite 6
Cheshire, CT 06410
203-272-1117
Disability Served: all

This company develops a skills training and assessment system designed to provide occupational information in electronic format.

Dickey Engineering
3 Angel Road
North Reading, MA 01864
508-664-2010
Disability Served: physically disabled

This company manufactures a call switch activated by body movement as well as a page-turning device.

Digital Equipment Corporation
146 Main Street
Maynard, MA 01754-2572
508-493-5111
Disability Served: vision

This company manufactures speech synthesizers compatible with many computer systems.

Dimango Products
7258 Kensington Road
Brighton, MI 48116
313-486-0770
Disability Served: physically disabled

This company manufactures a remote switch.

DiRAD Technologies Inc.
14 Computer Drive East
Albany, NY 12205
518-438-6000
Disability Served: hearing

This company develops a telecommunication program that enables companies with phone menu systems to accommodate callers with hearing impairments.

Discovery Data Systems Ltd.
3251 Old Lee Highway, Suite 104
Fairfax, VA 22030
703-385-0300
Disability Served: all

This company develops management information software programs for rehabilitation programs.

Don Johnston Developmental Equipment
PO Box 639
Wauconda, IL 60084-0639
847-526-2682, 800-999-4660
Disability Served: all

This company manufactures switches, communication boards, software programs, and much more.

Douglas Sorenson
5937 Portland Avenue South
Minneapolis, MN 55417
612-866-1661
Disability Served: communication

This company manufactures a scanning communication system controlled by switches.

DPI Services, Inc.
151 Martinvale Lane
San Jose, CA 95119
408-629-3700, 800-374-2140
Disability Served: hearing

This company develops the ESL Tutor, a language tutorial program that assists deaf individuals whose primary language is American Sign Language to learn English.

Dragon Systems Inc.
320 Nevada Street
Newton, MA 02160
617-965-5200, 800-443-7077
Disability Served: vision

This company produces a speech recognition system for IBM-compatible personal computers.

Dufco Electronics Inc.
2847 North Business Park Avenue
Fresno, CA 93727-1328
800-456-8168
Disability Served: all

This company manufactures switches.

Dunamis Inc.
3423 Fowler Boulevard
Lawrenceville, GA 30244
770-279-1144, 800-828-2443
Disability Served: all

This company develops software programs, such as an expanded keyboard modification program, graphics program, prereading tutorial programs, and more.

Duncan Institute
Public Domain Library
New Port Richey, FL 34653-4511
813-848-0413
Disability Served: learning disabled

The Institute produces an academic tutorial software program.

DuPage Easter Seal Assistive Technology Center
830 South Addison Avenue
Villa Park, IL 60181
630-620-4433
TDD: 630-620-4436
Disability Served: all

DuPage Easter Seal provides evaluations, various types of therapy, and equipment loans (e.g., mobility devices). Also offered are adapted computers and augmentative communication. A sliding fee scale is available for training of people in DuPage County.

Duxbury Systems, Inc.
435 King Street
Littleton, MA 01460
508-486-9766
http://world.std.com/~duxbury/
Disability Served: vision

This company produces software for Braille word processing and translation software.

Dvorak International
PO Box 44
Poultney, VT 05764-0044
802-287-2343
http://www.dvorakint.org
Disability Served: physically disabled

This organization promotes the use of the Dvorak keyboard layouts, including the single-hand layouts.

Dynacomp Inc.
178 Phillips Road
Webster, NY 14580
716-671-6160
Disability Served: learning disabled

This company develops a reading tutorial and graphics program for individuals with dyslexia and related disorders.

E & IS SignWare
206 Angie Drive
Cedar Falls, IA 50613
Disability Served: hearing

This company produces games and programs designed to teach American Sign Language.

E. David & Associates
Small Computer Systems
Storrs, CT 06268
860-429-1785
Disability Served: all

This company develops arithmetic flash cards for persons unable to type on a standard keyboard and a modified game program designed to teach vocabulary and spelling.

Easter Seals & Lehigh Valley Microcomputer
PO Box 333
Kulpsville, PA 19443
215-368-7000
Disability Served: all

This company, in conjunction with Easter Seals, develops software programs for children with disabilities. Products include cognitive skills tutorial programs, visual tracking skills development programs, keyboard modification programs, and speech training programs.

Easy Home Control
4931 Edsal Drive
Lyndhurst, OH 44124
216-381-9700
TTY/TDD: 800-750-0750
Disability Served: all

This company manufactures switch-controlled telephones and the Remote Ability Switch Adapter, which is designed to convert ability switches into wireless units.

Ebsco Curriculum Materials
PO Box 1943
Birmingham, AL 35201

205-991-1208, 800-633-8623
Disability Served: all

This company develops a variety of products and programs for children with disabilities of all kinds, including Blissymbol flash-cards, a sign language practice program, writing programs for the developmentally disabled, study guides, handwriting programs, and more.

Echo Consulting Services Inc.

PO Box 540
Center Conway, NH 03813-0540
603-447-5453, 800-635-8209
Disability Served: all

This company manufactures the Human Service Information Systems (HSIS) and Fund Accounting Series, clinical management programs designed to provide assistance to clinicians.

Echo Speech Corp.

6460 Via Real
Carpinteria, CA 93013
805-684-4593
Disability Served: vision

This company develops speech synthesizers for computers.

Eden Toys, Inc.

812 Jersey Avenue
Jersey City, NJ 07310
201-656-3331, 800-443-4275
Disability Served: all

This company manufactures a touch-activated stuffed animal.

Edmark Corporation

PO Box 97021
Redmond, WA 98073-9721
425-556-8400, 800-362-2890
http://www.edmark.com
Disability Served: learning disabled

This company develops and publishes children's educational software. The software is intended to develop self-esteem, higher-level thinking, and problem-solving skills.

Education TURNKEY Systems Inc.

256 North Washington Street
Falls Church, VA 22046
703-536-2310
Disability Served: learning disabled

This company develops software programs designed to track data on special education students.

Educational Activities, Inc.

1937 Grand Avenue
Baldwin, NY 11510
516-223-4666, 800-645-3739
http://www.edact.com
Disability Served: learning disabled

This company develops language skills training programs for older children and adults.

Educational Audiology Programs Inc.

1077 South Gilpin Street
Denver, CO 80209
303-777-0740
Disability Served: learning disabled

This company manufactures the Natural Language Processing Program, a language structure practice program.

Educational Software Institute

4213 South 94th Street
Omaha, NE 68127
402-592-3300, 800-955-5570
http://www.edsoft.com
Disability Served: all

This company provides an educational software catalog containing approximately 8,000 titles.

Educational Technology International

PO Box 64188
Virginia Beach, VA 23464
757-523-5680
Disability Served: all

This company designs a series of reading tutorial software programs.

Edutainment Catalog

PO Box 21330
Boulder, CO 8030

303-444-3700, 800-338-3844
http://www.edutainco.com
Disability Served: all

This company provides educational and entertainment software for both IBM compatible and Macintosh systems.

Edutek Corporation

415 Cambridge, #4
Palo Alto, CA 94306
650-325-9965
Disability Served: all

This company produces hand/eye coordination programs designed to train perception and coordination.

Edward Burns

School of Education and Human Development
Binghamton, NY 13901
607-777-2000
Disability Served: all

The School develops an educational game software program designed to provide practice in the use of switches.

Ekeg Electronics Co. Ltd.

PO Box 46199
Vancouver, BC Canada
604-857-0820
Disability Served: all

This company manufactures a variety of keyboards for people with disabilities, including expanded keyboards, expanded keyboards for automatic telephones, and more. The company also produces a communication training aid.

EMAC

5020 Brandin Court
Fremont, CA 94538-3140
800-821-0806, ext. 2222
Disability Served: physically disabled

This company manufactures the Silhouette Trackball, a trackball that emulates mouse cursor control.

ENABLE

Schneier Communication Unit
Syracuse, NY 13208
315-455-7591
TDD: 315-45-1794
http://www.enable1.org
Disability Served: communication

This organization provides assessment, training, therapy, and support for about 1,000 children and adults with disabilities and their families each year. Among the services provide are augmentative communication, adapted computer access, ergonomics, seating and positioning, splinting and bracing, environmental modifications, and adaptive equipment.

Engineering Consulting

583 Candlewood Street
Brea, CA 92621
714-671-2009
Disability Served: vision

This company manufactures the Maxi-Screen, a computer monitor screen magnifier.

Envirotrol Association

6575 Burger Drive SE
Grand Rapids, MI 49546-7209
616-940-0122
http://home.earthlink.net/~trwood/envirotrol/home.html
Disability Served: physically disabled

This nonprofit organization utilizes volunteers to adapt devices for special needs. It offers user-friendly and affordable controls and equipment. It is also a funding source for persons with limited resources. Included are: telephones, televisions, VCRs, radios, cassettes, CD remote controls, nurse calls for health care facilities, and chime help calls for home use.

Epilepsy Foundation of America

4351 Garden City Drive, Suite 406
Landover, MD 20785
301-459-3700, 800-332-4050
Disability Served: physically disabled

The Foundation manufactures a program designed to teach children about epilepsy.

Equal Access Computer Technology, Inc.
39 Oneida Road
Acton, MA 01720
978-263-6437
Disability Served: physically disabled

This company manufactures switches for those who have difficulty using ordinary switches.

Ergo-Eeze, Ltd.
PO Box 32908
Phoenix, AZ 85064-2908
602-222-8553
Disability Served: all

This company manufactures and distributes an ergonomic lumbar support device that attaches to a chair and a keyboard wrist support device.

Ergonomics Unlimited
422 Larkfield Center, #251
Santa Rosa, CA 95403-1408
707-544-3020
Disability Served: all

This company manufactures a keyboard wrist support.

ErgonomiXX
2813 University Boulevard West
Kensington, MD 20895
301-933-3747
Disability Served: all

This company has developed a comprehensive ergonomic keyboard-trackball combination specifically designed to alleviate the stresses that frequently result in repetitive-motion injuries.

Essex Electronics, Inc.
1130 Mark Avenue
Carpinteria, CA 93013
805-684-7601
http://www.keyless.com
Disability Served: vision

This company manufactures keypad-based, access control systems, including Braille keypads for the blind, keypads with LED readback for the deaf, and illuminated keypads with large buttons for the sight impaired.

EVAS CompuSight
PO Box 371
Westerly, RI 02891
401-596-3155, 800-872-3827
Disability Served: vision

EVAS is the distributor of various computer training cassettes and voice input systems for computers.

Exceptional Teaching Aids, Inc.
20102 Woodbine Avenue
Castro Valley, CA 94546
800-549-6999
http://www.exceptionalteaching.com
Disability Served: vision

This company sells teaching aids for the blind and visually impaired, as well as others with special needs.

FDLRS/South—Enabling Technologies Lab
Dade County Public Schools
Miami, FL 33165
305-274-3501
Disability Served: vision

This company develops educational programs with voice output capabilities for students with visual impairments.

Fellows Manufacturing
1789 Norwood Avenue
Itasca, IL 60143
630-893-1600, 800-945-4545
Disability Served: all

This company manufactures a pen-shaped cursor control device that emulates mouse control as well as a trackball designed to emulate a mouse.

First Byte
19840 Pioneer Avenue
Torrance, CA 90503
310-793-0610
http://www.fbyte.com
Disability Served: all

This company develops text-to-speech synthesis technology. Products cater to those with low vision and/or speech impairments.

Flanagan and Company Adaptive Devices

6832 Mokelumne Avenue
Oakland, CA 94605
510-638-3898
Disability Served: all

This company manufactures the All-Flex Switch, a wobble switch that can be twisted into any position.

Fliptrack Learning Systems

2055 West Army Trail Road, #100
Addison, IL 60101-1478
630-790-1117, 800-222-3547
Disability Served: all

This company develops and produces computer tutorial audiocassettes. Programs covered in the company's tapes include Pagemaker, WordPerfect, Microsoft Word, Lotus 1-2-3, and basic computer operation.

Floppy Enterprise

PO Box 366
Menomonie, WI 54751
715-235-2288
Disability Served: all

This company develops a series of prereading tutorial software programs.

Florida New Concepts Marketing, Inc.

PO Box 261
Port Richey, FL 34673-0261
727-842-3231
http://www.gulfside.com/compulenz/
Disability Served: vision

This company manufactures and distributes Compu-Lenz, a magnifier combined with a glare filter. When placed in front of a computer monitor, it magnifies character size while reducing glare and enhancing contrast.

Forte Communications Inc.

1050 East Duane Avenue, Suite J
Sunnyvale, CA 94086
408-876-5432, 800-331-3903
Disability Served: all

This company makes a wireless keyboard and a wireless mouse.

Franklin Electronic Publishers

One Franklin Plaza
Burlington, NJ 08016
609-386-2500, 800-525-9673
Disability Served: vision

This company produces voice output dictionaries, thesauruses, and tutorial software programs.

Freelance Communications

PO Box 1895
Upland, CA 91785
Disability Served: all

This company develops a keyboard modification software program.

FTG Data Systems

10801 Dale Street, Suite J-2
Stanton, CA 90680
714-995-3900, 800-962-3900
Disability Served: all

This company produces alternative input devices for computers in pen form.

Futura Wave Communications

7209 Cipriano Spring Drive
Lanham, MD 20706
301-552-4405
Disability Served: hearing

This company develops communication software programs that work with TDD/ASCII translation modems. The programs allow the user to save conversations, store phone numbers, and use the computer as an answering machine.

GenoVation Inc.

17741 Mitchell
North Irvine, CA 92714
714-833-3355
Disability Served: all

This company manufactures a keyboard with logically controlled, lighted keys.

Geoffrey Domowicz
2359 Rice Avenue
Lake City, PA 16423
814-774-9503
Disability Served: all

This manufacturer offers Call-For-Assistance, a call signal that produces an auditory or visual output to signal for assistance.

Glenn Weil
4139 Paramount Boulevard, Trailer 11
Pico Rivera, CA 90660-1674
310-692-4939
Disability Served: all

This company manufactures custom-made, plastic keyboard guards for computers or typewriters.

GNNETCOM Inc.
77 Northeastern Boulevard
Nashua, NH 03062
603-598-1100, 800-826-4656
http://gnnetcom.com
Disability Served: all

This company makes telephone headsets.

Greystone Digital Inc.
PO Box 1888
Huntersville, NC 28078
800-249-5397
http://www.bigkeys.com
Disability Served: all

This company makes BigKeys, a computer keyboard with large keys for PCs and Macintosh computers. Greystone also sells related educational and assistive-technology computer products.

Gus Communications Inc.
1006 Lonetree Court
Bellingham, WA 98226
360-715-8580
Disability Served: communication

This company develops augmentative communication software programs and touch screens.

GW Instruments
35 Medford Street
Somerville, MA 02143
617-625-4096
Disability Served: communication

This company develops speech and sound analysis software programs.

GW Micro, Inc.
310 Racquet Drive
Ft Wayne, IN 46825
219-483-3625
Disability Served: vision

This company produces voice output software programs, large-print programs, Braille text translation programs, voice output database management programs, voice output word processing programs, speech synthesizers, and screen-reading programs for persons with limited vision.

Hach Associates, Inc.
4994-D Indiana Avenue
Winston-Salem, NC 27106
800-624-7968
http://www.computersforkids.com
Disability Served: all

This company provides assistive technology to special needs individuals throughout the United States. Products include a wide variety of educational software and hardware, including switches, keyboards, mice, and switch interfaces.

Handykey Corporation
141 Mt Sinai Avenue
Mt Sinai, NY 11766
516-474-4405, 800-638-2352
Disability Served: all

This company manufactures a combination mouse pointer and keyboard that can be manipulated with one hand.

Harding & Harris Inc.

PO Box 1599
Orem, UT 84057
Disability Served: communication

This company designs a software program that evaluates speech conditions and a word catalog for use by speech therapists.

Hartley Courseware

9920 Pacific Heights Boulevard, Suite 500
San Diego, CA 92121-4330
800-247-1380
Disability Served: all

This company produces educational software programs to enhance the K-12 classroom learning experience.

Health Care Keyboard Company

North 61 West 15150 Wingwan Drive
Menomenee Falls, WI 53501
414-252-3282
Disability Served: all

This company makes modified computer keyboards.

Hello Direct, Inc.

5893 Rue Ferrari
San Jose, CA 95138
408-972-1990, 800-444-3556
http://www.hellodirect.com
Disability Served: hearing

This company offers telephone amplifiers for persons who are hard of hearing.

Henter Joyce Inc.

2100 62nd Avenue North
St Petersburg, FL 33702
813-528-8900, 800-336 5658
Disability Served: vision

This company manufactures voice output computer programs for persons with low vision, including a form processor, a screen reading program, and a vocabulary tutorial program.

Herzog Research

1433 East Broadway
Tucson, AZ 85719
520-792-2550
http://HerzogKeyboarding.com
Disability Served: all

This company has developed a quick and easy way to learn computer keyboarding. The Herzog System uses HubKey Sensors, a new sensory invention for the keyboard that provides accurate hand positioning, facilitates range of motion, and prevents errors caused by hand drift, hand pull-off, and hand contortions. The Herzog System also uses new Fast Tract Learning.

Hexagon Products

PO Box 1295
Park Ridge, IL 60068
847-692-3355
Disability Served: vision

This company designs software programs to accommodate persons with limited vision. Products include word processing programs with enlarged text and Braille tutorial programs.

Hexamedia

1309 rue St Louis
Ville St Laurent, QC H4L 2P4 Canada
514-748-7733
Disability Served: vision

This company manufactures a speech synthesizer and screen reading program that can speak French.

HFK Software

68 Wells Road
Lincoln, MA 01773
617-259-0059
Disability Served: vision

This company designs software programs to assist persons with low vision. Programs include large-print programs and voice output word processing programs.

High Tech Intelligence Inc.

1602 S. Parker Road, Suite 312
Denver, CO 80231
303-695-0609
Disability Served: physically disabled

This company manufactures a voice input controlled computer system that allows voice control over electrical devices.

Hooleon Corporation

260 Justin Drive
Cottonwood, AZ 86325
602-634-4503, 800-937-1337
Disability Served: vision

This company manufactures keyboard overlays to accommodate persons with limited vision.

Howtek Inc.

21 Park Avenue
Hudson, NH 03051
603-882-5200
Disability Served: vision

This company manufactures a Braille computer printer called the Pixelmaster.

HumanWare, Inc.

6245 King Road
Loomis, CA 95650
916-652-7253, 800-722-3393
http://www.humanware.com
Disability Served: vision, learning disabled

This company provides adaptive technology to people who need equal access due to blindness, low vision, and/or learning disabilities.

Hypertek

PO Box 5703
Derwood, MD 20855-0703
301-216-9836
Disability Served: physically disabled

This company manufactures an environmental control system that is programmed through a computer.

IBM Corporation

Special Needs Systems
Boca Raton, FL 33432
561-982-9099
Disability Served: all

This company manufactures keyboard modification programs, keyboard overlays, TDD emulation programs, voice output programs, and various tutorial programs.

Ideamatics, Inc.

1806 T Street, NW
Washington, DC 20009
202-667-9495, 800-247-4332
Disability Served: all

This company designs a telecommunication program card that allows the computer to act as a telephone.

IMPX

8801 Governor's Row
Dallas, TX 75247
214-688-4433
Disability Served: vision

This company manufactures an optical character recognition program for computers.

In Touch Systems

11 Westview Road
Spring Valley, NY 10977
914-354-7431, 800-332-6244
http://www.magicwandkeyboard.com
Disability Served: physically disabled

This company manufactures the Magic Wand Keyboard, a miniature computer keyboard with built-in mouse, which is designed to give full computer access to anyone with limited or no hand/arm movement.

Independence Engineering

1206 Jackson Street
La Porte, IN 46350
219-324-7018
Disability Served: all

This company makes a mouse emulator device called the Turtle. It is designed for persons who have difficulties pressing mouse buttons.

Individualized Rehabilitation Programs

615 East State Street
Long Beach, NY 11561-2442
516-889-3011
Disability Served: head/brain injury

This company designs rehabilitation tutorial software programs for persons with brain injuries. The company also produces a computerized vocational assessment program used in insurance rehabilitation environments.

Industrial Innovations, Inc.

10789 North 90th Street, Top Floor
Scottsdale, AZ 85260-6727
602-860-8584
Disability Served: all

This company manufactures a modified keyboard.

Infogrip Inc.

1145 Eugenia Place, Suite 201
Carpinteria, CA 93013
805-566-1049, 800-397-0921
Disability Served: physically disabled

This company manufactures one-hand keyboard interfaces.

Information Services Inc.

28 Green Street
Newbury, MA 01951
978-463-3399, 800-659-3399
http://www.is-inc.com
Disability Served: learning disabled, physically disabled

This company develops and markets Write Away, a software writing tool for children and adults who have difficulty with writing and/or oral communication. Write Away offers a multisensory approach to learning through features such as word prediction, speech synthesis/feedback, and multiple access modes.

Information Strategies Inc.

1200 East Campbell Road, #108
Richardson, TX 75081-1963
214-234-0176
Disability Served: all

This company makes a mouse emulator that is a touchscreen that plugs into a serial mouse port.

Innocomp

26210 Emery Road, Suite 302
Warrensville Heights, OH 44128
216-464-3636, 800-382-8622
http://www.sayitall.com
Disability Served: communication

This company manufactures and distributes products for augmentative and alternative communication.

Innovation Management Group, Inc.

21550 Oxnard Street, Suite 300
Woodland Hills, CA 91367
818-346-5381, 800-889-0987
http://www.IMGPresents.com
Disability Served: all

This company publishes My-T-Mouse, My-T-Mouse for Kids, and My-T-Soft AT on-screen keyboards with macro buttons and option word prediction. Joystick-To-Mouse runs Windows from any joystick. The Magnifier is magnification software with cursor crosshair, and JAMBox is a switch adapter for joysticks.

Innovative Designs Inc.

PO Box 2577
Santa Clara, CA 95055
408-985-9255
Disability Served: all

This company designs a word prediction software program.

Institute on Applied Technology

Fegan 9, The Children's Hospital
Boston, MA 02115
617-735-7870
Disability Served: communication

The Institute makes a portable speech synthesizer for use with computers.

Instructional/Communications Technology
10 Stepar Place
Huntington Station, NY 11746
516-549-3000
Disability Served: all

This company develops reading tutorial software programs, reading assessment programs, vocabulary tutorial programs, and cognitive skills tutorial programs.

Intelligent Peripheral Devices, Inc.
20400 Stevens Creek Boulevard, Suite 300
Cupertino, CA 95014
888-274-0680
http://www.alphasmart.com
Disability Served: all

This company manufactures and sells the Alphasmart 2000, a keyboard that lets students enter and edit text, then transfer it easily to a Macintosh or PC for formatting and printing.

IntelliTools
5221 Central Avenue, Suite 205
Richmond, CA 94804
510-528-0670, 800-899-6687
Disability Served: all

This company develops mouse emulator software programs and academic tutorial programs.

Interactive Learning Materials
150 Croton Lake Road
Katonah, NY 10536
914-232-4682
Disability Served: communication

This company develops speech therapy software programs.

Interface Systems International
PO Box 20415
Portland, OR 97220
503-256-3214
Disability Served: vision

This company designs voice output screen review computer programs.

InvoTek, Inc.
700 West 20th Street-ENRC
Fayetteville, AR 72701
501-575-7659
Disability Served: all

This company manufactures a keyboard interface, a voice-activated speaker phone, and an eye-controlled communication board.

Iscan Inc.
PO Box 382076
Cambridge, MA 02238-2076
617-868-5353
Disability Served: all

This company manufactures an on-screen keyboard program controlled by eye gaze and a pen-shaped cursor control interface that emulates a mouse.

J. E. Stewart—Teaching Tools
PO Box 15308
Seattle, WA 98115
425-486-4510
Disability Served: developmentally disabled

This company provides software for planning and instructional materials to teach community sign reading and vocational skills.

J. J. Hoefer
5200 West 68
Shawnee Mission, KS 66208
913-262-7440
Disability Served: vision

This company manufactures a Braille tutorial program for sighted Braille transcribers.

Jeff Weiss
3015 South Tyler Street
Little Rock, AR 72204
501-666-6552
Disability Served: vision

This company designs voice output game programs, voice output word processing programs, and voice output utility programs for persons with limited vision.

Jesana Ltd.

979 Saw Mill River Road
Yonkers, NY 10710
914-376-2894, 800-443-4728
Disability Served: all

This company supplies adapted devices or equipment and capability switches for children with physical and/or developmental disabilities.

Jims Instruments Mfg. Inc.

3703 Rohret Road
Iowa City, IA 52240
319-351-3429
Disability Served: physically disabled

This company manufactures head-mounted optical pointers.

Job Oriented Training, Inc.

60 Bishop Drive
Fredericton, NB E3C 1B2 Canada
506-459-2656
Disability Served: all

This company develops a math skills tutorial software program.

John Halleck

University of Utah Computer Center
Salt Lake City, UT 84112
801-581-6802
Disability Served: physically disabled

The Center provides on-screen keyboard computer programs.

John Monarch

525 Pawnee Trail
Frankfort, KY 40601
502-695-1761
Disability Served: vision

This company makes an audio output device for blind computer users that beeps to indicate activity over the serial port.

Joseph L. Terpenning

25 Rose Hill Park
Cornwall, NY 12518
914-534-4023
Disability Served: all

This company designs a skill-building software program.

Jostens Learning Corporation

9920 Pacific Heights Boulevard, #100
San Diego, CA 92121-4330
800-422-4339
Disability Served: vision

This company makes a speech synthesizer for computers.

Judy Lynn Software, Inc.

PO Box 373
East Brunswick, NJ 08816
908-390-8845
http://www.castle.net/~judylynn
Disability Served: physically disabled

This company produces single-switch software for PCs for cognitive age levels of nine months to five years.

Kansys Inc.

PO Box 1070
Lawrence, KS 66044-8070
913-843-0351, 800-279-4880
Disability Served: vision

This company develops Braille text translation software programs, address database programs, voice output software programs, and audio output computer utility programs to assist computer users with low vision.

Kennedy Day School Program

Franciscan Children's Hospital
Boston, MA 02135-3680
617-254-3800
Disability Served: all

This program manufactures a math tutorial software program and a keyboard modification program.

Kensington Microware Limited

2855 Campus Drive
San Mateo, CA 94403
650-572-2700, 800-535-4242
Disability Served: all

This company manufactures a trackball that emulates mouse functions.

Kenwood USA
PO Box 22745
Long Beach, CA 90801
562-639-4200
Disability Served: all

This company manufactures a hardware interface package that allows Kenwood receivers to be controlled via a computer.

Key Tronic Corp.
PO Box 14687
Spokane, WA 99214
509-928-8000, 800-262-6006
Disability Served: all

This company designs modified keyboards.

Keyboard Technology, Ltd.
824 East Rand Road, #271
Arlington Heights, IL 60004
847-392-0514
Disability Served: all

This company manufactures keyboard overlays and educational software programs.

Kidsview Software, Inc.
PO Box 98
Warner, NH 03278
603-927-4428, 800-542-7501
Disability Served: learning disabled

This company specializes in large-character software for the visually impaired, special needs student, and young children. Their line of software includes word processing, math, and game programs.

Kinetic Designs Inc.
14231 Anatevka Lane SE
Olalla, WA 98359
206-857-7943
Disability Served: vision

This company manufactures keyboard modification programs, Morse code interface programs, and a text enlargement program.

Kurzweil Applied Intelligence, Inc.
411 Waverly Oaks Road
Waltham, MA 02154
781-893-5151
Disability Served: physically disabled

This company provides a speech recognition system designed for persons who have difficulty using a standard keyboard.

KY Enterprises
3039 East Second Street
Long Beach, CA 90803
562-433-5244
Disability Served: physically disabled

This company provides adaptive products for operation of household recreational devices.

Laetare Solutions
2409 Belair Drive
Bowie, MD 20715
888-HOORAY-4
TTY/TDD: 301-249-0099
Disability Served: all

This company distributes augmentative communication products (Dyna Vox, Digi Vox, etc.) as well as switch and alternate computer access products from a variety of manufacturers.

Langer Biomechanics Group
21 East Industry Court
Deer Park, NY 11729
800-645-5520
Disability Served: all

This company manufactures a gait analysis system software program.

Language Analysis Lab—SALT Program
University of Wisconsin—Madison
1500 Highland Avenue
Madison, WI 53705
608-263-6791
http://www.waisman.wisc.edu/salt/
Disability Served: all

The Lab develops computer programs for analyzing language transcripts.

Laureate Learning Systems, Inc.
110 East Spring Street
Winooski, VT 05404-1898
802-655-4755
http://www.llsys.com
Disability Served: developmentally disabled

This company creates educational software for people with special needs.

Lawrence Erlbaum Associates Inc.
365 Broadway
Hillsdale, NJ 07642
201-666-4110, 800-926-6579
Disability Served: communication

This company develops a series of speech analysis software programs.

Lawrence Productions, Inc.
1800 South 35th Street
Galesburg, MI 49053-0458
800-421-4157
http://www.lpi.com
Disability Served: all

This company publishes educational software, including programs appropriate for children with special needs and for secondary students with learning and mental disabilities.

LC Technologies Inc.
9455 Silver King Court
Fairfax, VA 22031
703-385-7133, 800-393-4293
Disability Served: physically disabled

This company manufactures a cursor control interface for computers that is controlled by eye movement.

LeapFrog
2608 Ninth Street
Berkeley, CA 94710
510-704-3777
Disability Served: all

This company makes a prereading tutorial software program.

Learn PC
5101 Highway 55
Minneapolis, MN 55422
612-544-4500, 800-532-7672
Disability Served: all

This company develops a personal computer training system using a combination of manuals, videotapes, and practice software.

Learning Company
6493 Kaiser Drive
Fremont, CA 94555
510-792-2101, 800-852-2255
Disability Served: learning disabled

This company develops educational software programs geared toward children with learning disabilities. Products include the Reader Rabbit series, Super Solvers, and Treasure series.

Lefthanded Computer Keyboards, Inc.
354 Eisenhower Parkway
Livingston, NJ 07039
800-50-LEFTY
Disability Served: physically disabled

This company manufactures a left-handed computer keyboard to facilitate computer users with limited or no use of the right hand or arm.

Leithauser Research
4649 Van Kleeck Drive
New Smyrna Beach, FL 32169
904-423-0705
Disability Served: physically disabled

This company develops a software program designed to allow the user to input text via a mouse or trackball rather than by a standard keyboard.

Less Gauss, Inc.
187 East Market Street, Suite 160
Rhinebeck, NY 12572-1727
914-876-5432, 800-872-1051
http://www.lessgauss.com
Disability Served: vision

This company manufactures computer-related ergonomic products, including magnifiers, screens, wrist supports, foot rests, and back supports.

Lexia Learning Systems Inc.

11A Lewis Street
PO Box 466
Lincoln, MA 01773
800-435-3942
http://www.lexialearning.com
Disability Served: learning disabled

This company manufactures developmental award-winning reading-skills-assessment programs for use on Windows and Macintosh computers.

Life Science Associates

1 Fenimore Road
Bayport, NY 11705
516-472-2111
Disability Served: all

This company develops tutorial software programs.

Lind Electronic Design

6414 Cambridge Street
St Louis Park, MN 55426-4420
612-927-6303
Disability Served: all

This company develops portable battery packs for computers.

Linemaster Switch Corp.

Plaine Hill Road
Woodstock, CT 06281
203-974-1000
Disability Served: all

This company manufactures a number of foot switches.

Lingraphicare America

3600 West Bayshore Road, Suite 202
Palo Alto, CA 94303
650-842-7444, 800-332-4913
Disability Served: communication

This company manufactures the Lingraphica, a direct selection communicator for persons unable to communicate through speech.

Logitech Inc.

6505 Kaiser Drive
Fremont, CA 94555
510-795-8500, 800-231-7717
Disability Served: all

This company manufactures a cordless mouse, an ergonomically designed mouse, optical character recognition scanners, and numerous trackballs.

Lorin Software

PO Box 32854
Orlando, FL 32804
407-872-3245
Disability Served: vision

This company develops software programs for persons with low vision, including Braille reading tutorial programs, Braille math tutorial programs, graphics programs, and a typing tutorial program.

Lovejoy Electronics

35 Garrison Street
Portland, ME 04102
207-774-9421
Disability Served: all

This company manufactures a light-activated joystick emulator for computers.

MacKay Associates

6439 Boxelder Drive
Lincoln, NE 68506
402-486-3550
Disability Served: learning disabled

This company develops software programs, including a program designed to produce reports on students in special education and a program designed to create Individualized Education Programs for students.

MacLaboratory Inc.

314 Exeter Road
Devon, PA 19333
610-688-3114
Disability Served: communication

This company designs assessment and intervention software for persons with motor or cognitive impairments.

MacSema
1690 SW Western Boulevard
Corvallis, OR 97333-4108
541-757-1638
Disability Served: all

This company develops a voice input program where speech replaces the use of a keyboard or mouse.

Magic Laboratories Inc.
1733 Woodside Road, Suite 315
Redwood City, CA 94061
650-368-9498, 800-368-6244
Disability Served: communication

This company develops a communication board used in conjunction with a personal computer.

Malachi Ltd.
13 Colonial Drive
Mendon, MA 01756-1328
508-478-2838
Disability Served: vision

This company manufactures Sam, an environmental control unit that is voice activated.

Marblesoft
12301 Central Avenue NE, Suite 205
Blaine, MN 55434
612-755-1402
http://www.winternet.com/~marble
Disability Served: all

This company manufactures early learning and special needs educational software.

MASTERY Rehabilitation Systems, Inc.
105 Bala Avenue
Bala Cynwyd, PA 19004
610-664-2025, 800-859-2828
http://www.Esteps.com
Disability Served: all

This company manufactures Essential Steps, a cognitive orthotic designed to foster self-sufficiency.

Matias Corporation
600 Rexdale Boulevard, Suite 1204
Rexdale, ON M9W 6T4 Canada
416-749-3124, 888-663-4263
http://www.matiascorp.com
Disability Served: all

This company offers Half-QWERTY, software that allows a regular keyboard to function as a one-handed keyboard at speeds upwards of sixty-four words per minute.

Mayer-Johnson Company
PO Box 1579
Solana Beach, CA 92075-1579
619-550-0084, 800-588-4548
http://www.mayer-johnson.com
Disability Served: communication

This company produces books and software for use in augmentative communication and special education. Materials are geared toward people who are not able to speak.

McDowell-Craig
13146 Firestone Boulevard
Norwalk, CA 90650
562-773-3451
Disability Served: physically disabled

This company manufactures adaptive office equipment, including adjustable-height computer tables and work stations, keyboard platforms, monitor stands, and ergonomic chairs.

McIntyre Computer Systems
22809 Shagbark
Birmingham, MI 48025
313-645-5090
Disability Served: physically disabled

This company manufactures a trackball and joystick used as mouse alternatives and an on-screen keyboard modification program.

MDEX, Inc.
346 Rheem Boulevard, Suite 205
Moraga, CA 94556
800-344-6339
TTY/TDD: 800-888-6339
Disability Served: hearing

This company manufactures a TDD emulation communication program for persons with hearing impairments. The device is linked to a personal computer.

MECC Minnesota Educational Computing Co.
6160 Summit Drive North
Minneapolis, MN 55430-4003
612-569-1640, 800-685-MECC
Disability Served: all

This company develops educational software programs designed to teach children various skills, including arithmetic, letters of the alphabet, telling time, problem solving, and more.

Med Assist Inc.
1116A 8th Street, Suite 112
Manhattan Beach, CA 90266
310-515-7588
Disability Served: physically disabled

This company provides support for people in need of environmental control units and computer access systems.

Med Labs, Inc.
28 Vereda Cordillera
Goleta, CA 93117
805-968-2486, 800-968-2486
http://hometown.aol.com/medlabsinc
Disability Served: physically disabled

This company manufactures call-signal devices for calling a hospital nurse, electronic muscle stimulators, and portable alarms.

Medical Equipment Distributors
Medical Services Department
Lubbock, TX 79423
806-793-8421, 800-253-4134
Disability Served: all

This company manufactures a variety of switches and a word processing program.

Mensys Company
850 Pierre Dertrand, Suite 230
Vanier, QC J1N 3K8 Canada
418-682-3088
http://www.mensysqc.com
Disability Served: all

This company designs a keyboard modification software program.

Merritt Computer Products Inc.
5565 Red Bird Center Drive, Suite 150
Dallas, TX 75237
214-339-0753
Disability Served: all

This company makes a keyboard protector.

Mertt Software
13635 Gamma Road
Dallas, TX 75244
214-385-2353
Disability Served: all

This company designs a drawing software program.

Mextel Inc.
159 Beeline Drive
Bensenville, IL 60106
630-595-4146
Disability Served: physically disabled

This company manufactures an expanded keyboard modification program for computers.

Micro Ed
PO Box 24750
Edina, MN 55424
612-929-2242
Disability Served: all

This company designs a reading tutorial program for computers.

Micro Video Corporation
210 Collingwood, Suite 100
Ann Arbor, MI 48107-7357
734-996-0626, 800-537-2182
Disability Served: communication

This company produces a speech training software program.

Microflip, Inc.

11211 Petworth Lane
Glenn Dale, MD 20769-2017
301-262-6020
TDD: 301-262-6020
http://www.microflip.com
Disability Served: hearing

This company develops and manufactures TTY/TDD modems and software, as well as signaling devices for the hard of hearing.

Microlog Corporation

20270 Goldenrod Lane
Germantown, MD 20876
301-428-3227, 800-926-3227
Disability Served: hearing

This company manufactures a telecommunication program for the computer that enables the computer to act as a telephone system for the hearing impaired.

Microsoft Corporation

One Microsoft Way
Redmond, WA 98052
425-454-2030, 800-876-4726
Disability Served: all

Microsoft makes keyboard modification programs, trackballs to emulate standard mouse controls, and voice output programs.

Microspeed Inc.

5005 Brandin Court
Fremont, CA 94538-3140
510-490-1403
Disability Served: physically disabled

This company develops a number of computer trackballs designed to emulate mouse control.

Microsystems Software Inc.

600 Worcester Road
Framingham, MA 01701
508-626-8511, 800-828-2600
Disability Served: all

This company designs a number of computer products for persons with disabilities, including a computer-controlled phone system, keyboard modification programs, voice output programs, Morse code interface programs, and screen magnification programs.

MicroTalk Software

337 South Peterson Avenue
Louisville, KY 40206
502-832-3471
Disability Served: vision

This company designs software programs for persons with low vision. Products include a voice output screen review program, a Braille translation program, and a voice output word processing program.

MicroTouch Systems Inc.

300 Griffin Brook Park
Methuen, MA 41844
508-694-9900, 800-866-6873
Disability Served: all

This company offers touch screens and touch-activated tablets that emulate mouse controls.

Midwest Health Programs Inc.

Box 3023
Urbana, IL 61801
217-367-5293
Disability Served: hearing

This company designs an American Sign Language tutorial software program.

Mind Play

160 West Fort Lowell Road
Tucson, AZ 85705
520-888-1800
http://www.mindplay.com
Disability Served: learning disabled

This company produces curriculum-based software for special needs learners.

Misco

PO Box 399
Holmdel, NJ 07733
732-264-8200
Disability Served: all

This company offers computer supplies and accessories.

MRF Adaptive Resources Inc.

248 Farmview Lane
Mount Joy, PA 17552
717-653-6807, 800-249-4687
Disability Served: physically disabled

This company manufactures an environmental control unit program designed to allow control through a computer program and a computer-controlled telephone system.

Multimedia Designs Inc.

10 Woodcutter Court
Palm Harbor, FL 34683
888-353-3996, 727-786-3317
http://www.multimediadesigns.com
Disability Served: physically disabled

This company manufactures Multimedia Max, a voice-activated computer system which controls lights and electrical appliances, telephones, fax machines, door openers, window openers, thermostats, and more.

Myna Coporation

529 Main Street
Boston, MA 02129
617-242-7051
Disability Served: vision

This company makes voice output notebook computers for persons with visual impairments.

NanoPac, Inc.

4823 South Sheridan Road, Suite 302
Tulsa, OK 74145-5717
918-665-0329, 800-580-6086
http://www.nanopac.com
Disability Served: vision, physically disabled

This company provides computer-related assistive technology for those with blindness, low vision, and mobility disabilities.

National Association for the Deaf

814 Thayer Avenue
Silver Spring, MD 20910
301-587-1788
TTY: 301-587-1789
http://www.nad.org
Disability Served: hearing

The Association is the nation's largest organization safeguarding the accessibility and civil rights of 28 million deaf and hard of hearing Americans in education, employment, health care, and telecommunications. The NAD Publications Department produces "The NAD Broadcaster," its national newspaper, "The Deaf American Monograph." and various books.

National Institute for Rehab Engineering

PO Box T
Hewitt, NJ 07421
201-853-6585
Disability Served: vision

The Institute develops computer aids for persons with low vision, including screen magnifiers, large-print word processors, speech synthesizers, and a key lock for keyboards.

newAbilities Systems, Inc.

470 San Antonio Road, Suite G
Palo Alto, CA 94306
650-988-8889, 800-829-8889
Disability Served: physically disabled

This company manufactures an environmental control unit that is controlled by the touch of the tongue.

Nintendo of America Inc.

4820 150th Avenue NE
Redmond, WA 98052
425-882-2040
Disability Served: physically disabled

This company manufactures a cursor control interface device that allows persons with disabilities to play Nintendo games via a chin-activated joystick.

Nisus Software

990 Highland Drive, Suite 312
Solana Beach, CA 92075
619-481-1477, 800-922-2993
Disability Served: all

This company develops a keyboard modification software program.

North American Mercantile

292 Chicopee Row
Groton, MA 01450
508-448-3004
Disability Served: all

This company makes a keyboard caddy, which attaches to a standard keyboard and can hold a mouse, trackball, or joystick.

Northgate Computer Systems Inc.

7075 Flying Cloud Drive
Eden Prairie, MN 55344
612-943-8181, 800-548-1993
Disability Served: all

This company manufactures a modified keyboard that allows the user to change the configuration of the keyboard.

nVIEW

11835 Canon Boulevard
Newport News, VA 23606
757-873-1354, 800-736-8439
Disability Served: all

This company develops a wireless keyboard that allows remote control of computers.

NXi Communications, Inc.

3191 South Valley Street, Suite 205
Salt Lake City, UT 84109
801-466-1258
TTY/TDD: 801-466-0453
Disability Served: hearing

This company manufactures modems designed for text telephone use.

Oakland Schools

Communication Enhancement Center
Waterford, MI 48328
810-858-1901
Disability Served: communication

The Center develops a picture dictionary containing more than 600 symbolic language pictures and a reading tutorial software program.

Office Systems for the Visually or Physically Impaired

1822 North Wood Street
Chicago, IL 60622
800-253-4391
Disability Served: all

This organization provides workplace accommodation assistance, including training, demonstration of products, and implementation of systems.

Ohm/Electronics

746 Vermont Street
Palatine, IL 60067
847-359-5500
Disability Served: all

This company manufactures a game port for computers.

Olduvai Corp.

9200 South Dadeland Boulevard, Suite 525
Miami, FL 33156
800-822-0772
Disability Served: vision

This company develops optical character recognition software for computer scanners.

Omnichron

1438 Oxford
Berkeley, CA 94709
510-540-6455
Disability Served: vision

This company develops a voice output screen reading program for computers.

OMS Development

610 Forest Avenue, #8
Wilmette, IL 60091-1714
847-251-5787
Disability Served: all

This company manufactures an on-screen keyboard program, a word prediction software program, a mouse emulator program, and a voice output program.

Optimum Resource Inc.
5 Hiltech Lane
Hilton Head, SC 29926
803-689-8000, 800-327-1473
Disability Served: all

This company develops educational software programs including the Stickybear series.

Origin Instruments Corporation
854 Greenview Drive
Grand Prairie, TX 75050
972-606-8740, 800-280-3751
http://www.orin.com
Disability Served: all

This company manufactures computer access devices, including HeadMouse for Desktops and HeadMouse for Portables.

OT's Computer
21409 SE 268th Street
Maple Valley, WA 98038
206-432-2583
Disability Served: all

This company develops a computer program designed to assess perceptual deficits.

Pa Da Enterprises
8785 Martz-Paulin Road
Franklin, OH 45005
513-746-9487
Disability Served: all

This company manufactures a modified, oversized keyboard.

Pacific Data Systems
PO Box 1947
Burbank, CA 91507-1947
818-899-6077
Disability Served: all

This company develops a keyboard modification program in which the mouse is programmed to execute keyboard commands.

Pacific Psychological Services
1933 Jadwin Avenue
Richland, WA 99352
800-523-4915
Disability Served: all

This company develops software programs designed to assess vocational interests.

Parrot Software
PO Box 1139
State College, PA 16804
814-237-7282, 800-727-7681
Disability Served: all

This company develops reading and language tutorial software programs.

PC Compatibles
55 Valley View
Cappaqua, NY 10514
914-238-7818
Disability Served: all

This company manufactures a lapboard designed for a keyboard and a keyboard wrist support.

Peal Software
c/o Dr Laura Meyers
Playa del Rey, CA 90293
310-551-8585
Disability Served: all

This company develops language tutorial programs, literacy programs, and voice output programs for students with physical and mental disabilities.

PennStar Support Group
Box 213
Lewisburg, PA 17837-0213
717-523-1155
Disability Served: all

This company develops software programs designed to assist special education instructors by creating Individual Education Plans (IEPs).

Penny & Giles Computer Products
163 Pleasant Street
Attleboro, MA 02703
508-226-3008
Disability Served: all

This company manufactures joysticks and trackballs that emulate mouse controls.

Perfect Solutions
12657 Coral Breeze Drive
West Palm Beach, FL 33414
561-790-1070, 800-726-7086
Disability Served: all

This company develops a laptop computer with built-in software programs that word process, keep track of appointments, store telephone numbers and addresses, and more.

Peripheral Technologies Inc.
1109 Hillcrest Road
Narberth, PA 19072
215-667-2190
Disability Served: vision

This company makes a speech synthesizer for computers.

Personal Computer Resources
145 Webster Street, #D
Hanover, MA 02339-1228
617-871-5396
Disability Served: all

This company develops software programs that teach communication skills and output voice.

Personal Data Systems Inc.
100 West Rincon Avenue, Suite 103
Campbell, CA 95008
408-866-1126, 800-426-4832
Disability Served: vision

This company manufactures a speech synthesizer that converts alphanumeric text to speech to accommodate the visually or reading impaired.

PESCO International
21 Paulding Street
Pleasantville, NY 10570
800-431-2016
http://www.pesco.org
Disability Served: all

This company manufactures and sells SAGE, PESCO System 2000, and the Compute-A-Match System, which assesses an individual's aptitudes, reasoning, math skills, language aptitude, interests, temperaments, work attitude, ethics, and learning styles. (These products are available in Braille, large print, and Spanish.) The system then matches these assessments to appropriate training.

Phillip Rot, Inc.
PO Box 128
Indian Rocks Beach, FL 33785
727-593-2700, 800-255-9085
http://www.phillirot.com
Disability Served: all

This company develops more than ninety educational software programs and book programs in the areas of life skills, academic skills, and vocational and applied academic skills.

Phone TTY Inc.
202 Lexington Avenue
Hackensack, NJ 07601-4043
201-489-7889
Disability Served: hearing

This company manufactures aids for the hearing impaired. Products include doorbell signalers, telephone ring signalers, specialized alarm clocks, TDD emulation software programs, and more.

Phonic Ear Inc.
3880 Cypress Drive
Petaluma, CA 94954-7600
707-769-1110, 800-227-0735
Disability Served: hearing

This company makes items for the hearing impaired, including amplification systems, keyboard interface programs, and electronic communication aids.

Polytel Computer Products Corporation

1287 Hammerwood Avenue
Sunnyvale, CA 94089
408-745-1540
Disability Served: all

This company manufactures a modified keyboard and an expanded keyboard.

Power Translation Co.

11500 Statesville Road
Huntersville, NC 28078
704-875-2138
Disability Served: all

This company manufactures a voice input environmental control unit that can control electrical appliances.

Precedent Systems Inc.

PO Box 31478
Seattle, WA 98103
800-444-3454
Disability Served: all

This company develops a software program that automates report writing for therapists as well as an office management software program designed for physical therapy and rehabilitation facilities.

Premtech Corporation

4357-A Park Drive
Norcross, GA 30093
770-925-2700
Disability Served: all

This company manufactures an anti-glare screen magnifier for computer monitors and a trackball that emulates mouse controls.

Prentke Romich Company

1022 Heyl Road
Wooster, OH 44691
330-262-1984, 800-262-1984
http://www.prentrom.com
Disability Served: all

This company provides communication devices for people who are nonspeaking. The company also provides computer access products for people who are not able to use a standard keyboard.

Pres Air Trol Corporation

1009 West Boston Post Road
Mamaroneck, NY 10543
914-698-2026, 800-431-2625
http://www.presair.com
Disability Served: all

This company makes a variety of switches, among them foot switches and pneumatic and electric air bellows.

Pro-Team Products, Inc.

1800 Star-Batt Drive
Rochester Hills, MI 48309
810-853-2375, 800-314-3754
Disability Served: all

This company manufactures a keyboard wrist support for computer users who need to relieve wrist and arm stress while typing.

Productivity Software International

211 East 43rd Street, #2202
New York, NY 10017-4707
212-967-8666, 800-533-7587
Disability Served: physically disabled

This company manufactures a software program that allows computer keyboards to be used by one finger or mouthstick. Another program this company offers is an abbreviation expansion program.

Programming Concepts Inc.

5221 McCullough
San Antonio, TX 78212
210-824-5949, 800-594-4263
Disability Served: all

This company develops educational programs and games designed to teach behavior skills, independent living skills, health skills, eating skills, money skills, speaking skills, and more.

Programs That Work
19 Palmer Drive
Sayville, NY 11782-2823
516-563-7296
Disability Served: all

This company designs a software program that creates Individual Education Plan (IEP) reports. It is designed primarily for teachers.

Psychological Corporation
555 Academic Court
San Antonio, TX 78204
210-299-1061
Disability Served: all

This company manufactures communication software programs.

Psychological Software Services, Inc.
6555 Carrollton Avenue
Indianapolis, IN 46220
317-257-9672
http://www.neuroscience.cnter.com/
Disability Served: head/brain injury

This company develops and markets rehabilitation software for use in clinical or educational settings. The software is used to rehabilitate the cognitive skills compromised from head injury, stroke, tumor, and problems associated with learning disabilities.

Quartet Technology Inc.
52 Davis Road
Tyngsboro, MA 01879
508-692-9313
Disability Served: all

This company manufactures voice-controlled environmental control units that can be used to operate appliances, telephones, lights, and other household items.

R. J. Cooper & Associates
24843 Del Prado, Suite 283
Dana Point, CA 92629
949-661-6904, 800-752-6673
http://www.rjcooper.com
Disability Served: all

This company develops control-switch training programs, speech-training programs, game programs, and trackballs.

R/COM Inc.
5116 25th Avenue NE
Seattle, WA 98105
206-443-9325
Disability Served: all

This company designs software programs for managing the operation of medical rehabilitation facilities.

Radio Shack
1500 One Tandy Center
Ft Worth, TX 76102
817-390-3011
Disability Served: all

This company manufactures electronic goods, including telephones, calculators, phone flashers, cassette recorders, switches, and more.

Raised Dot Computing
408 South Baldwin
Madison, WI 53703
608-257-9595, 800-347-9594
http://www.rdcbraille.com
Disability Served: vision

This company produces a software program for Braille translation.

Rapidtext
230 Newport Center Drive, Suite 250
Newport Beach, CA 92660
714-644-6500
http://www.rapidtext.com
Disability Served: hearing

This company offers a full line of captioning services, including real-time captioning for the classroom, seminars, meetings, and television. Rapidtext also offers closed or open captioning for videos. Captioning software and hardware are also sold.

RC Systems Inc.
121 West Winesap Road
Bothell, WA 98012
206-672-6909
Disability Served: all

This company develops voice output software programs and speech synthesizer cards for computers.

RDL Inc.
1758 Empire Central
Dallas, TX 75235
214-630-3965, 800-688-1758
Disability Served: physically disabled

This company supplies the home health care industry with a Power Door system that automatically unlocks, opens, holds open, closes, and relocks doors for the physically challenged.

REACH Inc.
890 Hearthstone Drive
Stone Mountain, GA 30083
404-292-8933
Disability Served: all

This company manufactures various switches and accessories to modify computer keyboards by locking down specified keys.

Reflection Technology
230 Second Avenue
Waltham, MA 02154
781-890-5905
Disability Served: vision

This company manufactures a large-print display system for personal computers.

Rehabilitation Consultants Inc.
PO Box 43254
Birmingham, AL 35243-0254
205-967-9798
http://www.oakes.org
Disability Served: all but substance abuse and mentally disabled

This company provides rehabilitation and safety/technical consultation for life-care planning, pain management, wheelchair accessibility, industrial safety, and catastrophic injury.

Rehabilitation Technology Services
2305 Carlisle Drive
Champaign, IL 61820
217-398-4543
Disability Served: vision

This company develops a typing tutorial program for blind individuals.

Research Press
2612 North Mattis Avenue
Champaign, IL 61822
217-352-3273
Disability Served: all

This company produces books, videocassettes, and software in the area of developmental disabilities.

Robert J. Sbordone
7700 Irvine Center Drive, Suite 750
Irvine, CA 92718
714-753-7711
Disability Served: all

This company manufactures a cognitive skills assessment program for computers.

Roberts Book Mark Co.
3038 North Federal Highway, Building H
Ft Lauderdale, FL 33306
954-563-6155
http://members.aol.com/~roberts98/index1.html
Disability Served: physically disabled

This company distributes a book holder/reading aid.

Robo Systems Corporation
408 South State Street, #4
Newtown, PA 18940-1947
215-750-6990
Disability Served: all

This company develops computer-aided design software programs.

RolControl Products
6750 Worth Way
Camarillo, CA 93012
805-386-4191
Disability Served: physically disabled

This company develops controls for powered wheelchairs, switches, and kits to convert manual wheelchairs to powered wheelchairs.

Ronald S. McCuiston

5795 Adelyn Road
Pensacola, FL 32504
850-476-8916
Disability Served: all

This manufacturer develops keyboard modification software programs.

RoseSoft Inc.

PO Box 70337
Bellevue, WA 98007
425-562-0225
Disability Served: all

This company develops a keyboard enhancement software program.

Royal Data Systems

Route 8, Box 53-G
Morganton, NC 28655
704-433-5909, 800-843-9750
Disability Served: learning disabled

This company produces a reading tutorial software program designed to print text with reversed characters and numbers. Teachers can use the software for instructing students with dyslexia.

Ruth Huebner MS OTR

2302 Liberty Lane
Janesville, WI 53545
608-752-3977
Disability Served: all

This therapist designs an Individual Education Plan (IEP) that evaluates and determines treatments for occupational therapy patients.

Safe Reading & Computer Box Co.

4407 Swinson Road
Rhodes, MI 48652
517-689-6369
http://www.mesrelief.com
Disability Served: all

This company manufactures boxes for persons who are chemically sensitive, including a computer box for persons who are chemically sensitive to the radiation emitted from computers, a reading box for persons who are chemically sensitive to book, magazine, or newspaper print, and a sauna box for persons who are chemically sensitive to sauna treatments, or need to detoxify.

Safko International Inc.

Lon Safko
PO Box 1479
Chandler, AZ 85244-1479
602-731-9805
Disability Served: all

This company manufactures a computer-based environmental control unit.

SAIA-Burgess Electronics Inc.

1335 Barclay Boulevard
Buffalo Grove, IL 60089
847-215-9600
http://www.saia-burgess-usa.com
Disability Served: all

This company manufactures microswitches.

SARA Systems, Inc.

PO Box 4007
Wichita, KS 67204-0007
800-872-7279
Disability Served: all

This company develops a keyboard modification software program.

Scholastic Software

2931 East McCarty Street
Jefferson City, MO 65102
800-392-2179 (MO), 800-541-5513
Disability Served: all

This company develops reading tutorial software programs, spelling tutorial programs, and voice output word processing programs.

See-Sign Productions

15 Bluebill Avenue, Suite 1104
Naples, FL 33963
941-598-3067
Disability Served: hearing

This company develops sign language tutorial programs for children and for persons with developmental disabilities.

SEMCO

1833 North 20th Street
Sheboygan, WI 53081
414-458-2065
http://www.excel.net/business/quadjoy~mouse.htm
Disability Served: physically disabled

This company manufactures a computer mouse for quadriplegics. The mouse can be mounted to the computer workstation and activated through sip and puff maneuvers.

Sensible Software Inc.

20200 East 9-Mile Road, #150
St Claire Shores, MI 48080-1791
313-774-7215
Disability Served: vision

This software company develops a voice output spell checker and dictionary.

SET Inc.

3205 Spyglass Drive
Vancouver, WA 98684-3724
360-944-2029
Disability Served: all

This company manufactures personal amplification systems, speech synthesizers, and computer headphone sets so persons with hearing and communication disabilities can listen to and create sounds for playback through a computer.

Shea Products Inc.

1721 West Hamilton Road
Rochester Hills, MI 48309
810-852-4940
Disability Served: communication

This company manufactures a portable scanning communicator and a portable electronic communication aid with voice output.

Sher Mark Products Inc.

11 Ramleh Road
Mt Kisco, NY 01549
914-241-6262
Disability Served: vision

This company manufactures a glare reduction magnification screen that fits over computer screens.

Sign Enhancers, Inc.

1320 Edgewater NW, Suite B10
Salem, OR 97304
503-370-9721, 800-767-4461
Disability Served: hearing

This company develops a sign language dictionary program, an interactive sign language software program, and a sign language training videotape.

SkiSoft Publishing Corporation

1644 Massachusetts Avenue, Suite 79
Lexington, MA 02173
781-863-1876, 800-662-3622
Disability Served: vision

This company manufactures a word processing software program for people with limited vision.

Skools Inc.

40 Fifth Avenue, Suite 15A
New York, NY 10011
212-674-1150, 800-545-4474
http://www.kinderlink.com
Disability Served: physically disabled

This company manufactures a wheelchair-accessible computer work station designed for children.

Slipstream Solutions

9583 South Corsair
Conifer, CO 80433
800-321-7685
Disability Served: all

This company develops an Individual Education Plan (IEP) creation program for computers.

Slosson Educational Publications, Inc.

PO Box 280, 538 Buffalo Road
East Aurora, NY 14052
716-652-0930, 888-756-7766
http://www.slosson.com
Disability Served: all

This company offers an extensive product line that includes testing and assessment materials, learning enhancement materials, books, games, videos, cassettes, and computer software. These products are intended for use by professionals, psychologists, teachers, counselors, students, and parents.

Smith Kettlewell Eye Research Institute

2318 Fillmore Street
San Francisco, CA 94115
415-345-2000
Disability Served: vision

The Institute develops light sensors, computer accessories for blind persons, dark probes designed to detect light, educational devices, and electronic orientation systems (Talking Signs).

SOFT X

Traxler Enterprises
Milwaukee, WI 53210
414-445-5925
Disability Served: vision

This company designs a voice output check register software program and a voice output filing program.

Softac Corporation

23 Sunset Road
Winchester, MA 01890
617-721-1010
Disability Served: vision

This company manufactures a mouse emulator and large-print software program.

Software Designs

4594 East Lake Circle North
Littleton, CO 80121
303-220-8682
Disability Served: all

This company develops software programs, including student tracking programs and Individual Education Plan (IEP) creation programs.

Software for Sam

2971 53rd Street SE
Auburn, WA 98092-8310
253-735-6350
Disability Served: vision

This company develops software for blind or visually impaired children for education or communication purposes.

Software Research Corp.

4252 Commerce Circle
Victoria, BC V8Z 4M2 Canada
250-727-6522
Disability Served: communication

This company designs a speech analysis computer program and a speech training program.

Southern Calif Research Group

PO Box 593
Moorpark, CA 93020
805-529-2082
Disability Served: all

This company manufactures switch adapters for computers, disk loading systems, and other hardware for Apple computers.

Southern Microscope

225 North Main Street
Graham, NC 27253
910-570-1101, 800-888-8555
Disability Served: all

This company develops academic assessment and report programs.

Spec Tech

200 North Emerson Avenue, Suite B
Greenwood, IN 46143
317-782-4346
Disability Served: all

Spec Tech represents manufacturers of different types of adaptive equipment, including communication aids, computer equipment, and controls.

Special Learning Ed Software

PO Box 16322
Minneapolis, MN 55416
612-926-5820
Disability Served: all

SLED manufactures a spelling tutorial program for computers.

Speller Teller Communications

Al Kalashian
West Allis, WI 53227
414-327-4051
Disability Served: communication

This company makes a variety of switches and communication boards.

SRA

155 North Wacker Drive
Chicago, IL 60606
312-984-7000
Disability Served: all

This company develops software programs designed to teach basic skills and concepts to children.

SRA

Macmillan/McGraw-Hill
Backlick, OH 43004-0543
800-843-8855
Disability Served: all

This company develops educational software programs.

Steck-Vaughn Company

PO Box 26015
Austin, TX 78755
800-531-5015
Disability Served: all

This company develops language training programs and personal skills training programs.

Stephen Blache, PhD.

Department of Communication Disorders
Carbondale, IL 62901
618-453-4301
Disability Served: communication

The Department develops a software program designed to assess and analyze children's articulation errors.

Stoelting

620 Wheat Lane
Wood Dale, IL 60191
630-860-9700
http://www.stoeltingco.com
Disability Served: all

Among the items offered by this company are a mirrored device for hand-eye coordination development, a sensory integration evaluation system, and a skills training evaluation program.

StrateCision

475 Hillside Avenue
Wellesley, MA 02181
781-453-1938
Disability Served: all

This company develops a computer program called Healthcommand. The program is a medical tracking record for families and reminds families of necessary immunizations and exams.

Subtle Impact Software, Inc.

7195 Sand Trap Drive
Colorado Springs, CO 80925
719-382-5437
Disability Served: hearing

This company produces a software program designed to teach sign language.

Sunburst Communications
101 Castleton Steet
Pleasantville, NY 10570
914-747-3310, 800-628-8897
Disability Served: all

This company develops software programs, including writing skills programs, math tutorial programs, typing tutorial programs, and more.

Sunset Software
9277 East Corrine Drive
Scottsdale, AZ 85260
602-451-0753
Disability Served: all

This company develops educational software programs.

Super Impact Images
RR 1, Box 67
Warriors Mark, PA 16877-9708
Disability Served: vision

This company develops a large-print computer program.

Switch in Time
101 Clay Street
Cambridge, MA 02140
617-354-6577
Disability Served: all

This company manufactures a music composition program for computers.

Symbol Graphics
1047 West Sixth Street
Corona, CA 91720
909-736-4040, 800-736-4045
Disability Served: vision

This company develops a Braille graphics software program.

Synergy
412 High Plain Street, Suite 19
Walpole, MA 02081
508-668-7424
http://www.speak-withus.com
Disability Served: physically disabled

This company develops a portable voice output computer that can be attached to a wheelchair.

Syntha Voice Computers Inc.
125 Gailmont Drive
Hamilton, ON L8K 4B8 Canada
416-578-0565
Disability Served: vision

This company manufactures portable voice output computers, large-print software programs, and speech synthesizer programs.

Talking Computers Inc.
4301 Fairfax Drive, #1034
Arlington, VA 22203-1627
Disability Served: vision

This company develops a Braille reference guide for WordPerfect as well as computer training audiocassettes.

Talktronics Inc.
27341 Eastridge Drive
El Toro, CA 92630
714-768-4220, 800-421-7668
Disability Served: vision

Talktronics manufactures speech synthesizers for computers.

Tapeswitch Corp. of America
100 Schmitt Boulevard
Farmingdale, NY 11735
516-694-6312
htttp://www.tapeswitch.com
Disability Served: all

This company manufactures a variety of switches, sensing bumpers, safety/sensing mats, light curtain safety systems, touch pads, foot/hand/grip switches, and interface controllers.

TASH International Inc.
Unit 1, 91 Station Street
Ajax, ON L1S 3H2 Canada
905-686-4129, 800-463-5685
http://www.tashint.com
Disability Served: physically disabled

Assistive Technology

This company manufactures and markets assistive technology devices for people with physical disabilities. It has been in operation since 1979.

Teachers Institute for Special Education

2947 Bayside Court
Wantagh, NY 11793
516-781-2020
Disability Served: all

This company develops typing instruction software programs.

Technology Assessment Program

Gallaudet University
Washington, DC 20002
Disability Served: hearing

The Program develops a telecommunication software program that allows communication between home computers and text telephones.

Technology for Language & Learning

5 Tameling Road
East Rockaway, NY 11518
516-625-4550
Disability Served: all

This company produces public domain software for children and adults with special needs.

Teddy Bear Software

c/o Maleta Blessing
Gladewater, TX 75647-4941
903-845-4244
Disability Served: developmentally disabled

Teddy Bear Software produces drivers education software to assist mentally handicapped and learning disabled individuals with passing driver's license tests.

Telesensory Corporation

455 North Bernardo Avenue
Mountain View, CA 94039
650-960-0920, 800-804-8004
Disability Served: vision

This company manufactures a number of items to assist persons with limited vision. Products include low vision reading systems, Braille computer terminals, large-print programs, Braille translators, tactile reading systems, TDD systems and voice output programs.

Tell 'Em Ware

1714 Olson Way
Marshalltown, IA 50158
Disability Served: all

This company develops public domain educational software programs for persons with disabilities.

The Co/Op

135 Beaver Street
Waltham, MA 02154
781-890-0700, 800-543-3000
Disability Served: all

This company designs software programs that produce Individual Education Plans (IEPs) as well as student tracking programs.

The Lighthouse Catalog

36-20 Northern Boulevard
Long Island City, NY 11101
800-829-0500
http://www.lighthouse.org
Disability Served: vision

This nonprofit organization seeks to overcome vision impairment through rehabilitation services, education, and research. The Lighthouse Catalog offers assistive devices for sale.

The Sword Company

PO Box 176
Comptche, CA 95427-0176
707-937-4298
Disability Served: all

This company develops a keyboard expansion software program and word processing program.

Thought I Could

107 University Place, Suite 4D
New York, NY 10003
212-673-9724
Disability Served: vision

This company manufactures a voice output calculator program for Macintosh computers.

TIGER Communication Systems, Inc.

328 Main Street East, Suite 514
Rochester, NY 14604-2115
716-454-5134, 800-724-7301
Disability Served: all

This company designs a voice output program of symbolic language pictures, communication boards, and keyguards for communication devices.

Tiger Electronics Inc.

980 Woodlands Parkway
Vernon Hills, IL 60061
847-913-8100
Disability Served: communication

This company develops speech analysis software programs.

TRAIN Inc.

Neshaminy Plaza, Suite 101
Ben Salem, PA 19020
215-632-5900
Disability Served: learning disabled

This company develops a software program designed to diagnose and evaluate learning disabilities.

TriTek Corp.

5263 Stewart Road
Sumerduck, VA 22742
540-439-3690
http://www.tritekcorp.com
Disability Served: all

This company develops and sells tools of science that can be used by people with severe mobility deficits. The PC-Scope is a computer-controlled microscope that can be operated without limb mobility using voice-activated commands or a trackball for microscopists with partial limb mobility.

Typewriting Institute for the Handicapped

3102 West Augusta Avenue
Phoenix, AZ 85051
602-939-5344
Disability Served: physically disabled

This company sells computer keyboards and typewriters designed for typists who use only one hand.

UCLA Microcomputer Project

1000 Veteran Avenue, Room 23-10
Los Angeles, CA 90095
310-825-4821
Disability Served: all

A variety of educational software programs are offered by the Project, including programs designed to teach cognitive skills and prereading skills.

Ultraflo Corporation

310 Industrial Lane
Sandusky, OH 44870
419-626-8182, 800-760-5629
http://ultraflo.com
Disability Served: all

This company manufactures Ultraflo, a do-it-yourself, one-line, temperature-controlled, push-button plumbing system designed to help people with disabilities turn on and off water with ease.

United Educational Services Inc.

PO Box 1099
Buffalo, NY 14224
716-668-7691, 800-458-7900
Disability Served: communication

This company manufactures communication aids, including speech training programs, symbolic language tutorial programs, and more.

Universal Learning Technology

39 Cross Street
Peabody, MA 01960
508-538-0036
TTY/TDD: 508-538-3110
http://www.unilearn.com
Disability Served: learning disabled

This company makes products designed to make curriculum material accessible for all levels of learners. Products include Ultimate Reader, Ultimate Kid Books, Ultimate Caption Works, and Quick Caption for Word.

University of Michigan Software

Intellectual Properties Office
Ann Arbor, MI 48109
734-936-0435
Disability Served: all

The University develops a software program designed to test and improve short-term memory.

Valpar International Corp.

2450 West Ruthrauff
Tucson, AZ 85705
520-293-1510, 800-528-7070
Disability Served: all

This company designs a software program that assesses vocational interests and aptitude.

Van Duerr Industries

426 Broadway, Suite 207
Chico, CA 95928
916-893-1596
http://www.vanduerr.com
Disability Served: all

This company manufactures products for people with disabilities.

Versatron Corp.

103 West North Street
Healdsburg, CA 95488
707-433-3000
Disability Served: all

This company develops a foot-operated mouse for computers.

Vertex System Corp.

705 Lakeview Plaza, Suite J
Worthington, OH 43085
614-846-3427
http://www.vertexsoftware.com
Disability Served: all

This company develops a software program designed for clinical management tasks of rehabilitation facilities.

Vision Aid Systems, Inc.

PO Box 1369
Greenwood, IN 46142
317-888-0323, 800-765-7483
Disability Served: vision

Vision Aid Systems, Inc. represents manufacturers who provide adaptive equipment, specifically computer equipment, for those suffering from low vision and/or blindness.

VistaMed

1315 Pembina Highway
Winnipeg, MB R3T 5S3 Canada
204-949-7676, 800-563-7676
Disability Served: all

This company makes a software program designed to evaluate seating systems.

Visuaide 2000 Inc.

955 rue D'Assigny
Longueuil, QC J4K 5C3 Canada
514-463-1717
Disability Served: vision

This company develops a voice output software program.

ViziFlex Seels Incorporated

16 East Lafayette Street
Hackensack, NJ 07601
201-487-8080
Disability Served: all

This company develops a keyboard wrist support.

VME Technologies, Inc.

5202 Westland Boulevard
Baltimore, MD 21227
410-455-6395
Disability Served: physically disabled

This company makes a blink detection switch that allows persons with disabilities to control their environments.

Vocational Research Institute
1528 Walnut Street, Suite 1502
Philadelphia, PA 19102
215-875-7387, 800-874-5387
http://www.vri.org
Disability Served: all

This company develops career-assessment systems (interest and aptitude testing).

Voice Connexion
17971 Skypark Circle, Suite F
Irvine, CA 92714
714-261-2366
Disability Served: vision

This company develops voice input systems for computers and a voice-activated environmental control unit program.

Vort Corporation
PO Box 60132
Palo Alto, CA 94306
650-322-8282
Disability Served: all

This company designs developmental assessment software programs for instructors and other professionals.

VRRI—Vocational & Rehabilitation Research
3304 33rd Street NW
Calgary, AB T2L 2A6 Canada
403-284-1121
Disability Served: all

This company develops software programs for perceptual training, cognitive skills training, Blissymbol training, and math skills training.

Waveco
PO Box 1331
Palmetto, FL 34220
941-723-2229, 800-261-8132
Disability Served: all

This company manufactures a gel-filled keyboard wrist support.

West Virginia Research and Training Center
806 Allen Hall
Morgantown, WV 26506
304-293-5313
Disability Served: all

The Center develops a series of software programs designed to provide clinical management for rehabilitation facilities.

WEST—Work Evaluation Systems Technology
22741 North Highway 1
Ft Bragg, CA 95437
Disability Served: all

This company develops work stations that measure range of motion and physical strength and dexterity.

Western Center for Microcomputers Inc.
1259 El Camino Real, PMB 275
Menlo Park, CA 94025
650-855-8064
http://home.earthlink.net/~thecatalyst/
Disability Served: vision

This company produces a speech synthesizer for use with computers.

Western Psychological Services
12031 Wilshire Boulevard
Los Angeles, CA 90025-1251
310-478-2061, 800-648-8857
http://www.wpspublish.com
Disability Served: all

This company designs tests and software programs that assess and evaluate persons with developmental disabilities, evaluate a child's development, and train students with speech disabilities.

WesTest Engineering Corporation
1470 North Main Street
Bountiful, UT 84010
801-292-7379
Disability Served: all

This company designs joysticks that emulate mouse and keyboard controls.

William K. Bradford Publishing Co.
310 School Street
Acton, MA 01720
Disability Served: all

This company designs a keyboard modification program for children.

Woodsmith Software
Route 3, Box 550A
Nashville, IN 47448
812-988-2137
Disability Served: vision

This company produces a large-print software program for persons with low vision.

World Communications
245 Tonopah Drive
Fremont, CA 94539
510-656-0911
Disability Served: all

This company develops software programs. Products include word processing programs, on-screen keyboard programs, word prediction programs, and keyboard modification programs.

Wrist-Eze Products, Inc.
54 Woodcut Lane
Roslyn Heights, NY 11577-2324
516-484-5792
Disability Served: all

This company manufactures a keyboard wrist support for computer users.

XEROX Adaptive Technology
9 Centennial Drive
Peabody, MA 01960
508-977-2000
Disability Served: vision

This company develops optical character recognition scanning systems to assist persons with low vision.

Xpert Software
8865 Polland Avenue
San Diego, CA 92123
619-268-0112
Disability Served: all

This software company develops keyboard expansion programs that allow the user to define macros.

Daily Living Aids

These companies manufacture, sell, or distribute daily living aids, which may include home management aids, personal care items such as utensils or clothing, seating and cushions, therapeutic aids, orthotics, and more.

A & E Industries Inc.
525 South Seventeenth Street
Belleville, IL 62226
618-233-6176
Disability Served: all

This company manufactures a back support for toilets.

A+H International Products, Inc.
Shoreline Square Tower
301 East Ocean Boulevard, Suite 1010
Long Beach, CA 90802
562-435-1011, 800-455-4345
Disability Served: all

This company manufactures a wireless signal transmitter for children so parents can keep track of their location.

A-Solution, Inc.
2928 Ghiradelli NE
Albuquerque, NM 87106-1750
505-256-0115
Disability Served: physically disabled

This company manufactures and markets a retrofit, handicapped-accessible window operator called Window Ease.

AA Sales Inc.

PO Box 996
Lake Zurich, IL 60047-0996
847-726-7520
Disability Served: all

This company manufactures a combination walker and transfer lift as well as an elbow and knee splint.

AAA Healthcare Equipment

41967 State Route 39
Wellsville, OH 43968
216-532-1509, 800-331-8042
Disability Served: all

This company makes adjustable commodes, foot stools, crutches, and walkers.

Abilitations by Sportime International

One Sportime Way
Atlanta, GA 30340
800-850-8603
Disability Served: all

This company provides pediatric equipment for the restoration of physical ability, including movement, exercise, sensory, aquatics, and positioning equipment.

Ability Building Center

1911 14th Street NW
PO Box 6938
Rochester, NY 55901
Disability Served: all

This company manufactures access signs.

Able Table Co.

Weir Enterprises
227 Fern Street
Santa Cruz, CA 95060
408-425-5767
Disability Served: all

This company manufactures overhead bookholders designed to raise books to eye level.

Able Walker Inc.

1122 Fir Avenue, Building C-2
Blaine, WA 98230
360-299-3444, 800-663-1305
Disability Served: physically disabled

This company manufactures a folding, wheeled walker.

ABLEDATA

8455 Colesville Road, Suite 935
Silver Spring, MD 20910
301-608-8998, 800-227-0216
TTY/TDD: 301-608-8912
http://www.abledata.com
Disability Served: all

ABLEDATA is an electronic database of assistive technology and rehabilitation equipment listing more than 23,000 products from more than 2,500 companies.

Accelerated Learning System

1315 Apple Avenue
Silver Spring, MD 20910
301-587-8686
Disability Served: all

This company makes devices for measuring stress, treating high blood pressure, migraines, and tension headaches using biofeedback devices.

Access Elevator Technology

8230 Ronda Drive
Canton, MI 48187
313-455-9172
Disability Served: all

This company builds a home elevator.

Access Industries, Inc.

4001 East 138th Street
Grandview, MO 64030
816-763-2840, 800-925-3100
Disability Served: physically disabled

This company manufactures a wide array of lifts and residential elevator systems.

Access Remodeling, Inc.
PO Box 60027
Potomac, MD 20859-0027
301-983-0131
Disability Served: physically disabled

This company designs and implements solutions to architectural barriers for the disabled.

Access Specialties and Products, Inc.
Division of Mobile Care, Inc.
211 Beeline Drive, #3
Bensenville, IL 60106
630-766-2304, 800-8-LEVERS
Disability Served: all

This company manufactures door handle levers.

Access to Recreation
8 Sandra Court
Newbury Park, CA 91320-4302
800-634-4351
http://www.accesstorecreation.com
Disability Served: physically disabled

This is a mail order company specializing in exercise and recreation equipment for the physically challenged.

Access With Ease
PO Box 1150
Chino Valley, AZ 86323
602-636-9469
Disability Served: all

This company makes an extension for tool handles, such as rakes, brooms, and shovels.

Access-Able Designs, Inc.
2851 Elderwood Road
Salem, OR 24153
503-389-7530
Disability Served: physically disabled

This company manufactures shower and toilet transfer benches.

Accessible Designs—Adjustable Systems, Inc.
94 Columbus Road
Athens, OH 45701
740-593-5240
http://www.ad-as.com
Disability Served: all

This company manufactures accessible computer furniture, library furniture, rehab furniture and equipment, kitchen cabinets, and sinks.

Accessible Work Systems, Inc.
2295 County Road 292
Bellevue, OH 44811
419-483-4872, 800-344-9301
Disability Served: all

This company manufactures accessible office equipment, including motorized storage shelves, file cabinets, height-adjustable work stations, and vertical outlet extensions.

ACCESSories
426 Broadway, Suite 207
Chico, CA 95928
800-497-2003
Disability Served: physically disabled

This company makes door threshold ramps.

Accidental Accessories
15 Bridge Street
Carthage, NY 13619
315-493-2658
Disability Served: all

This company makes carrying accessories for wheelchairs, walkers, and crutches, as well as arm slings, aprons, and lap robes.

Accu-Back
1475 East Del Amo Boulevard
Carson, CA 90746
310-639-7992, 800-272-8888
Disability Served: all

This company manufactures back and wrist support cushions.

Achievement Products Inc.
PO Box 9033
Canton, OH 44711
330-453-2122, 800-373-4699
Disability Served: all

This company manufactures innovative mobility, seating, and positioning equipment for children with special needs. A wide range of adapted furniture, early stimulation products, ADL, and products for people with Alzheimer's disease and related dementias is available. Call for a free catalog.

Acor
18530 South Miles Road
Cleveland, OH 44128
216-662-4500, 800-237-2267
Disability Served: all

Acor makes orthotics, orthopedic footwear, and orthotic shoe inserts.

Action Lift Chairs
PO Box 126
Richfield, WI 53076
414-628-4178
Disability Served: physically disabled

This company manufactures a seat lift recliner.

Action Products Inc.
22 North Mulberry Street
Hagerstown, MD 21740
301-797-1414, 800-228-7763
Disability Served: all

This company manufactures flotation pads for chairs and beds as well as hand exercisers.

Activa Brand Products Inc.
36 Fourth Street
West Royalty Industrial Park
Charlottetown, PE C1E 1B0 Canada
800-565-0263
http://www.advantajet.com
Disability Served: diabetes

This company makes a needle-free jet injector for delivery of insulin to persons with diabetes (in which insulin is deliverd by noninvasive means, producing a result in which insulin is absorbed faster and in which less insulin is often required).

Activeaid Inc.
101 Active Road
Redwood Falls, MN 56283
800-533-5330
http://www.activeaid.com
Disability Served: physically disabled

This company manufactures assistive devices for the bathroom, including commode and shower chairs, bath and shower benches, and shower wheelchairs for rehabilitation purposes.

ADA Compliance Specialists
26525 Lucinda
PO Box 4735
Mission Viejo, CA 92690
714-348-2786
Disability Served: all

This company manufactures nonslip floor coverings.

ADA Enterprises
PO Box 768
9 Abbey Lane
Middleboro, MA 02346
508-947-9880
Disability Served: hearing

This company manufactures a combination smoke alarm and strobe light designed for persons with hearing impairments.

Adamo Industries, Inc./WALKERALLS
1182 Pallwood Road
Memphis, TN 38122
901-682-1123, 800-682-7702
http://www.walkeralls.com
Disability Served: physically disabled

This company manufactures and distributes aids for daily living.

Adams Rite Manufacturing Co.
4040 Capitol Avenue
PO Box 1301
City of Industry, CA 91749
310-699-0511
Disability Served: all

This company manufactures door handles and push bars.

Adapt-A-Lap
44 Main, Suite 513
Champaign, IL 61820
217-356-2300, 800-419-2354
Disability Served: all

This company manufactures an adjustable, portable easel that can support a book or magazine without being held by the reader.

Adaptability
PO Box 515
Colchester, CT 06415-0515
203-537-3451, 800-243-9232
Disability Served: all

This company manufactures more than 300 daily living and home health care aids, including commodes, restraints, tables, orthotics and support systems, recreational items and games, clothing and dressing aids, canes, eating utensils, and much more.

Adaptive Design Shop
12847 Point Pleasant Drive
Fairfax, VA 22033
800-351-2327
http://www.adaptivedesignshop.com
Disability Served: cerebral palsy, physically disabled

This company designs and builds pediatric bath chairs and toilet supports for those with significant balance problems.

Adaptive Engineering Ltd.
419 34th Avenue SE
Calgary, AB T2G 1V1 Canada
403-243-9400, 800-448-4652
Disability Served: physically disabled

This company manufactures portable wheelchair lifts.

Adaptive Fashions Inc.
5641 Bartlett Boulevard
Mound, MN 55364
612-473-5945
Disability Served: all

This company manufactures clothing for men and women.

Adaptogs, Inc.
PO Box 339
201 North Washington
Otis, CO 80743
303-246-3761, 800-535-8247
Disability Served: all

This company manufactures adaptive clothing for men and women.

Adjusta Inc.
1901 Kiowa Road
Bennett, CO 80102
303-644-4160
Disability Served: all

This company makes an adjustable shower head.

Adlib Inc.
5142 Bolsa Avenue, Suite 106
Huntington Beach, CA 92649
714-895-9529
Disability Served: physically disabled

This company manufactures daily living aids, including beverage holders for wheelchairs, sock aids, door knob turners, mouthsticks, hairbrushes, dressing sticks, and writing and typing aids.

Adrian's Closet
PO Box 9930
Rancho Santa Fe, CA 92067
800-831-2577
Disability Served: physically disabled

This company provides adaptive clothing and accessories for children and young adults with limited mobility.

Advanced Mobility Systems Corporation
621 Justus Drive
Kingston, ON K7M 4H5 Canada
613-384-7460
Disability Served: all

This company makes a positioning chair for persons who need positioning of the legs and hips.

Aequitron Medical Inc.
14800 28th Avenue North
Minneapolis, MN 55447
612-557-9200, 800-497-4979
Disability Served: all

This company makes ventilators and apnea respiration monitors.

Aeromotive Manufacturing Co.
PO Box 2678
Kalamazoo, MI 49003
616-381-1242, 800-999-8559
Disability Served: all

This company makes a ceiling-mounted adjustable suspension cable.

AES Corporation
285 Newbury Street
PO Box 2093
Peabody, MA 01960
508-535-7310
Disability Served: all

This company makes an emergency alert system that uses the telephone lines to send messages.

AFW Company of North America
201 North Union Street
Olean, NY 14760
716-372-2935
Disability Served: physically disabled

This company manufactures swimming aids for persons with disabilities, including access stairs and ramps, swimming pool shower chairs, rails, and movable swimming pool floors.

Age Appropriate Puzzles By Cheryl
7756 Winding Way
Fair Oaks, CA 95628
916-961-3507
Disability Served: all

This company manufactures wooden puzzles.

Aging Technologies Inc.
420 Fairman Road
PO Box 12232
Lexington, KY 40581-2232
606-231-1738
Disability Served: physically disabled

This company manufactures elevators for wheelchair users.

Aiphone Health Care Systems
1700 130th Avenue NE
PO Box 90075
Bellevue, WA 98009
425-455-0510, 800-692-0200
http://www.aiphone.com
Disability Served: hearing, physically disabled

This company manufactures the Aiphone Freedom Environment Control System (ECS), which helps those persons who have limited ability to move around. This "sip 'n' puff" system allows immobile users to control everyday devices such as lights, heating and cooling systems, sound systems, motorized beds, room-to-room or door-answering intercoms, and any other device that is activated by a relay, switch, or infrared control.

Air Beds Inc.
1815 Grant Street
Santa Clara, CA 95050
408-727-8563
Disability Served: all

This company manufactures air flotation mattresses.

Air Lift Oxygen Carriers
1212 Kerr Gulch
Evergreen, CO 80439
303-526-4700, 800-776-6771
http://www.airlift.com
Disability Served: oxygen-dependent individuals

Air Lift manufactures carriers for portable and cylinder oxygen systems including backpacks, fanny packs, shoulder carriers, wheelchair/walker/scooter carriers, and a universal conserving device pouch.

Air Techniques Inc.
11438 Z Cronridge Drive
Owings Mills, MD 21117
410-356-9941
Disability Served: all

This company manufactures air purification systems.

Aircast Incorporated
PO Box 709
Summit, NJ 07902-0709
800-526-8785
Disability Served: all

This company manufactures orthotics and support braces.

Akron-Cleveland Home Medical Services Co.
489 West Exchange Street
Akron, OH 44302
330-376-2135
Disability Served: all

This company makes a seat and back support system.

Al Len Pattern Company
1931 Perry Highway
Fredonia, PA 16124
412-475-3708
Disability Served: all

This company manufactures a faucet wrench.

Alagold Corporation Inc.
1920 South Court Street
PO Box 4959
Montgomery, AL 36103
334-834-6900
Disability Served: all

This company manufactures support pillows, mattress and pillow protectors, wheelchair cushions, and lap desks.

Alexander Industries
PO Box 32
Cuyahoga Falls, OH 44222-0032
216-928-2153, 800-345-7341
Disability Served: all

This company manufactures cervical pillows, bed trays, decubitus pads, and therapeutic hosiery.

Alimed Inc.
297 High Street
Dedham, MA 02026
617-329-2900, 800-225-2610
Disability Served: all

This company offers more than eighty items, including cushions, supports, orthotics, lapboards, copy stands, computer accessories, decubitus pads, and more.

All Orthopedic Appliances
1801 West Nabor Road
PO Box 388
Marlow, OK 73055
405-658-5436, 800-327-3288
Disability Served: all

This company manufactures orthotics, splints, and supports.

Allied Medical
690 South Mendenhall
Memphis, TN 38117
901-683-3543, 800-422-2126
Disability Served: all

This company manufactures support cushions and seating systems, including foam in-placc seating systems, vacuum-molded seating systems, and lower back support cushions.

Allmilmo Corporation
PO Box 629
70 Clinton Road
Fairfield, NJ 07006
201-227-2502
Disability Served: physically disabled

This company manufactures accessible kitchens.

Allyn Air Co.
18 Millstream Road
Woodstock, NY 12498
914-679-2051
Disability Served: physically disabled

This company manufactures wheelchair air cushions.

Alpha Protech Inc.
903 West Center Street, Building E
North Salt Lake, UT 84054
801-298-3240, 800-527-7689
Disability Served: all

This company manufactures decubitus pads and fleece bed pads, wheelchair accessories, and elbow and heel protectors.

Alsto Company
PO Box 1267
Galesburg, IL 61401
309-343-6181, 800-447-0048
Disability Served: all

This company manufactures gardening accessories, including carts, kneelers, hose extenders, trimmers, pruners, and trowels.

AlumiRamp Inc.
90 Taylor Street
Quincy, MI 49082
517-639-8777, 800-800-3864
http://www.inmax.com/alumiramp
Disability Served: physically disabled

This company manufactures modular aluminum access ramps for vehicle and home use.

Am Fab Inc.
A Bissell Healthcare Company
2525 Miller Road
Kalamazoo, MI 49001
616-385-2938, 800-432-6322
Disability Served: all

This company manufactures overbed tables and side rails for hospital beds.

Amana Refrigeration Inc.
2800 220th Trail
Amana, IA 52204
319-622-5511, 800-843-0304
http://www.amana.com
Disability Served: all

This company manufactures electric ranges.

AmbuTech
Division of Melet Plastics Inc.
670 Golspie Street
Winnipeg, MB R2K 2V1 Canada
204-663-3340
Disability Served: physically disabled

This company manufactures an adjustable cane.

Amcest Corporation
1017 Walnut Street
Roselle, NJ 07203
800-631-7370
Disability Served: all

This company manufactures a personal emergency alert system.

American Airless
7302 E. Alondra Boulevard
Paramount, CA 90723
800-248-4737
http://www.americanairless.com
Disability Served: physically disabled

This company manufactures foam core tires and airfree tires and tubes for pneumatic wheelchair tires.

American Art Clay Co. Inc.
4717 West 16th Street
Indianapolis, IN 46222
317-244-6871, 800-428-3239
http://www.amaco.com
Disability Served: all

This company manufactures an electric potter's wheel that is wheelchair accessible.

American Bidet Company
Box 1500
Hollywood, FL 33022
800-US-BIDET
Disability Served: all

This company manufactures bidets.

American Craftsmen, Inc.
PO Box 484
Coffeyville, KS 67337
316-251-3340, 800-835-0687
http://amcrafts.com
Disability Served: all

This company manufactures rocking chairs.

American Dream International
210 Division Street
Kingston, PA 18704
717-288-5561, 800-839-9025
Disability Served: physically disabled

This company manufactures an electronic seat lift for recliners.

American Ergonomics Corp.
PO Box 2848
Sausalito, CA 94966
415-332-5635, 800-332-5635
Disability Served: all

This company manufactures ergonomic office chairs.

American Health Care Apparel Ltd.
334 Church Street
Easton, PA 18042
610-250-0584, 800-252-0584
Disability Served: physically disabled

This company provides clothing and footwear to aid the caregiver in dressing and undressing those restricted in mobility.

American Health Manufacturing Company
205 West Main
Hill City, KS 67642
913-674-2139, 800-982-1866
Disability Served: back injury

This company manufactures a home traction orthosis for lower back conditions.

American Health Specialties Inc.
5521 Greenville Avenue, Suite 104-837
Dallas, TX 75206
214-696-9251
Disability Served: physically disabled

This company manufactures crutch cushions for handgrips and underarm sections as well as pads for walker handgrips.

American Innovations Inc.
PO Box 671
Buckingham, PA 18912
215-345-9579
Disability Served: physically disabled

This company manufactures carrying accessories for walkers, wheelchairs, and crutches.

American Medical Alert Corporation
3265 Lawson Boulevard
Oceanside, NY 11572
800-645-3244
http://amacalert.com
Disability Served: all

This company makes an emergency alert system activated by pushing a button on a pendant worn by the user. Activation allows two-way communication with the alert center.

American Medical Industries
330 1/2 East Third Street
Dell Rapids, SD 57022
605-428-5501
http://ezhealth.com
Disability Served: all

This company manufactures a line of health care products called EZ-SWALLOW that assist individuals with limited strength and mobility to crush, split, and store their medication.

American Olean Tile Company
1000 Cannon Avenue
PO Box 271
Lansdale, PA 19446-0271
215-855-1111
Disability Served: all

This company manufactures nonslip floor tiles and tactile floor surfaces designed to alert persons with low vision.

American Plastics Marketing Group

1902 Progress Avenue
Columbus, OH 43207
614-445-8818, 800-870-8811
Disability Served: all

This company makes a light switch extension to accommodate wheelchair users who have difficulty reaching standard light switches.

American Standard Inc.

PO Box 6820
Piscataway, NJ 08855
800-442-1902
Disability Served: all

American Standard manufactures toilets, including tall toilets.

Americare

3950-A Nebraska Street
Newportville, PA 19056
215-781-0430, 800-220-CARE
Disability Served: vision

This company manufactures a waterproof sheet and mattress pad.

Ameritech Information Industry Services

Infochannel Multimedia Systems
350 North Orleans, Floor 3
Chicago, IL 60654
800-298-2926
Disability Served: all

This company manufactures an audio and visual messaging system.

Ames Division Mile Laboratories

PO Box 70
Elkhart, IN 46515
800-348-8100
Disability Served: diabetes

This company manufactures blood sugar test strips.

AMI, Inc.

PO Box 808
Groton, CT 06340-0808
860-536-3735, 800-248-4031
Disability Served: all

This company manufactures the Aqua PT, a dry hydrotherapy, massage therapy, and dry heat therapy machine.

Amick Manufacturing Co.

12737 Woodcrest Plaza, #1188
Omaha, NE 68137-3234
402-895-2091
Disability Served: all

This company manufactures a suspension system with a body support harness designed for ambulation training.

Amoena Corporation

1955 West Oak Circle
Marietta, GA 30062-2249
800-726-6362
Disability Served: all

This company manufactures prosthetic breast forms.

Ampco Products Inc.

PO Box 4190
Hialeah, FL 33014
305-821-5700
Disability Served: physically disabled

This company manufactures wheelchair-accessible bathroom cabinets.

Anaco Inc.

909 5th Avenue NE
Brainerd, MN 56401
218-829-8488
Disability Served: all

Anaco manufactures portable whirlpools.

Andermac Inc.

2626 Live Oak Highway
PO Box 1594
Yuba City, CA 95992-1594
916-674-8450, 800-824-0214
Disability Served: all

This company manufactures sitz baths and magnification mirrors.

Angel Hands, Inc.

PO Box 1117
Lynnwood, WA 98046-1117
206-672-8602
Disability Served: physically disabled

This company manufactures carrying accessories for crutches, canes, walkers, and strollers.

Ann Morris Enterprises Inc.

890 Fams Court
East Meadow, NY 11554-5101
516-292-9232, 800-454-3175
Disability Served: all

This company manufactures tactile kitchen scales, button battery testers, tactile thermometers, and other products for the hearing and vision impaired.

Anna-Dote, Inc.

40 Pullam Drive
West Middlesex, PA 16159
412-346-6132
Disability Served: physically disabled

This company manufactures and distributes support cushions for wheelchairs and geriatric chairs.

Ansa Bottle Company Inc.

1200 South Main Street
Muskogee, OK 74401
918-687-1664, 800-527-1096
Disability Served: all

This company manufactures an easy-to-hold baby bottle with a hole in the middle.

Anthros Medical Group

807 East Spring
Highland, KS 66035
913-442-3551, 800-258-0782
Disability Served: physically disabled

This company manufactures bath and shower chairs, shower stretchers, and adjustable walkers.

Apex Medical Corporation

800 South Van Eps Avenue
PO Box 1235
Sioux Falls, SD 57104
605-332-6689, 800-328-2935
Disability Served: all

This company makes health care aids, including pill organizers, medicine spoons, nitroglycerine tablet holders, and forehead thermometers.

Apollo Corporation

PO Box 219
Somerset, WI 54025
715-247-5625
Disability Served: all

This company manufactures portable bathtubs.

Apollo Light Systems Inc.

352 West 1060 South
Orem, UT 84058
801-226-2370, 800-545-9667
http://www.apollolight.com
Disability Served: all

This company manufactures lighting systems for the treatment of seasonal affective disorder.

Aqua Glass Corporation

PO Box 412
Industrial Park
Adamsville, TN 38310
800-632-0911
Disability Served: physically disabled

This company manufactures and distributes bathing fixtures, including a complete line of products for the physically challenged.

AquaSoothe International, Inc.

2808 Concord Lake Road
Kannapolis, NC 28083
800-223-1008
Disability Served: all

This company manufactures a therapy whirlpool.

AquaTec Health Care Products LP

PHP-ICM Building
1003 International Drive
Oakdale, PA 15071-9223
412-695-2122
Disability Served: all

This company manufactures hydraulic bath lifts for children and adults.

Aquatic Access Inc.

417 Dorsey Way
Louisville, KY 40223
502-425-5817, 800-325-5438
http://www.aquatic-access.com
Disability Served: physically disabled

This company manufactures water-powered lifts, providing people with disabilities access to in-ground and above-ground pools, spas, and therapy tanks.

Aquatic Development Group

PO Box 648
1 Aquatic Center
Cohers, NY 12047
518-783-0038
Disability Served: all

This company builds swimming pool stairs.

Aquatic Exercise Association

PO Box 1609
Nokomis, FL 34274-1609
813-486-8600
Disability Served: all

The Association produces aquatic exercise video and audio tapes.

Arch/EEZ Institute for Back Health, Inc.

1011 East Ginter Road
Tucson, AZ 85706
520-889-3997, 800-326-2724
Disability Served: all

This company manufactures a gravity traction system.

Architectural/Augmentative Designs

PO Box 17
Niwot, CO 80544-0017
303-652-3175
Disability Served: communication

This company manufactures a carrying case for communication aids.

ArcMate Manufacturing Corp.

637 South Vinewood Street
Escondido, CA 92029-1926
760-489-1140, 888-637-1926
Disability Served: physically disabled

This company manufactures reaching and gripping devices for the home. Products include the EZ Reacher, a reaching aid, the Dress EZ, a dressing aid, and many more.

Arcola Mobility

51 Kero Road
Carlstadt, NJ 07072
201-507-8500, 800-272-6521
Disability Served: physically disabled

This company provides wheelchair lifts, ramps, stairlifts, platform lifts, and accessible and paratransit vehicles to the disabled.

Area Access, Inc.

8117 Ransell Road
Falls Church, VA 22042
703-573-2111, 800-333-AREA
http://www.areaaccess.com
Disability Served: physically disabled

This company sells, rents, and installs scooters, stairlifts, and residential elevators. Installation of wheelchair lifts in commercial buildings and private residences is provided. Area Access also sells hand controls, van lifts, and lowered-floor minivans.

Arimura International

507 Walker Avenue
Baltimore, MD 21212-2624
410-433-2832
Disability Served: all

This company manufactures a card that can be used for personal identification, security, and door access. The card can be detected without removing it from a pocket or bag.

Aris Isotoner Gloves Inc.

11 Cayadutta Street
Gloversville, NY 00120
518-725-4369
Disability Served: all

This company manufactures gloves.

Aristoplay

450 South Wasner Road
Ann Arbor, MI 48103
734-995-4353, 800-GR8-GAME
http://www.aristoplay.com
Disability Served: all

This company manufactures educational board and card games for ages four and up.

Arjo Century Inc.

8130 Lehigh Avenue
Morton Grove, IL 60053
847-967-0360
Disability Served: physically disabled

This company manufactures a number of lifts, including pool lifts and bath lifts, bath and shower cabinets and chairs, portable bathtubs, and whirlpools.

Arnco AR Nelson Company Inc.

38-35 Crescent Street
Long Island City, NY 11101
718-361-0180, 800-377-6625
Disability Served: all

This company manufactures hand rails.

Artec Inc.

PO Box 25103
Greenville, SC 29616
803-288-2111, 800-445-0234
Disability Served: all

This company manufactures orthotics for the lower back and rocking attachments for wheelchairs.

Arvee Medical Inc.

730 East Michigan Avenue
Battle Creek, MI 49017
616-965-1423, 800-537-9941
Disability Served: all

This company manufactures an infant respiration monitor.

Ascension

3526 East Fort Lowell Road
Tucson, AZ 85716
520-881-3993, 800-459-0400
http://www.wheelchairlift.com
Disability Served: physically disabled

This company manufactures a portable wheelchair lift that enables people with disabilities to access stages and platforms in public facilities.

Ascension International Inc.

1975 Seneca Road
Eagan, MN 55122
612-452-0600
Disability Served: all

This company manufactures a fiberglass whirlpool.

ASI American Specialties Inc.

441 Saw Mill River Road
Yonkers, NY 10701
914-476-9000
Disability Served: physically disabled

This company manufactures grab bars for bathrooms, shower and tub seats, mirrors, and towel dispensers.

ASKO Inc.

1161 Executive Drive West
Richardson, TX 75081
214-644-8595
http://askousa.com
Disability Served: physically disabled

This company manufactures dishwashers, clothes washers, and clothes dryers designed to accommodate persons with physical disabilities.

Assist Equip, Inc.
PO Box 1558
Levelland, TX 79336
806-894-5700, 800-654-9664
http://www.ncmedical.com
Disability Served: physically disabled

This company manufactures transferring devices such as the Pivot Pole.

Astro Nautics Company Inc.
162 San Lazard Avenue
Sunnyvale, CA 94086-5209
408-736-9215
Disability Served: all

This company manufactures an elevated toilet seat.

AT's Freedom Factory
PO Box 641473
San Jose, CA 95164
408-259-1122
Disability Served: physically disabled

This company manufactures mono-skis and adult tricycles.

Atlantic Rubber Products, Inc.
3065 Cranberry Highway
East Wareham, MA 02538
800-585-0446 (MA), 800-695-0446
http://www.atlrubber.com
Disability Served: all

This company makes nonslip floor coverings.

Audio Book Contractors, Inc.
PO Box 40115
Washington, DC 20016
202-363-3429
Disability Served: all

This company produces unabridged classic books on cassettes.

Audiotone Inc.
4120 Olson Memorial Highway
Golden Valley, MN 55422
612-520-9723, 800-757-8055
Disability Served: hearing

This company makes hearing aids.

Autofold Inc.
208 Coleman Street
PO Box 1063
Gardner, MA 01440-1063
508-632-0667
Disability Served: vision

This company manufactures canes.

Aviano USA-Wheelchair Clothing
1199 Avenida Acaso, Suite K
Camarillo, CA 93012
805-484-8138
Disability Served: all

This company manufactures clothing for men and women, including exercise and workout apparel.

Avionix Medical Devices
PO Box 9669
Midland, TX 79708
915-689-0222, 800-627-8914
Disability Served: all

This company manufactures neuromuscular and transcutaneous electrical nerve stimulators.

Award Brush Co.
12212 51st Avenue NE
Marysville, WA 98271
206-659-7272
Disability Served: all

This company makes a long-handled bathing brush.

B Stout Company
367 New Road
Southampton, PA 18966
215-364-1017
Disability Served: all

This company makes Velcro fasteners.

Baby Look Co.
1817 Amherst Street NE
Grand Rapids, MI 49503
616-454-2229
Disability Served: all

This company manufactures and distributes a visual stimulation product for the physically impaired and infants.

Baby Tenda Corp.
123 South Belmont Boulevard
Kansas City, MO 64123
816-231-2366
http://babytenda.com
Disability Served: all

This company manufactures feeding and play tables for children and an adjustable crib.

BabySmart
5 Foxchase Drive
Watchung, NJ 07060
908-756-1555, 800-756-5590
Disability Served: all

This company manufactures skin care wipes for persons with physical disabilities.

Back Ease Inc.
PO Box 5283
Louisville, KY 40205
502-458-2000
http://www.ameraccess.com
Disability Served: all

This company manufactures back support cushions.

Backco Products
11160 Zodiac Lane
Box 59373
Dallas, TX 75229
214-241-8363, 800-545-3533
Disability Served: all

This company manufactures a gravity traction system.

Backsaver Products Co.
Division of Nepsco Inc.
53 Jeffrey Avenue
Holliston, MA 01746
508-429-5940, 800-251-2225
Disability Served: back injury

This company manufactures back aids, including support cushions, footrests, pillows, recliner chairs, and positioning chairs.

Bag Lady (The)
PO Box 531
West Stockbridge, MA 01266
413-499-4534, 800-248-5239
Disability Served: physically disabled

This company manufactures carrying accessories for wheelchairs, crutches, walkers, and canes.

Bailey Manufacturing Co.
118 Lee Street
Lodi, OH 44254
800-321-8372
Disability Served: all

This company offers more than seventy-five therapeutic aids, ranging from training stairs to parallel bars.

Balfour Inc.
PO Box 77077
4905 Koger Boulevard
Greensboro, NC 27407-2639
910-852-2030, 800-262-2404
Disability Served: all

This company manufactures slippers for men, women, and children.

Ball Dynamics International Inc.
1616 Glenarm Place, Suite 1900
Denver, CO 80202
303-893-0532, 800-752-2255
Disability Served: all

This company manufactures therapeutic inflatable balls and exercise equipment designed for therapeutic and rehabilitative activities.

Ballert International Inc.
3645 Woodhead Drive
Northbrook, IL 60062-1816
847-480-0390, 800-345-3456
Disability Served: all

This company offers orthotics, prosthetics, support cushions, wheeled walkers, and dynamometers.

Baltimore Therapeutic Equipment Co.

7455-L New Ridge Road
Hanover, MD 21076-3105
410-850-0333, 800-331-8845
Disability Served: all

This company develops therapeutic activities and products, including cognitive rehabilitation evaluation machines, electronic motion evaluation systems, work simulator exercisers, and eye-hand coordination activities.

Bard Patient Division

Patricia West Bartlett
111 Spring Street
Murray Hill, NJ 07974
908-277-8000
Disability Served: all

This company offers wound care products, catheters and drainage bags, and skin care products.

Barrier Free Access Systems Inc.

339 Wardlaw Avenue
Winnipeg, MB R3L 0L5 Canada
204-475-9500
Disability Served: physically disabled

This company manufactures a wheelchair ramp.

Barrier Free Lifts Inc.

PO Box 4163
Manassas, VA 22110
703-361-6531, 800-582-8732
Disability Served: physically disabled

This company manufactures battery-operated overhead lifts.

Baseline Corporation

700 South Buckout Street
Irvington, NY 10533
914-591-8341, 800-835-5002
Disability Served: all

This company manufactures massager units, exercise equipment, exercise weights, hot and cold packs, dynamometers, and goniometers to measure range of motion.

Bassmatic

PO Box 7117
Canton, OH 44705
330-455-3983
Disability Served: physically disabled

This company manufactures a fishing-reel adapter for hand amputees.

Bath Ease Inc.

3815 Darston Street
Palm Harbor, FL 34685
813-786-2604
Disability Served: all

This company makes a fiberglass bathtub and shower cabinet.

Bathe-Eez

224 Summit Road
PO Box 365
Springfield, PA 19064
215-328-0802
Disability Served: physically disabled

This company manufactures bathtub inserts that provide body support for children with disabilities.

Bathroom Gem

512 Grand Avenue
Chariton, IA 50049
515-279-4057, 800-453-8880
Disability Served: physically disabled

This company manufactures a roll-in shower unit.

Battle Creek Equipment Company

307 West Jackson Street
Battle Creek, MI 49017-2385
616-692-6181, 800-253-0854
Disability Served: all

This company manufactures products including the Thermophore Automatic Moist Heat Packs, cervical pillows, Pedlar Exerciser, and fitness and massage products.

Bauerfeind USA Inc.

2100 Barrett Park Drive, #508
Kennesaw, GA 30144-3673
800-423-3405
Disability Served: all

This company manufactures support cushions, splints, and orthotics.

Beatrice M Brantman, Inc.

207 East Westminster
Lake Forest, IL 60045
847-615-8890, 800-232-7987
Disability Served: physically disabled

This company makes transfer boards with sliding seat chairs.

Becker Industries, Inc.

6 Highway 140 South
PO Box 386
Kingsley, IA 51028-0386
712-378-2069
Disability Served: all

This company markets three assistive technology products: the Scooter Transfer Board, the Freedom Lap Tray, and the Convertible Lap Tray/Desk.

Bed Check Corporation

PO Box 170
Tulsa, OK 74101
800-523-7956
Disability Served: all

This company manufactures a wandering patient alert system, an alarm unit to prevent wheelchair falls, and a wheelchair lever to facilitate one-handed propulsion.

Bed Handles, Inc.

4825 South Tierney Drive
Independence, MO 64055
800-725-6903
http://www.bedhandles.com
Disability Served: all

This company manufactures bed handles and travel handles.

Bell-Horn

451 North Third Street
PO Box 3408
Philadelphia, PA 19123
215-627-2773
Disability Served: all

Bell-Horn makes canes, walkers, support pillows, and braces.

Bema USA Inc.

2015 Weaver Park Drive
PO Box 4280
Clearwater, FL 33518
813-446-2362
Disability Served: all

This company manufactures inflatable hand exercisers, float swim aids that provide buoyancy, inflatable support pillows, inflatable exercise pads, and inflatable therapy balls.

Bemis Manufacturing Co.

300 Mill Street
PO Box 910
Sheboygan Falls, WI 53085-0901
414-467-4621, 800-558-7651
http://www.BemisMfg.org
Disability Served: all

This company manufactures Quality Lift and Medic-Aid toilet seats for home healthcare and commercial applications. These seats contain DuraGard, an antimicrobial agent, and fit round and elongated bowls.

Beneficial Designs, Inc.

5858 Empire Grade
Santa Cruz, CA 95060
831-429-8447
http://www.beneficialdesigns.com
Disability Served: physically disabled

This engineering and design firm works toward universal access through research, design, and education. The company develops and markets technologies for daily living, vocational, and leisure activities and provides design, consultation, and product-testing services.

Berel Health Products, Inc.
6932 Gettysburg Pike
Ft Wayne, IN 46804
219-436-3172, 800-648-1453
Disability Served: all

This company manufactures a dental floss holder that can be used with one hand.

Bernina Sewing Machines
70 Orchid Drive
Salt Lake City, UT 84054
Disability Served: all

Bernina manufactures sewing machines.

Bernlit Enterprises Inc.
2840 Pine Road
Huntington Valley, PA 19006
215-781-9522
Disability Served: all

This company manufactures a paraffin bath for use in therapy.

Besam Inc.
171 Twin Rivers Drive
East Windsor, NJ 08520
609-443-5800, 800-752-9290
Disability Served: all

This company manufactures powered door operators.

Best Manufacturing Co.
1202 North Park Avenue
PO Box 577
Montrose, CO 81402-0577
970-249-2378, 800-235-2378
http://www.bestsigns.com
Disability Served: vision

This company manufactures Braille and tactile architectural signage.

BEST Orthopedic Products
2356-B Springs Road NE
Hickory, NC 28601
704-256-1933, 800-344-5279
Disability Served: all

This company manufactures support pillows and wrist and hand splints.

Beta Industries
707 Commercial Avenue
Carlstadt, NJ 07072
201-939-2400, 800-BSCREEN
Disability Served: all

This company produces a powered door operator.

Betta Medical, Inc.
547 West 9560 South
Sandy, UT 84070
801-568-1781
Disability Served: all

This company manufactures a baby bottle designed to prevent the flow of milk or formula into the auditory tube and thus reduce the risk of the baby developing an ear infection during feeding times.

Better Health Inc.
PO Box 18200
Knoxville, TN 37928
800-233-2569
Disability Served: all

This company makes leg extenders for beds.

Better Sleep Inc.
57 Industrial Road
Berkeley Heights, NJ 07922
Disability Served: all

This company manufactures pillows, support cushions, leg rests, reachers, nonslip bath and shower mats, and portable beds.

Bike Track, Inc.
RFD #1, Box 247
Wayside Road
Woodstock, VT 05091
888-663-8537
http://www.biketrack.com
Disability Served: physically disabled

This company produces recycled plastic surfacing tile to improve the quality and durability of ramp surfaces.

Bikeland
233 North Main at High Street
Oshkosh, WI 54901
920-235-3121
Disability Served: all

This company manufactures small carts that attach to bicycles or adult tricycles that can hold children and goods.

Bil Jax Construction/Rental
595 East Lugbill Road
Archbold, OH 43502
419-445-8915
Disability Served: all

This company designs elevating platforms that lift persons straight up.

Bio Concepts Inc.
2424 East University Drive
Phoenix, AZ 85034
602-267-7854, 800-421-5647
Disability Served: all

This company manufactures custom-made elastic pressure garments, ready-made pressure gloves, and gel for use with elastic pressure garments.

Bio Medical Supply Co.
43-15 Bell Boulevard
Bayside, NY 11361
212-229-0202, 800-358-8883
Disability Served: back injury

This company manufactures a lower back orthosis.

Bio Stimu Trend Corp.
14851 NW 27th Avenue
Opa Locka, FL 33054
305-688-4647
Disability Served: all

This company manufactures garments with built-in electrodes for pain management and nerve stimulation.

Biocompression Systems Inc.
736 Gotham Parkway
Carlstadt, NJ 07072
201-939-0716
Disability Served: all

This company manufactures hyper-baric sleeves to treat edema and other conditions.

Bioenergetics Inc.
200 Industrial Boulevard
Birmingham, AL 33211
205-941-2110, 800-433-2627
Disability Served: all

This company manufactures wet suit vests designed to be worn when exercising or running in water.

Bioflex Corporation
736 Kenwick Road
Columbus, OH 43209
614-236-8079, 800-552-3539
Disability Served: all

Bioflex manufactures garments with built-in electrodes for transcutaneous electrical nerve stimulation treatment.

Biologics
PO Box 307
Indian Rocks Beach, FL 34635
813-821-9685
Disability Served: all

This company manufactures an air flotation bed mattress.

Biomark Inc.
PO Box 340
Edmonds, WA 98020
206-745-9200, 800-633-3034
Disability Served: all

This company manufactures reusable hot and cold gel packs.

Biomedical Systems
2464 West Port Plaza Drive
St Louis, MO 63146
314-576-6800, 800-877-6334
Disability Served: all

This company makes an inflatable pillow designed to prevent pressure sores caused by extensive bed rest.

Biomet Inc.
PO Box 587
Warsaw, IN 46580-0587
219-267-6639
Disability Served: all

This company manufactures a shoulder harness to immobilize the arm and shoulder area.

Biosig Instruments Inc.
PO Box 860
Champlain, NY 12919
514-733-3362
Disability Served: all

This company manufactures biofeedback units and pulse monitors.

Biosources International Inc.
PO Box 3868
Napa, CA 94558
707-944-0645
Disability Served: all

This company manufactures a stethoscope with an amplifier.

Biotech Ltd.
18 North State Street
Elgin, IL 60123
847-608-8490, 800-526-2158
Disability Served: all

This company makes foam seat cushions and supports.

Black and Decker
US Household Products Group
6 Armstrong Road
Shelton, CT 06484-4797
203-926-3000
Disability Served: all

This company manufactures household appliances and goods, including toasters, can openers, food choppers, mixers, and security power-failure lights.

Bobrick Washroom Equipment Inc.
11611 Hart Street
North Hollywood, CA 91605-5882
818-764-1000
http://www.bobrick.com
Disability Served: all

This company provides washroom accessories and toilet partition products for nonresidential building washrooms.

Body Care, Inc.
315 Gilmer Ferry Road
Ball Ground, GA 30107
800-858-9888
Disability Served: back injury

This company manufactures orthopedic soft goods.

Body Glove
530 Sixth Street
Hermosa Beach, CA 90254
213-374-4074, 800-523-1757
Disability Served: all

Body Glove manufactures wrist and knee supports made of neoprene.

Bodyline Comfort Systems
3730 Kori Road
Jacksonville, FL 32257
904-262-4068, 800-874-7715
Disability Served: all

Among the items this company manufactures are mattress pads, lower back support braces, support pillows, and rib belts.

Bodylog Inc.
120 Kisco Avenue
Mt Kisco, NY 10549
914-273-6480, 800-233-2911
Disability Served: all

This company manufactures biofeedback units.

Bodypoint Designs, Inc.
80 South Washington, #303
Seattle, WA 98104
206-621-9648, 800-547-5716
Disability Served: all

This company manufactures switch mounting hardware and seating hardware.

Boehringer Mannheim Corp.
PO Box 50100
9115 Hague Road
Indianapolis, IN 46250
317-845-2000, 800-858-8072
Disability Served: diabetes

This company manufactures aids for diabetics, including blood glucose test strips and monitors.

Bogen Photo Corp.
PO Box 506
Ramsey, NJ 07446-0506
201-818-9500
Disability Served: all

Bogen manufactures a camera mount for wheelchairs and tables.

Books On Tape
PO Box 7900
Newport Beach, CA 92658
800-626-3333
Disability Served: all

This company produces books on audiocassette tapes.

Bossert Specialties, Inc.
PO Box 15441
Phoenix, AZ 85060
602-956-6637, 800-776-5885
http://www.bossertspecialties.com
Disability Served: vision

This company offers a full line of products for the visually impaired, including electronic read/write systems, and services all makes of such equipment.

Boston Music Company
172 Tremont Street
Boston, MA 02111
617-426-5100
Disability Served: all

This company produces music lesson books for the piano.

BPS Architectural Products Inc.
10816 Fallstone Road, Suite 505
Houston, TX 77099
713-568-9945, 800-255-9513
Disability Served: physically disabled

This company manufactures accessible vanity systems and wardrobes.

Brace Mates
627 Carwile Road
Rustburg, VA 24588
804-332-5591
Disability Served: all

This company produces liners for patients who wear orthopedic body braces.

Bradley Corporation
PO Box 309
9101 Fountain Boulevard
Menomonee Falls, WI 53051
414-251-6000
Disability Served: all

This company manufactures bath aids and accessories, including wall grab bars, mirrors, shower and bath seats, faucets, and one-hand hand dryers.

Brandt Industries Inc.
4461 Bronx Boulevard
Bronx, NY 10470
718-994-0800, 800-221-8031
Disability Served: all

This company manufactures tubular steel furniture, IV stands, footstools, heatlamps, and sunlamps.

Breathing Aids Limited
PO Box 62-D
Dolton, IL 60419
708-238-7222
Disability Served: all

This company manufactures a breathing mask that supplies air warmed by body temperature rather than outside air.

Brewer
13901 Main Street
PO Box 159
Menomenee Falls, WI 53051
414-251-9530, 800-558-8777
Disability Served: all

Brewer makes bath equipment, including commode chairs and shower chairs. The company also makes step stools for commercial and hospital use.

Briggs Plumbingware Inc.
4350 West Cypress
Tampa, FL 33607
813-878-0178
Disability Served: physically disabled

This company builds commercial accessible bathrooms and tall toilets.

Bright Ideas Inc.
PO Box 8714
Wichita, KS 67208-0714
316-686-1450, 800-215-4472
Disability Served: vision

This company manufactures incontinence pads for children.

Brio
North 120 West 18485 Freistadt Road
Germantown, WI 53022
414-250-3240, 800-558-6863
Disability Served: all

Brio makes tactile tic-tac-toe games.

British American Medical, Inc.
27111 Aliso Creek Road, #115
Aliso Viejo, CA 92656-3366
800-866-1187
Disability Served: vision

This company manufactures blood glucose test strips, glucose analyzers, and insulin syringes for visually impaired diabetics.

Brocar Products Inc.
PO Box 68024
Cincinnati, OH 45206
800-827-1207
Disability Served: all

This company manufactures a safety cover for pipes and valves to protect wheelchair users from injury.

Brookstone Company
5 Vose Farm Road
Peterborough, NH 03458
603-924-9541, 800-926-7000
Disability Served: all

This company manufactures aids for daily living, gardening tools, and other handy devices.

Brown Engineering Corporation
289 Chesterfield Road
Westhampton, MA 01027
413-527-1800, 800-726-4233
Disability Served: all

This company manufactures support rails for beds.

Brown Medical Industries
481 South 8th Avenue East
Hartley, IA 51346
712-728-2269, 800-843-4395
Disability Served: all

This company manufactures Seal Tight, a waterproof sheath designed to keep casts and bandages dry while bathing.

Bruce Medical Supply
411 Waverly Oaks Road
Waltham, MA 02154
781-894-6262, 800-225-8446
Disability Served: all

This company manufactures stoma covers, puncture devices for conducting blood tests, and wound care products.

Bruno Independent Living Aids, Inc.

1780 Executive Drive
PO Box 84
Oconomowoc, WI 53066
414-567-4990, 800-882-8183
http://www.bruno.com/
Disability Served: physically disabled

This company manufactures wheelchair and scooter lifts for cars, trucks, and vans. It also produces battery-powered scooters and stairlifts.

Buck and Buck Inc.

3111 27th Avenue South
Seattle, WA 98144-6502
800-458-0600
http://www.buckandbuck.com
Disability Served: physically disabled

This company manufactures a full line of clothing and footwear for men and women who are either living in a nursing facility or receiving home health care.

Buddy Products

1350 South Leavitt Street
Chicago, IL 60608
312-733-6400, 800-886-8688
Disability Served: physically disabled

This company manufactures adaptive office products and equipment, including desktop organizers and telephone accessories.

Builders Brass Works Corporation

3447 Union Pacific Avenue
Los Angeles, CA 90023
213-269-8111, 800-533-6229
Disability Served: physically disabled

This company provides door handles, panic bars, and handicap signs.

Burke Mobility Products

PO Box 1064
Mission, KS 66222
913-722-5658, 800-255-4147
Disability Served: physically disabled

This company manufactures three-wheeled scooters and a reclining chair with a seat lift.

Bushline

PO Box 527
New Tazewell, TN 37825-0527
615-626-5246, 800-620-1682
Disability Served: physically disabled

This company manufactures a chair with a powered elevating seat.

BWN Industries

2311 East Locust Center
Ontario, CA 91761
800-772-1616
Disability Served: all

This company develops automatic doors.

C & C Dynamics

PO Box 711701
San Diego, CA 92171-1701
619-576-0173
Disability Served: physically disabled

This company manufactures electronic sliding patio door operators and sliding window operators, and distributes entry door operators.

C & H Distributors Inc.

400 South Fifth Street
PO Box 04499
Milwaukee, WI 53204
414-271-2250
Disability Served: all

This company manufactures rolling carts and height-adjustable work bench legs and tables.

C. Beil Designs

5435 North Artesian Avenue
Chicago, IL 60625
773-509-0995
Disability Served: physically disabled

This company manufactures aids for reading, including book and newspaper holders and page turners.

Cadwell Laboratories, Inc.

909 North Kellogg
Kennewick, WA 99336
509-735-6481, 800-245-3001
Disability Served: all

This company manufactures EMG (electromyogram) feedback units and accessories.

Camp International, Inc.

744 West Avenue
PO Box 89
Jackson, MI 49204-0089
517-787-1600, 800-492-1088
Disability Served: all

This company manufactures casts, support systems and stabilizers, carrying accessories for walkers, and therapeutic compression stockings.

Campbell-Childs, Inc.

400 Industrial Circle
White City, OR 97503
503-826-6511, 800-446-7233
Disability Served: physically disabled

This company manufactures prosthetic feet for children and adults.

Canadian Hearing Society

271 Spadina Road
Toronto, ON M5R 2V3 Canada
416-964-9595
TTY/TDD: 416-964-0023
http://www.chs.ca
Disability Served: hearing

CHS provides services that enhance the independence of deaf, deafened, and hard-of-hearing people and encourage the prevention of hearing loss.

Canoe Creek Rehabilitation Products, Inc.

2508 Collins Road
Pittsburgh, PA 15235
800-753-1788
http://www.canoe-creek.com
Disability Served: multiple sclerosis

This company manufactures the Stable Slide self-feeding support.

Canyon Products Inc.

10173 Croydon Way
Sacramento, CA 95827
916-361-1687, 800-221-5499
Disability Served: physically disabled

This company manufactures wheelchair accessories, including wheelchair upholstery, wheelchair battery accessories, wheels, carrying accessories for wheelchairs, and wheel locks. This company also makes support cushions and seats.

Caolo & Bieniek Associates, Inc.

435 Cottage Street
Springfield, MA 01104-4005
800-309-2255
Disability Served: all

This company develops a software program that identifies architectural barriers in buildings and produces a graphical floor plan.

Capri Plastics Theraco Division

Capri Plastics
1801 SE Industrial Road
PO Box 705
Brainerd, MN 56401
218-829-1796, 800-843-7226
http://www.plasticsnet.com/mbr/capri
Disability Served: all

This company manufactures and distributes portable whirlpool baths.

Captek—Science Products

Box 888
Southeastern, PA 19399
800-888-7400
Disability Served: vision

This company provides electronic aids and adaptations for the visually impaired.

Carderock Limited

PO Box 4061
Rockville, MD 20850
301-342-9390
Disability Served: physically disabled

This company makes an accessible bathtub with a whirlpool unit.

Cardinal Manufacturing Co.

1055 East 52nd Street
PO Box 55223
Indianapolis, IN 46205
317-283-4175
Disability Served: all

This company produces a laryngectomy filter.

Cardio Systems Inc.

PO Box 29923
Dallas, TX 75229
214-242-2164, 800-527-0443
Disability Served: physically disabled

This company manufactures air flotation mattresses.

Cardon Rehabilitation Products

8001 Jane Street
Thornhill, ON L4X 2C1 Canada
905-761-7868
Disability Served: vision

This company manufactures a plastic writing template to accommodate persons with visual impairments.

Care Electronics Inc.

5741 Arapahoe Road, Suite 2A
Boulder, CO 80303
303-444-2273
Disability Served: all

This company manufactures a wandering patient monitoring system.

Care Products Inc.

158 North Main Street
Florida, NY 10921
914-651-3332, 800-446-5206
Disability Served: physically disabled

This company manufactures covers for walker handgrips and crutches.

Carex Health Care Products

PO Box 20260A
Newark, NJ 07101
201-824-7637, 800-526-8051
Disability Served: physically disabled

This company manufactures walkers and bath aids.

Carica Inc.

155-176th Street, #208
Surrey, BC V4P 1M7 Canada
604-538-1401
Disability Served: all

This company manufactures reaching aids that allow individuals to grab items without bending over, stooping, etc. This company also makes a toilet seat attachment that provides a larger seating area.

Caring Concepts

469 7th Avenue, 14th Floor
New York, NY 10018
800-321-2856
http://www.caringconcepts.com
Disability Served: physically disabled

This company designs and manufactures assistive apparel for men and women.

Caring Products International, Inc.

250 Park Avenue, 19th Floor
New York, NY 10177
212-599-2888
Disability Served: vision

This company manufactures incontinence aids for adults and children.

Carolyn's Low Vision Products

1415 57th Avenue West
Bradenton, FL 34207
800-648-2266
http://www.carolynscatalog.com
Disability Served: vision

This mail order catalog features more than 700 visual aids and hearing helpers.

Cascade Designs Inc.

4000 1st Avenue South
Seattle, WA 98134
206-583-0583, 800-527-1527
Disability Served: physically disabled

This company develops support cushions.

Casio Incorporated
PO Box 7000
Dover, NJ 07801
201-361-5400
Disability Served: all

Casio manufactures communication aids, clocks, and watches.

CC-M Productions
8512 Cedar Street
Silver Spring, MD 20910
301-588-4095, 800-453-6280
http://www.CC-M.com
Disability Served: physically disabled

This company produces Armchair Fitness videos, a four-video series of exercise and fitness workouts.

CD Denison Orthopaedic
220 West 28th Street
Baltimore, MD 21211
410-235-9645
Disability Served: all

This company manufactures custom ortheses and prostheses for children and adults.

CD Sparling Co.
498 Farmer Street
Plymouth, MI 48170
313-455-3121
Disability Served: physically disabled

This company manufactures a variety of grab bars for use in bathrooms.

Cemco
20235 Olinda Trail North
Marine on St Croix, MN 55047
612-433-3374
Disability Served: vision

This company makes a syringe magnifier so persons with low vision can better see the graduation scales on syringes.

Centec Orthopedics
742 Pancho Road
Camarillo, CA 93012-8576
805-484-2600, 800-521-0601
Disability Served: all

This company makes an ankle orthosis that uses gel support.

Center for Rehabilitation Technology
Georgia Institute for Technology
Atlanta, GA 30332-0156
404-894-4960
http://www.arch.gatech.edu/crt/
Disability Served: physically disabled

This company manufactures and develops adaptive office products, including mail opening devices, copy holders, desk accessories, and keyboard trays.

Central Specialties Ltd.
1122 Silver Lake Road
Cary, IL 60013
847-639-3900
Disability Served: all

This company manufactures a low clothes bar for closets in hotels, motels, and other facilities.

Century Products Co.
9600 Valley View Road
Macedonia, OH 44056-2096
216-468-4379
Disability Served: all

This company manufactures a variety of car seats for children.

Cepco
21515 Parthenia Street
Canoga Park, CA 91304
818-998-7315
Disability Served: hearing

This company develops an environmental control unit and a home security unit.

CF Wood Industries Inc.
7021 West Augusta Avenue, Suite 108
Glendale, AZ 85303
602-939-0570
Disability Served: physically disabled

This company manufactures wheelchair accessories, such as a drink holder, shopping baskets, trays, and oxygen tank holders.

Chattanooga Corporation
PO Box 489
4717 Adams Road
Hixson, TN 37343-9903
615-870-2281, 800-592-7329
Disability Served: all

This company manufactures a number of therapeutic aids.

Chempath Inc.
115 Poplar Loop
Flatrock, NC 28731
800-843-4743
Disability Served: physically disabled

This company manufactures a polyethylene grid designed to support and protect grassy areas from erosion and damage caused by heavy traffic.

Chenbe Inc.
Sit Right Baby
PO Box 3275
Yuba City, CA 95992
916-671-3947, 800-525-9755
Disability Served: all

This company manufactures an abductor for a high chair that is designed to prevent a child from sliding forward in the seat.

Chicago Faucet Company
2100 South Nuclear Drive
Des Plaines, IL 60018
847-694-4400
Disability Served: physically disabled

This company manufactures a lever faucet handle to facilitate persons with limited hand dexterity or strength.

Child's Play
3359 Collingwood SW
Wyoming, MI 49509
616-530-2471
Disability Served: all

This company manufactures children's clothing.

Childcraft
22 Kilmer Road
Edison, NJ 08817
908-572-6100, 800-631-5652
Disability Served: all

This company manufactures an inflatable ball used for developing large muscle coordination and teaching throwing and catching skills.

Children's Factory
245 West Essex
St Louis, MO 63122
314-821-1441
Disability Served: all

This company manufactures aids for developing and practicing fine motor dressing skills for children, as well as foam play blocks and shoes for practicing lacing and bow tying.

Chrono Art
9175 Poplar Avenue
Cotati, CA 94928
707-795-1834
Disability Served: vision

This company manufactures a telephone cutoff switch and a chiming clock activated by touch.

CHS International
PO Box 21067
550 39th Avenue NE
Columbia Heights, MN 55421
612-788-0204, 800-878-4550
Disability Served: all

This company manufactures orthoses, braces, and support pillows and cushions.

CIL Publications & Audiobooks
c/o Visions
120 Wall Street, 16th Floor
New York, NY 10005
212-425-2255, 888-CIL-8333
http://www.cilpubs.com
Disability Served: vision

CIL audiobooks are self-study tapes designed for use by persons experiencing vision loss or who are blind. CIL teaching manuals are textbooks providing lesson plans for use by instructors of people who are blind or visually impaired.

Cindy Lift Products, Inc.
7220 Governors West
Huntsville, AL 35806
205-837-6575
Disability Served: physically disabled

This company manufactures a transfer lift.

Citadel Asphalt Systems Inc.
9241 Citadel Court
St Louis, MO 63123
314-638-3888
Disability Served: all

This company manufactures parking area and pavement markers with the international symbol of access.

CJ Rush Inc.
189 Milner Avenue
Agincourt, ON M1S 3R1 Canada
416-291-2551
Disability Served: physically disabled

This company manufactures a revolving door large enough to accommodate wheelchairs and a powered door closer.

Clairson International
650 Southwest 27th Avenue
Ocala, FL 34474
800-227-8319
http://www.closetmaid.com
Disability Served: all

This company produces vinyl-coated wire shelving.

Clark Medical Products Inc.
1333 Matheson Boulevard East
Mississauga, ON L4W 1R1 Canada
905-238-6163, 800-889-5295
http://www.clarkmedical.com
Disability Served: physically disabled

This company manufactures products for the bathroom, including a wall grab bar, an elevating toilet seat lift, a bathtub seat, and a hydraulic bath lift.

Claypool Classics, Inc.
820 South Green Bay Road
Lake Forest, IL 60045
847-234-4092
Disability Served: all

This company sells casual clothing designed for men and women who cannot get dressed easily. Daytime clothes, some sleepwear, and underwear are offered. The items are designed with special attention to closure and room for movement. They are produced in washable fabrics.

Clyde Fox
11107 Dulcet Avenue
Northridge, CA 91326
818-360-3573
Disability Served: physically disabled

This company manufactures a spring-loaded billiard cue.

CME Medical Equipment Corporation
1130 Donamy Glen
Scotch Plains, NJ 07076
908-561-0906
Disability Served: all

This company manufactures aids for daily living, including reaching devices.

COARC
PO Box 2, Route 217
Mellenville, NY 12544
518-672-4451
http://www.coarc.org
Disability Served: developmentally disabled

This company manufactures carrying accessories for walkers and wheelchairs. It provides a wide range of services to persons of all ages with disabilities.

Cobblecrete

205 West 2000 South
Orem, UT 84058
801-224-6662, 800-798-5791
Disability Served: physically disabled

This company manufactures a surface mat designed to warn persons of construction or other hazards.

Coburn Optical Industries Inc.

4606 South Garnett Road, Suite 200
Tulsa, OK 74146
918-665-1815, 800-252-8761
Disability Served: vision

This company manufactures magnifiers.

Cochlear Corporation

61 Inverness Drive East, Suite 200
Englewood, CO 80112
800-523-5798
http://www.cochlear.com
Disability Served: hearing

This company manufactures cochlear implants, which are designed for a safe, reliable, effective treatment for severe to profound hearing loss in adults and profound hearing loss in children as young as eighteen months.

Collis Curve Catalog

302 North Central Avenue
Brownsville, TX 78521-5530
800-298-4818
Disability Served: all

This company provides a therapeutic toothbrush designed for limited range brushers and assisted brushing. The toothbrush fits over the teeth for easy placement and allows for a thorough cleaning in thirty seconds.

Colopast Corporation

1955 West Oak Circle
PO Box 8300
Marietta, GA 30062
770-281-8400, 800-533-0464
http://www.us.colopast.com
Disability Served: all

This company manufactures wound care products and ointments as well as urologicals and ostomy care products.

Coloplast Inc.

5610 West Sligh Avenue, Suite 100-C
Tampa, FL 33634
813-886-5634, 800-237-4555
Disability Served: all

This company manufactures incontinence aids and a decubitus ulcer dressing.

Colorado Giraffe

7235 South Steele Circle
Littleton, CO 80122-1940
800-346-5662
Disability Served: physically disabled

This company manufactures a door knob cover to accommodate persons with limited or no hand dexterity in opening doors.

Columbia Medical Manufacturing Corp.

PO Box 633
Pacific Palisades, CA 90272
310-454-6612, 800-454-6612
http://www.columbiamedical.com
Disability Served: physically disabled

This company provides products for children and adults with physical disabilities.

Columbus McKinnon Corporation—Mobility Products

140 John James Audubon Parkway
Amherst, NY 14228-1197
800-888-0985
http://www.industry.net/cm
Disability Served: physically disabled

This company manufactures lifting and transferring systems to assist people with disabilities in moving from chair to bed, chair to tub, and so on.

Comdial
1180 Seminole Trail
PO Box 7266
Charlottesville, VA 22906
804-978-2200
Disability Served: physically disabled

This company manufactures telephones with built-in speakerphones.

Comfort Creations, Inc.
PO Box 8588
Turnersville, NJ 08012
609-464-3131, 800-220-4045
Disability Served: all

This company manufactures ski attachments for walkers so the walkers can glide over surfaces such as carpet and grass.

Comfort Lift Corporation
Box 606
Remsen, IA 51050
712-786-2097
Disability Served: physically disabled

This company manufactures a patient lift for bedside use and a wheelchair with a removable seat.

Comfort Med
A Division of Comfort Sleeper Inc.
609 Interchange Drive SW
Atlanta, GA 30336-1603
404-841-0458, 800-527-3626
Disability Served: physically disabled

This company manufactures a variety of pillows, cushions, and orthotics.

Comfortex Inc.
PO Box 850
Winona, MN 55987
507-454-6579
Disability Served: physically disabled

Comfortex manufactures a foam mattress and a foam mattress overlay.

Comfy Back/Evans Inc.
1611 Lincoln Boulevard
PO Box 988
Venice, CA 90294
310-821-6400, 800-272-6639
Disability Served: all

This company manufactures a variety of back support cushions.

Commander Omni Company
301 Lodi Street
Hackensack, NJ 07602
800-526-4753
Disability Served: all

This company manufactures toilet seat cushions, back support cushions, wheelchair trays, walking cane tips, and other aids for daily living.

Communication Board (The)
Graley Marketing
15935 El Soneto Drive
Whittier, CA 90603
562-947-7848
Disability Served: all

Community Advocates, Inc.
PO Box 83304
Lincoln, NE 68501
402-486-3091
TTY/TDD: 402-486-3091
Disability Served: vision

This company sells measuring devices, Braille labelers, and other products for the blind and visually impaired.

Companion Products International
PO Box G
Milford, PA 18337-0208
717-686-4713, 800-258-6423
http://www.augcom.com
Disability Served: communication

This company develops and sells low-cost voice communicator devices for the speech impaired. It also provides communicator kits for building special voice devices.

Companion Walker Ltd.

1420 40th Avenue NE, Suite 4
Calgary, AB T2E 6L1 Canada
403-250-1888
http://www.companionwalker.com
Disability Served: physically disabled

This company designs and manufactures mobility aid products for senior citizens and the disabled. Products include wheelchairs, walkers, carriers, and canes.

Composite Medical Equipment

17310 Jackie Street
Ramona, CA 92065
619-788-0828
Disability Served: physically disabled

This company manufactures aids to prevent restless or disoriented patients from wandering off or falling and injuring themselves. The company also manufactures a transfer board.

CompuMed Inc.

One Pitchfork Road
Meeteetse, WY 82433
307-868-2555, 800-722-4417
Disability Served: physically disabled

This company makes switches and wheelchair hardware and accessories.

Computer Comfort Installation

1863 16th Street
West Linn, OR 97068-4408
503-650-5250
Disability Served: physically disabled

This company manufactures a height-adjustable computer table to accommodate wheelchair users.

Computer Instruments Corp.

99 Seaview Boulevard
Port Washington, NY 11050-4632
516-483-8200, 800-227-1314
Disability Served: all

This company manufactures heart rate monitors.

Comtek Communications Technology

357 West 2700 South
Salt Lake City, UT 84115
800-496-3463
Disability Served: hearing

This company manufactures amplification systems for the hard of hearing.

Concertina Group

PO Box 13558
Austin, TX 78711-3558
512-476-1259
Disability Served: physically disabled

This company offers wheelchair gloves.

Concord Elevator, Inc.

107 Alfred Kuehne Boulevard
Brampton, ON L6T 4K3 Canada
905-791-5555, 800-661-5112
Disability Served: physically disabled

This company manufactures and develops residential elevators and lifts.

Connector Set Toy Company

2800 Sterling Drive
PO Box 700
Hatfield, PA 19440-0700
215-997-7722, 800-KID-KNEX
Disability Served: all

This company manufactures building piece kits for children.

Conrad Carpenter

6531 SE Federal Highway, #A-109
Stuart, FL 34997-8334
561-221-7649
Disability Served: physically disabled

This company manufactures a cane holder.

Consumer Care Products Inc.

1446 Pilgrim Road
Plymouth, WI 53073
800-977-2256
http://www.consumercareinc.com
Disability Served: all

Consumer Care Products Inc. manufactures and distributes rehabilitation equipment for children and adults. Products include positioning and mobility equipment, fasteners, and do-it-yourself products.

Consumer Engineering Inc./Seavon Corp.

PO Box 060100
Palm Bay, FL 32906-0100
407-984-0179
Disability Served: all

This company develops a strobe light adapter that acts as an emergency flashing light when necessary.

Contour Fabricators Inc.

PO Box 56
4100 East Baldwin Road
Grand Blanc, MI 48439
313-695-2910
Disability Served: physically disabled

This company manufactures home health care aids, including seat cushions and supports.

Contour Form Products

12 North Diamond Street
PO Box 328
Greenville, PA 16125
412-588-4452, 800-223-8808
Disability Served: all

This company manufactures a knee orthosis designed to immobilize the knee and lower back orthoses.

Convaid

PO Box 4209
Palos Verdes, CA 90274
310-539-6814, 800-552-1020
http://www.convaid.com
Disability Served: physically disabled

This company manufactures mobile positioning systems for children and young adults. The chairs are lightweight and compact-folding, with non-wheelchair styling. Positioning, support, tilt, tilt/recline, and anatomic chairs are available.

Convatec

PO Box 4000
Princeton, NJ 08540
800-422-8811
Disability Served: all

Convatec makes a colostomy irrigation system.

Cooper Tools

PO Box 728
Apex, NC 27502
919-362-7510
Disability Served: physically disabled

This company manufactures self-opening scissors.

Corbin Architectural Hardware

225 Episcopal Road
PO Box 4003
Berlin, CT 06037
203-225-7411
Disability Served: all

This company, a division of Black & Decker, manufactures door locks and handles.

Cord-Mate, Inc.

74 Hickory Hill Road
Simsbury, CT 06070
203-651-3090, 800-922-7990
Disability Served: physically disabled

This company manufactures an emergency alert system to assist individuals who cannot get to a phone or are injured.

Cornell Communications, Inc.

4911 West Good Hope Road
Milwaukee, WI 53223-4840
414-351-4660, 800-558-8957
http://www.cornellinc.com
Disability Served: all

This company manufactures an emergency alert system designed for multistory buildings.

Corometrics Medical Systems, Inc.

61 Barnes Park Road North
Wallingford, CT 06492
203-265-5631, 800-243-3952
Disability Served: all

This company manufactures an apnea respiration and cardiac monitor for use with infants.

Cotterman Company

130 Seltzer Road
Croswell, MI 48422
810-679-4400, 800-552-3337
Disability Served: physically disabled

This company develops a portable elevating work platform.

Crane Plumbing/Fiat Products

1235 Hartrey Avenue
Evanston, IL 60202
847-864-9777
Disability Served: physically disabled

This company manufactures plumbing fixtures, including toilets, showers, tubs, and sinks.

Craner Cabinetry

3190 South 4140 West
West Valley City, UT 84120
801-966-1127
Disability Served: physically disabled

This company manufactures computer work stations adapted for computer users with disabilities.

Crazy Creek Products Inc.

1401 South Broadway
PO Box 1050
Red Lodge, MT 59068
406-446-3446, 800-331-0304
http://www.crazycreek.com
Disability Served: all

This company manufactures portable chairs and loungers equipped with padded seat and back supports.

Creations in Space

PO Box 508
Garfield, WA 99130
509-635-1547
Disability Served: physically disabled

This company manufactures carrying accessories for use with wheelchairs, walkers, and crutches. Products include crutch bags, backpacks for wheelchairs, beverage holders for wheelchairs, and more.

Creations in Wood Inc.

5843 East Brown
Fresno, CA 93727
209-294-1100
Disability Served: all

This company builds wood bedroom furniture that is wheelchair accessible.

Creations Unlimited, Inc.

8944 H Street
Omaha, NE 68127
402-592-9388
Disability Served: physically disabled

This company manufactures a shower stall with a built-in seat and a roll-in shower insert to accommodate wheelchairs.

Creative Adaptations

PO Box 36
Milton, NH 03851
603-652-7826
Disability Served: physically disabled

This company adapts bicycles for children with special needs.

Creative Industries

Medical Products Division
5366 Jackson Drive
La Mesa, CA 91942
619-469-5012, 800-748-5530
Disability Served: physically disabled

This company is the manufacturer of Grip Mate, a handle adapter.

Creative Rehabilitation Equipment

609 NE Schuyler Street
Portland, OR 97212
503-281-6747, 800-547-4611
Disability Served: physically disabled

This company specializes in seating systems and supports for wheelchairs.

Creative Shop, Inc.

PO Box 7
Leoma, TN 38468
615-852-2323
Disability Served: physically disabled

This company manufactures a bowling ball holder to accommodate bowlers in wheelchairs and a one-hand fishing reel and rod holder.

Crescent Corporation

PO Box 610987
Port Huron, MI 48061-0987
810-982-2783, 800-233-6506
Disability Served: physically disabled

This company manufactures aids for daily living, canes, walkers, and more.

Crestline Products, Inc.

PO Box 2108
Orlando, FL 32802-2108
407-859-6428
Disability Served: physically disabled

This company manufactures handgrip attachments and extensions for walkers.

Crutch Tote, Inc.

PO Box 211433
Salt Lake City, UT 84121-8433
801-943-7067
Disability Served: physically disabled

This company manufactures carrying caddies for use with walkers, crutches, wheelchairs, and scooters.

Cryo 2 Corporation

4106 Avenue D
PO Box 2078
Ft Pierce, FL 33450
305-465-6660, 800-327-0313
Disability Served: all

This company manufactures portable oxygen systems.

CSP Industries Inc.

4120 Delmar Avenue
Victoria, BC V8Z 4J6 Canada
250-479-1350
Disability Served: all

This company makes a collapsible cane with a built-in light for use at night. The light is visible for up to two miles away.

Custom Home Elevators of St Louis, Inc.

8582 St Charles Rock Road
PO Box 142725
St Louis, MO 63114-2725
314-423-1620, 800-783-1620
Disability Served: physically disabled

This company furnishes and installs stairway chairs, residential elevators, on-slope and vertical wheelchair lifts, small dumbwaiters, accessibility elevators, and barrier-free lifts.

Cybex

Division of Lumex
2100 Smithtown Avenue
Ronkonkoma, NY 11779-0903
516-585-9000
Disability Served: physically disabled

This company manufactures exercise and rehabilitation equipment, including isokinetic knee machines, isokinetic joint exercise systems, computers for exercise machines, cycle ergometers, and dynamometers.

DA Matot

1533 West Altgeld Street
Chicago, IL 60614
773-549-2177, 800-628-6832
Disability Served: physically disabled

This company manufactures residential elevators.

Dakon Corporation
1836 Gilford Avenue
New Hyde Park, NY 11040
516-775-5525
Disability Served: physically disabled

This company manufactures therapeutic equipment, including whirlpool baths, body immersion tanks, and resistive exercisers.

Dale Medical Products
7-11 Cross Street
PO Box 1556
Plainville, MA 02762
800-343-3980
Disability Served: physically disabled

This company manufactures orthotics and therapeutic aids, including abdominal binders, catheter tube holders, rib belts, wrist splints, and tracheostomy tube holders.

DANCO International Inc.
13354 McKinley Road
Chelsea, MI 48118
313-475-7994
Disability Served: physically disabled

This company manufactures the Oxford Pressure Monitor, a portable pressure evaluation system.

Danmar Products, Inc.
221 Jackson Industrial Drive
Ann Arbor, MI 48103
734-761-1990, 800-783-1998
http://www.danmarproducts.com
Disability Served: physically disabled

This company manufactures adaptive equipment, including seating and positioning equipment, helmets (for seizure or behavioral problems), flotation devices, and toileting aids.

Dazey Corporation
One Dazey Circle
Industrial Airport, KS 66031
913-782-7500
Disability Served: physically disabled

This company manufactures a knife sharpener that can be used with one hand and a plastic bag sealer.

Dean Rosecrans
PO Box 310
Nampa, ID 83651
208-467-4790, 800-522-4425
Disability Served: all

This company manufactures foam stoma filters, stoma shower shields, a cloth stoma cover, and a speech aid for persons who have lost the use of their larynxes.

Decoguard Products
PO Box 400
Muncy, PA 17756
717-546-5941, 800-233-8458
Disability Served: all

This company manufactures hand rails that can serve as bumper guards.

Delta Faucet Co.
Division of Masco Group
PO Box 40980
Indianapolis, IN 46280
317-848-1812
Disability Served: physically disabled

This company manufactures water temperature control monitors, lever handles for faucets, and controls for adjusting water flow volume.

Delta T Company
PO Box 473
Santa Clara, CA 95052
408-243-0241
Disability Served: physically disabled

This company develops a portable sensor that measures the pressure between skin and seat cushions.

Dermacare
Division of PSC Corporation
7651 National Turnpike
Louisville, KY 40214
502-368-1654, 800-626-4550
Disability Served: physically disabled

This company manufactures mattresses, cushions, and foam limb positioners.

Designabilities Inc.
PO Box 784
Millbury, MA 01527
508-865-0006
Disability Served: physically disabled

The Activity Chair and Table is an adjustable seating system for children.

Designs for Comfort Inc.
PO Box 8229
Northfield, IL 60093
847-446-9190, 800-443-9226
Disability Served: all

This company manufactures hair pieces and hats with hair pieces for women experiencing hair loss.

Designs For Vision Inc.
760 Koehler Avenue
Ronkonkoma, NY 11779
516-585-3300, 800-345-4009
Disability Served: vision

This company develops various lens systems for persons with low vision or specific visual problems.

Detecto
Division of Cardinal Scale Manufacturing
PO Box 151
Webb City, MO 64870
417-673-4631, 800-641-2008
Disability Served: physically disabled

This company manufactures various scales, including wheelchair scales, chair scales, and electronic in-bed scales.

DeVilbiss Company
PO Box 635
Somerset, PA 15501
814-443-4881
Disability Served: all

This company manufactures nebulizers, portable aspirators, air compressors, and oxygen concentrators.

Dewtronics
PO Box 308
Ghent, WV 25843-0308
304-787-9712
Disability Served: hearing, vision

This company manufactures a Braille telecaption system that allows deaf-blind persons to read television closed-captioning programs in Braille.

DFE Inc.
PO Box 725
Oklahoma City, OK 73101
405-232-2809
Disability Served: all

DFE manufactures a door security system that allows the user to answer the intercom at the door with a telephone.

DGS Corp.
4850 West Belmont Avenue
Chicago, IL 60641-4329
800-621-1260
Disability Served: all

This company manufactures access signs.

Diagnostic Ultrasound Corporation
PO Box 818
18109 NE 76th Street
Redmond, WA 98052
425-867-1348, 800-331-2313
Disability Served: physically disabled

This company manufactures ultrasound units designed to monitor bladder volume.

Dial A Hearing Screening Test
PO Box 1880
Media, PA 19063
800-222-EARS
Disability Served: hearing

This company provides automated hearing screening tests via telephone. Call the 800 number for instructions and a local test number.

Diestco Manufacturing Co.

PO Box 6504
Chico, CA 95927
530-893-3136, 800-795-2392
Disability Served: physically disabled

This company manufactures accessories for wheelchairs, scooters, and walkers. Products include canopies, backpacks, threshold ramps, cup holders, and lap trays.

Dillon Manufacturing Company, Inc.

6463 Warren Drive
Norcross, GA 30093
800-955-3556
Disability Served: physically disabled

This company manufactures colored arm slings for children.

Dipsters Corporation

265 Wyndcliff Road
Scarsdale, NY 10583
914-725-0225, 800-431-2660
Disability Served: physically disabled

This company manufactures heat packs, heat pads, resistance exercisers, and therapeutic weights.

Disability Management Systems, Inc.

Aquatic Therapy Products and Service
1403 East B Avenue
Plainwell, MI 49080
616-349-9049
Disability Served: all

This company makes a swimming aid that provides flotation.

Dixie USA Inc.

PO Box 55549
Houston, TX 77255
713-688-4993, 800-347-3494
Disability Served: physically disabled

This company manufactures a board designed to transfer persons from vehicles to chairs as well as a personal alarm.

Dixon Industries Inc.

Box 494
Coffeyville, KS 67337
316-251-2000
Disability Served: physically disabled

This company manufactures a hand-controlled riding lawnmower.

DJ Technical Sales Ltd.

2647 Kingsway
Vancouver, BC V5R 5H4 Canada
604-436-2694
Disability Served: physically disabled

This company manufactures a mounting kit for attaching communication devices to wheelchairs.

Don Johnston Inc.

1000 North Rand Road, Building 115
Wauconda, IL 60084
847-526-2682, 800-999-4660
http://www.donjohnston.com
Disability Served: all

This company provides products and services for those who struggle with reading and writing.

Donegan Optical Company

PO Box 14308
Lenexa, KS 66215
Disability Served: vision

This company manufactures magnifying lenses.

Dor-O-Matic

Division of Republic Industries, Inc.
7350 West Wilson Avenue
Harwood Heights, IL 60656-4786
708-867-7400, 800-543-4635
Disability Served: physically disabled

This company manufactures powered door operators.

Double K Products

915 West Lehigh Avenue
PO Box 1087
Englewood, CO 80150
303-781-4019
Disability Served: all

This company makes a portable tray that can attach to walkers, wheelchairs, or armchairs. The company also manufactures the necessary mounting hardware.

Doug Heir's Amusement Corporation

702 Park Boulevard
Cherry Hill, NJ 08002-3321
609-482-1474, 800-443-5725
Disability Served: physically disabled

This company manufactures an arcade-type basketball game accessible for wheelchairs, walkers, or chairs.

Dover Elevator Corp.

Elevator Division
PO Box 2177
Memphis, TN 38101
901-393-2110
Disability Served: all

This company manufactures a residential elevator.

Dr & Mrs Richard Wainerdi

PO Box 27067
Houston, TX 77227
Disability Served: physically disabled

The Wainerdis provide a matching service for amputees needing single shoes or gloves.

Dremel Manufacturing

4915 21st Street
Racine, WI 53406
414-554-1390
http://ww.dremel.com
Disability Served: all

Mr. A.J. Dremel invented the high-speed rotary tool in 1934. Dremel quality products include rotary tools, sanders, and scroll saws.

DresserMat

3500 52nd Street
Sacramento, CA 95820
916-454-2653
Disability Served: physically disabled

This company manufactures the Waterbed and DresserMat system, which consists of a waterbed frame and storage insert.

Drew Karol Industries, Inc.

PO Box 1066
Greenville, MS 38702-1066
601-378-2188
Disability Served: physically disabled

This company manufactures and distributes a toothbrush for persons with limited or no hand use.

Dri Pride

Division of Weyerhauser Company
PO Box 1198
Bowling Green, KY 42102
502-843-1070
Disability Served: vision

This company manufactures incontinence aids, including pants, pads, and diapers.

Driving Systems Inc.

16139 Runnymede Street
Van Nuys, CA 91406-2913
818-782-6793
Disability Served: physically disabled

This company manufactures wall grab bars for bathrooms, bath seats, an adapted driving control unit that enables drivers without the use of their right foot to drive standard vehicles, and a one-hand driving control system.

Dundee Mills Inc.

Healthcare Products
111 West 40th Street
New York, NY 10018
212-840-7200
Disability Served: physically disabled

This company manufactures incontinence aids, including a bed underpad, incontinence pants, and adult diapers. The company also manufactures adult bibs.

Duralife Inc.
195 Phillips Park Drive
South Williamsport, PA 17702
717-323-9743, 800-443-5433
http://www.duralife-usa.com
Disability Served: physically disabled

This company manufactures commode chairs, shower chairs, walkers, geriatric chairs, shower beds, and bath transfer benches.

Duro-Med Industries, Inc.
155 Polifly Road
Hackensack, NJ 07601
201-488-5055, 800-526-4753
Disability Served: all

This company manufactures a number of health care products, including orthopedic supports, daily living aids, and footcare products.

Dwight Pollock Sales
18 Padilla Court
Danville, CA 94526
800-801-5515
Disability Served: physically disabled

This company manufactures The Shower Cover Up, a laryngectomy shower shield designed to protect the stoma.

Dwyer Products Corporation
418 North Calumet Avenue
Michigan City, IN 46360-5019
219-874-5236, 800-348-8508
Disability Served: physically disabled

This company manufactures custom compact kitchens for the physically challenged. These kitchens are designed for applications where food storage and food preparation capabilities are required in a limited amount of space.

Dyn-Aura Engineering Labs Inc.
8057 Vickers Street
San Diego, CA 92111-1917
619-565-4922
Disability Served: hearing

This company manufactures a telephone adapter for hearing aids that eliminates feedback.

Dynamic Life Products
3215 East Hearn Road
Phoenix, AZ 85032
602-867-8243, 800-543-2572
Disability Served: physically disabled

This company manufactures the Bathboard, a portable device enabling easy entry and exit from a bathtub, as well as safe bathing or showering in a sitting position.

Dynamic Products Corp.
3860 Broadway Street
Grove City, OH 43123
Disability Served: physically disabled

This company manufactures Grip-Tac, a spray-on nonslip grip coating, and Dyna-Form-It, a custom molding rubber used for building up grips and handles.

Dynamic Systems, Inc.
235 Sunlight Drive
Leicester, NC 28748
828-683-3523
http://www.cheta.net/dsi
Disability Served: all

This company manufactures orthopedic foam seating for anyone requiring special seating. Products include SunMate foam cushions and sheets, Pudgee pads, Laminar cushions, and Liquid SunMate for Foam-in-Place Seating.

Dynasplint Systems Inc.
645 Baltimore Annapolis Boulevard, Suite 110
Severna Park, MD 21146-3923
410-544-9530, 800-638-6771
Disability Served: orthopedic

This company manufactures extension and flexion contracture splints designed to increase joint movement.

DynaVox Systems, Inc.
2100 Wharton Street, Suite 400
Pittsburgh, PA 15203
412-381-4883
http://www.dynavoxsys.com
Disability Served: communication

This company manufactures voice output communication boards.

DynaWave Corporation
2520 Kaneville Court
Geneva, IL 60134
630-232-4945
Disability Served: all

This company manufactures ultrasound units to promote healing and reduce pain.

DynOrthotics Inc.
8206 Leesburg Pike, Suite 404
Vienna, VA 22182
703-790-0200, 800-292-7223
Disability Served: all

This company develops and manufactures a variety of orthotics.

E Apparel Ltd.
250 Passaic Street
Newark, NJ 07104
201-481-3888, 800-309-3888
Disability Served: physically disabled

This company manufactures clothing and footwear.

E Z EM Inc.
7 Portland Avenue
Westbury, NY 11590
516-333-8230
Disability Served: all

This company manufactures a suspension mitt for use during shoulder arthroscopy.

E. L. Foust Co., Inc.
754 Industrial Drive
Elmhurst, IL 60126
630-834-4952, 800-225-9549
http://www.foustco.com
Disability Served: all

This company manufactures and sells air purifiers for the chemically sensitive. Products include water filters, face masks, specialty HVAC system filters, and books.

Eagle Marketing
5321 South Sheridan, #15
Tulsa, OK 74145
918-663-4477
Disability Served: all

This company manufactures Pagemate, a plastic copy holder for people requiring one-handed reading, adhesive line markers for marking lines in publications or books, and plastic overlays to eliminate glare on pages.

Earmark Inc.
1125 Dixwell Avenue
Hamden, CT 06514
203-777-2130
Disability Served: hearing

This company manufactures a number of products for the hard of hearing, including hearing aids and amplification systems.

Easy Motion Wood Splitter
PO Box 1285
Vestal, NY 13850
607-785-3962
http://www.woodwiz.com/woodwiz
Disability Served: all

This company manufactures a safe, easy-to-use log splitter for use by physically challenged individuals.

Ebco Manufacturing Co.
265 North Hamilton Road
Columbus, OH 43213
800-950-3226
http://www.OasisWaterCoolers.com
Disability Served: physically disabled

This company manufactures wheelchair-accessible water coolers and fountains.

EBM Corporation
2249 South Grout Road
Gladwin, MI 48624
517-426-6327
Disability Served: physically disabled

This company designs and manufactures various workstations and desks to accommodate persons with physical and/or visual disabilities. Products include an ergonomic desk, a fold-up computer work center, and an adjustable-height work table.

Eckstein Brothers, Inc.

4807 West 118th Place
Hawthorne, CA 90250
323-772-6113
Disability Served: hearing

This company manufactures a line of audiometers, a line of speech therapy and auditory training equipment, and desktop hearing amplifiers.

Econol Stairway Lift Corp.

2513 Center Street, Box 854
Cedar Falls, IA 50613
319-277-4777
Disability Served: physically disabled

This company manufactures assorted lifts for wheelchairs. Products include inclined wheelchair lifts, vertical lifts, home elevators, and dumb waiters.

EFCO/ROTOSWING Division

5405 NW 5th
Oklahoma City, OK 73127
405-942-8641
Disability Served: all

This company makes a mechanical, belt-driven, automatic door operator.

Ekco Houseware Company

9234 West Belmont Avenue
Franklin Park, IL 60131
847-678-8600
Disability Served: physically disabled

This company manufactures kitchen tools, including peelers, cheese slicers, bottle brushes, and jar openers.

Elcombe Systems Ltd.

603 March Road
PO Box 72099
Kanata, ON K2K 2M5 Canada
613-591-5678
Disability Served: all

This company manufactures the Mainstreet Messenger, an emergency alert system telephone designed for persons with visual, hearing, mobility, and dexterity disabilities.

Election Supplies Ltd.

Division of Business Records Corp.
1111 Mockingbird Lane, Suite 1400
Dallas, TX 75247
214-224-8618, 800-331-8683
Disability Served: all

This company produces products to assist those with disabilities to vote with ease. Products include a ballot magnifier for those with visual impairments, a flexible stylus for use in voting booths, and a handicapped adapter kit for voting.

Electone Inc.

PO Box 910
Winter Park, FL 32790
407-831-2555, 800-432-7483
Disability Served: hearing

Electone manufactures products for the hearing impaired, including behind-the-ear hearing aids, miniature hearing aids, and more.

Electric Fishing Reel Systems, Inc.

PO Box 20411
Greensboro, NC 27420
336-273-9101
http://www.elec-tra-mate.com
Disability Served: physically disabled

This company manufactures electric fishing reel drives designed to facilitate retrieval of fish for people with disabilities.

Electromedical Products Inc.

12591 Crenshaw Boulevard
Hawthorne, CA 90250
310-973-8931
Disability Served: physically disabled

This company manufactures the Alpha Stim 100, a neuromuscular stimulator.

Electronic Monitors Inc.
PO Box 1087
Euless, TX 76039
817-283-0859
Disability Served: all

This company manufactures an apnea respiration monitor.

Electronic Research Devices
9220 SW Barbur Boulevard, Suite 107
Portland, OR 97219
503-245-7241, 800-547-0366
Disability Served: physically disabled

This company manufactures electrical nerve stimulators.

Electronic Speech Enhancement, Inc.
1115 Ridge Road
St Louis, MO 63021
314-394-0770
Disability Served: communication

ESE manufactures an assistive speech device that processes the speaker's speech and clarifies it.

Elgin Exercise Equipment Corp.
270 Eisenhower Lane North, Unit 4A
Lombard, IL 60148
630-268-1000
Disability Served: physically disabled

This company manufactures pulley exercise units.

Eljer Plumbingware
100 Forbes Avenue, #850
Pittsburgh, PA 15222-1311
412-338-3330
Disability Served: physically disabled

This company manufactures plumbing fixtures and supplies, including bathtubs, faucets, handles, and showers.

Elkay Manufacturing Co.
2222 Camden Court
Oak Brook, IL 60521
630-574-8484
Disability Served: physically disabled

This company manufactures hot and cold water dispensers, kitchen sink accessories, and wheelchair-accessible water fountains.

Ellison Bronze Co.
125 West Main Street
Falconer, NY 14733
716-665-6522
Disability Served: physically disabled

This company manufactures an exterior door.

Elmers Weights Inc.
Division of Bollinger Healthcare
222 Airport Freeway
Irving, TX 75062
972-554-0458, 800-858-4568
Disability Served: physically disabled

This company manufactures weights and exercise equipment to accommodate people with disabilities.

Elra Industries Inc.
550 South Erie Highway
Hamilton, OH 45011
513-829-7387
Disability Served: all

This company manufactures the Shower Shield, a plastic protector designed to keep casts and bandages dry during bathing or showering.

Elsafe, Inc.
4303 Vineland Road, Suite F-15
Orlando, FL 32811
407-423-7233, 800-252-3004
Disability Served: physically disabled

This company manufactures a safe with keypad access.

Elyon, Inc.
PO Box 20548
Brandenton, FL 34203
813-758-2408, 800-435-5484
Disability Served: physically disabled

This company manufactures the Vari-Chair, an adaptive seating system; the Mobilizer, a mobile standing aid; Ad-Just, a spinal management system orthosis; and the Berryboot, a foot and ankle orthosis.

Elze Enterprises
300 South Meadow Drive, #15
Carson City, NV 89701
702-883-3967
Disability Served: all

This company manufactures a motorized file cabinet.

Embracing Concepts Inc.
40 Humboldt Street
Rochester, NY 14609
716-654-9090, 800-962-5542
Disability Served: all

This company manufactures cushions, seating accessories, and covers for electronic devices, such as keyboards, communication devices, and switches.

Empi Inc.
1275 Grey Fox Road
St Paul, MN 55112
800-328-2536
Disability Served: physically disabled

This company manufactures an electrical nerve stimulator.

Emsco Inc.
PO Box 151
Girard, PA 16417
814-774-3137, 800-458-0839
Disability Served: all

This company manufactures scrub brushes, easy-wring mops, and various sponges for housekeeping and bathing needs.

Enabling Technologies Inc.
2411 North Federal Boulevard
Denver, CO 80211
303-455-3578
Disability Served: physically disabled

This company manufactures a mono-ski for downhill skiing.

ENDURANCE Inc.
8830 Piney Branch Road, #212
Silver Spring, MD 20903
301-445-0851, 800-797-RAIN
Disability Served: all

This company manufactures raincoats and capes.

Eneslow The Foot Comfort Center
924 Broadway
New York, NY 10010
212-477-2300
Disability Served: physically disabled

This company designs, manufactures, fits, and modifies shoes and foot appliances as prescribed to lessen or eliminate painful and disabling conditions of the foot.

Enswell & Sabia Scoliometer
30 North Prospect
Red Bank, NJ 07701
201-747-4765
Disability Served: all

This company manufactures the Scoliometer, a measuring device for detecting scoliosis, and a cold pack for reduction of edema.

Enviro Med
Stacey French
509 La Cresta
Red Oak, TX 75154
214-617-8039
Disability Served: physically disabled

This company manufactures the Body Cooler System, a cooling vest designed to regulate body temperature and prevent heat stress.

Environmental Technologies Co.

2020 Meadowridge Road
PO Box 10395
Prescott, AZ 86301
800-757-0993
Disability Served: all

This company manufactures a variety of non-toxic cleaning clothes designed to clean without the use of chemical products.

Environmental Toys

PO Box 40962
San Francisco, CA 94140
415-601-1506
Disability Served: physically disabled

This company manufactures the Roller Board, a balance training device for those with physical disabilities.

Equipment Shop

PO Box 33
Bedford, MA 01730
800-525-7681
Disability Served: physically disabled

This company's catalog offers pediatric physical therapy equipment, including Tripp Trapp adjustable chairs, Airex mats, original "Pezzi" Gymnastik and Physioballs, feeding tools, books, videos, and tricycles with accessories.

Eschenbach

904 Ethan Allen Highway
Ridgefield, CT 06877
203-438-7471
http://www.eschenbach.com
Disability Served: vision

This company distributes vision aids to eyecare and rehabilitation professionals who then dispense these products to the visually impaired. Products include hand and stand magnifiers, telescopes, filters, and electronic reading devices.

Everest & Jennings Inc.

Division of Graham Fields
3601 Rider Trail South
Earth City, MO 63045
314-517-7000, 800-235-4661
Disability Served: physically disabled

This company manufactures more than 200 items for persons with physical disabilities, including wheelchairs, seat cushions, shower chairs, grab bars, and more.

Everett Assistive Resources Co.

PO Box 3353
Everett, WA 98203-8353
206-353-5680, 800-669-7371
Disability Served: hearing

This company manufactures a telephone adapter for hearing aid wearers. The adapter eliminates the feedback that occurs with hearing aids.

Evlo Plastics, Inc.

310 Industrial Lane
PO Box 2295
Sandusky, OH 44870
419-626-2430
Disability Served: all

This company manufactures the Handi Holder to make milk or juice cartons easier to pour for people with arthritis or impaired movement of the hands.

Exceptional Hearing Services

515 Northgate Drive, Suite D
San Rafael, CA 94903-3639
415-499-7766
Disability Served: hearing

This company manufactures an amplification system that works with radios and televisions.

Executive Coach Corporation

1003 Route 22
Fox River Grove, IL 60021
847-639-0575
Disability Served: physically disabled

This company provides mobility modifications of vehicles.

Exploring Concepts
PO Box 7035
Wilmington, NC 28406
910-397-2988, 800-278-8697
Disability Served: all

This company manufactures Tub-Craze, a set of foam letters, designed to teach the alphabet and spelling skills, that can adhere to tubs and tile and Fridg-Craze, magnetic letters.

Extend Incorporated
303 21st Street North
Moorhead, MN 56560
218-236-9686, 800-425-3837
Disability Served: physically disabled

This company manufactures door levers to replace round doorknobs.

Extensions for Independence
555 Saturn Boulevard, #B-368
San Diego, CA 92154
619-423-7709
Disability Served: physically disabled

This company develops a number of items to accommodate persons with physical disabilities, including adaptive work stations, desk lapboards, a motorized easel, telephone receiver holders, mouthsticks, computer disk loading systems, keyboard keylocks, and more.

Eyetronics
PO Box 252
Danielson, CT 06239
203-779-1076
Disability Served: vision

This company manufactures a magnifying lens that can accommodate large-size reading materials.

EZ Close—Fashionable Adaptive Clothing
6939 Reynolds Street
Pittsburgh, PA 15208
412-362-9940
Disability Served: physically disabled

This company manufactures adaptive trousers for both men and women.

EZ Fit Inc.
53-16 62nd Street
Maspeth, NY 11378
718-507-6664
Disability Served: physically disabled

This company produces underwear for men, women, and children with limited range of movement.

EZ On Products Inc. of Florida
500 Commerce Way West
Jupiter, FL 33458
407-747-6920, 800-323-6598
Disability Served: physically disabled

This company manufactures a vest restraint designed for children too big for car seats yet too small for standard seat belts.

EZMT Valve Co., Inc.
22260 Davenrich Street
Salinas, CA 93908-1011
408-484-1934
Disability Served: physically disabled

This company manufactures and sells urological supplies to the public and to distributors. Products manufactured include latex and vinyl collection leg bags and other related products.

Ezy Ramp Company
4502 North Armenia Avenue
Tampa, FL 33603
813-875-6302
Disability Served: physically disabled

This company manufactures a portable wheelchair ramp.

Face Guards, Inc.
PO Box 901
21 West Main Street
Salem, VA 24153
703-389-6999, 800-336-9683
Disability Served: all

This company manufactures face guards and helmets for youth.

Facilis, Ltd.
PO Box 832 R
Romeoville, IL 60441
815-886-4892
Disability Served: physically disabled

This company distributes products manufactured by various companies. Products include grab bars for bathtubs, canes, walkers, door handles, cups, and more.

Fairway King
3 East Main Street
Oklahoma City, OK 73104
405-528-8571, 800-222-1145
Disability Served: physically disabled

This company manufactures various tables, stools, and eating utensils.

Falcon Lock Ni Industries Inc.
PO Box 6119
Garden Grove, CA 92645
714-373-2880, 800-266-4456
Disability Served: physically disabled

This company manufactures door locks with lever handles.

Falcon Rehabilitation Products, Inc.
4404 East 60th Avenue
Commerce City, CO 80011
303-287-6808, 800-370-6808
Disability Served: physically disabled

This company manufactures the HiRider wheelchair and many other medical devices.

Falls Welding & Fabricating
608 Grant Street
Akron, OH 44311
800-231-6444
http://www.fwfmedicalproducts.com
Disability Served: physically disabled

This company manufactures carts for oxygen canisters and cylinder racks for wheelchairs.

Farberware
1500 Bassett Avenue
Bronx, NY 10461
718-863-8000
Disability Served: all

This company manufactures a variety of kitchen tools and appliances, including an electric peeler, a battery-operated can opener, electric skillets, convection ovens, indoor grills, and mixing bowls.

Fashion Ease
1541 60th Street
Brooklyn, NY 11219
718-871-8188, 800-221-8929
Disability Served: all

This company sells clothing and other products for people with incontinence.

Fellowes Worcester Division
PO Box 60
Belcamp, MD 21017
301-273-0330
Disability Served: all

This company manufactures wire desk accessories, book holders, computer accessories, and file trays.

Ferno Ille
70 Weil Way
Wilmington, OH 45177-9371
802-133-3766
http://www.ferno.com
Disability Served: all

This company manufactures and distributes lift and transfer products and a complete line of aquatic rehabilitation products.

Ferring Laboratories Inc.

75 Montebello Road
Suffern, NY 10901
914-368-2244
Disability Served: all

This company manufactures an infusion pump that dispenses medication intravenously.

Fibar Group

141 Halstead Avenue
Mamaroneck, NY 10543-2650
914-835-1511, 800-342-2721
Disability Served: all

This company offers a processed wood fiber surface.

Finger Tips

2965 Holly Springs Road
Marietta, GA 30062
770-977-3251
Disability Served: physically disabled

This company manufactures Yes U Can, a home exercise kit to develop motor coordination, and Kids Can Too, motor coordination activities for children ages three years and older.

First Years, Inc.

1 Kiddie Drive
Avon, MA 02322
508-588-1220, 800-225-0382
Disability Served: all

This company manufactures a visual stimulation mobile that attaches to infant cribs and other visual stimulation and eye-hand coordination toys.

Fishburne Enterprises Inc.

140 E. Stetson Avenue, Suite 319
Hemet, CA 92543
909-766-0843
Disability Served: vision

This company makes large-print embossed labels for persons with vision impairments who are unable to read Braille.

Fishburne International, Inc.

PO Box 706, Airport Road
Arden, NC 28704
704-684-3521, 800-553-8167
Disability Served: all

Fishburne develops a unit for schools and other facilities that keeps track of students' medication needs and reminds administrators to administer medication at appropriate times.

Fisher Scientific Company

711 Forbes Avenue
Pittsburgh, PA 15219
412-562-8300
Disability Served: physically disabled

This company builds a portable science work station to accommodate wheelchair users who wish to conduct lab work.

Fisher-Price, Inc.

636 Girard Avenue
East Aurora, NY 14052
716-687-3000, 800-432-5437
http://www.fpp.com
Disability Served: all

Fisher-Price manufactures toys and activities for children and infants that are designed to stimulate and enhance fine motor and eye-hand coordination skills. Products include blocks, puzzles, and touch-activated toys.

Fitness Equipment Company Inc.

PO Box 167
Clanton, AL 35045
205-755-4953, 800-826-3518
Disability Served: all

This company manufactures a treadmill.

Fitness To Go, Inc.

PO Box 266
Independence, MO 64051
800-821-3126
Disability Served: all

This company manufactures an exercise machine that provides resistance.

Fitter International Inc.
4515 1st Street SE
Calgary, AB T2G 2L2 Canada
403-243-6830, 800-348-8371
http://www.fitter1.com
Disability Served: all

Fitter supplies balance and fitness products, including balance boards, Power Web hand exercisers, Physio Toner resistance tubing, and more.

FJR Industries, Inc.
PO Box 968
Painesville, OH 44077
440-352-9333
Disability Served: all

This company manufactures a fishing rod holder.

FLA Orthopedics Inc.
5757 NW 158th Street
Miami Lakes, FL 33014
305-820-1900, 800-327-4110
Disability Served: all

This company makes a back support system that provides support during lifting activities.

Flaghouse
150 North MacQuesten Parkway
Mt Vernon, NY 10011
914-699-1900, 800-793-7900
Disability Served: all

Flaghouse manufactures a wide variety of therapeutic toys and aids for children, including developmental balls, scooter boards, tricycles, helmets, standing frames, balance boards, wheelchair swings, and games.

Fleetwood Furniture Co.
PO Box 1259
Holland, MI 49422-1259
800-257-6390
Disability Served: physically disabled

This company manufactures accessible work benches, height-adjustable tables and work stations suitable for school settings or other institutions, and bedside cabinets.

Flex Vision
2635 Cleveland Avenue, Suite #1
Santa Rosa, CA 95403
707-544-3020
Disability Served: all

This company makes a keyboard wrist support that attaches to a desk.

Flex-A-Bed, Inc.
4020 Long Beach Boulevard, Suite C
Long Beach, CA 90807-0500
562-426-7371, 800-421-2277
Disability Served: all

This company manufactures a motorized bed.

Flinchbaugh Company Inc.
390 Eberts Lane
York, PA 17403
717-848-2418, 800-326-2418
Disability Served: physically disabled

This company manufactures interior seat lifts and interior wheelchair stair lifts.

Floating Swimwear, Inc.
PO Box 30
Derby, KS 67037-0030
316-524-0444
http://www.floatingswimwear.com
Disability Served: all

This company makes a one-piece bathing suit that provides buoyancy and flotation assistance.

Florida Manufacturing Corp.
501 Beville Road
Daytona Beach, FL 32119
800-447-2372
http://home.att.net/~flamenco~flamenco
Disability Served: all

This company manufactures cervical collars and home traction equipment.

Florlift of New Jersey Inc.
41 Lawrence Street
East Orange, NJ 07017
973-429-2200
http://florlift.com
Disability Served: physically disabled

This company makes interior and exterior wheelchair lifts.

Flotation Systems Inc.
PO Box 5070
Syracuse, NY 13220
315-452-4502, 800-888-8529
Disability Served: all

This company makes a water flotation mattress.

Foam Products Inc.
4747 Bronx Boulevard
Bronx, NY 10470
718-324-8000, 800-283-4362
Disability Served: all

This company manufactures support cushions and pillows, decubitus pads, and mattresses.

Force 10
PO Box 4400
Allentown, PA 18105-4400
610-798-2200, 800-367-2310
Disability Served: all

This company manufactures braces and supports, including knee braces, heel inserts, and neoprene elbow pads.

Foundation for Fluency
9242 Gross Point Road, #305
Skokie, IL 60077
847-677-8280
Disability Served: communication

This company makes an assistive speech device designed to prevent and reduce stuttering.

Four Point Design
1575 Catamount Road
Fairfield, CT 06430
203-259-1174
Disability Served: hearing

This company manufactures personal amplification systems.

Fourth Dimension Instruments, Inc.
PO Box 376
Spring, TX 77373
713-288-9366
Disability Served: hearing

This company manufactures a flashing doorbell signaler for persons with hearing impairments.

FourX Products Inc.
PO Box 555
Millwood, NY 10546
914-762-3555
Disability Served: vision

This company makes an electronic bar magnifier for persons with low vision.

Fox Bay Industries, Inc.
4150 B Place NW, #101
Auburn, WA 98001
253-941-9155, 800-874-8527
http://www.foxbay.com
Disability Served: all

This company manufactures office and computer equipment, including ergonomic office chairs, keyboard wrist supports, keyboard trays, document holders, foot supports, and back support cushions.

Frame Technologies
W681 Pearl Street
Oneida, WI 54155
920-869-2979
http://www.frame-tech.com
Disability Served: communication

This company develops communication aids for children with speech disabilities.

Frank Stubbs Company Inc.
4518 Vanowen Street
Burbank, CA 91505
818-842-5137, 800-223-1713
Disability Served: all

This company manufactures arm slings, hemiplegic shoulder harnesses, and back support cushions.

Franklin Brass

PO Box 5226
Culver City, CA 90231
310-306-5944, 800-421-3375
Disability Served: all

This company manufactures grab bars, folding shower seats, and arm supports for toilets.

Fred Scott and Sons

1444 West Rand Road
Des Plaines, IL 60016
847-297-1603
Disability Served: physically disabled

This company manufactures an exterior wheelchair lift.

Freedom Designs Inc.

2241 Madera Road
Simi Valley, CA 93065
805-582-0077, 800-331-8551
Disability Served: physically disabled

This company offers more than sixty items, including support cushions and seats, solid seats, restraint systems, and mounting hardware for wheelchairs.

Freedom Laces Incorporated

2955 Canfield Road
Youngstown, OH 44511
330-533-9642
Disability Served: all

This company makes elastic shoe laces that do not need to be tied.

Freedom Machine, Inc.

PO Box 32453
Phoenix, AZ 85064-2453
602-735-7373
Disability Served: physically disabled

This company manufactures a weight exercise machine for wheelchair users.

Freedom Room Inc.

Box 33
Freeport, IL 61032
815-235-9116, 800-359-6178
Disability Served: all

This company manufactures an elevated toilet seat.

Freeman Manufacturing Co., Inc.

900 West Chicago Road
PO Box J
Sturgis, MI 49091
616-651-8248, 800-253-2091
http://www.freemanmfg.com
Disability Served: physically disabled

Freeman is an established manufacturer and worldwide supplier of orthopedic soft goods. Its products range in diversity from a full line of back-support garments and spinal braces to lower-limb prosthetic supplies. Freeman's 800 Center is open from 8:00 a.m. to 8:00 p.m. EST, Monday through Friday.

Frigidaire

c/o WCI
6000 Perimeter Drive
Dublin, OH 43017
614-792-4100
Disability Served: all

Frigidaire makes home appliances, including cooktops, air conditioners, and oven ranges.

Frohock-Stewart Inc.

455 Whitney Avenue
Northboro, MA 01532-0330
508-393-2543, 800-343-6059
Disability Served: all

This company manufactures bath aids and fixtures, including grab bars and safety rails, safety benches, elevated toilet seats, and transfer benches.

Front Row Experience

540 Discovery Bay Boulevard
Byron, CA 94514-9454
923-634-5710, 800-524-9091
http://www.frontrowexperience.com
Disability Served: all

This company manufactures children's games and motor coordination building activities. Products include balance beams, large foam shapes, foam balls, coordination ladders, tumbling mats, scooter boards, beanbag kits, rhythm stick kits, ribbon stick kits, and rubber-band ball kits.

Futuro Inc.

A Beiersdorf Company
5405 Dupont Circle, Suite A
Milford, OH 45150-2735
513-576-8000, 800-933-0214
Disability Served: all

Futuro manufactures a wide variety of wheelchairs as well as home health care aids, such as whirlpools, patient lifts, bedpans, toilet safety frames, shower and tub benches, walkers, crutches, support cushions, safety rails, and more.

G & T Manufacturing Inc.

17520 Lemon Street
Hesperia, CA 92345
619-244-2972
Disability Served: physically disabled

This company manufactures an interior wheelchair lift.

G. E. Miller Inc.

540 Nepperhan Avenue
Yonkers, NY 10701
914-969-4036, 800-431-2924
Disability Served: all

This company sells more than one hundred items for daily living and home health care. Products include height-adjustable commodes, walkers, crutches, shower chairs, grab bars, accessible tables, patient lifts, dressing aids, eating aids, protective helmets, child tricycles, wheelchair swings, and more.

Gaggenau USA Corporation

425 University Avenue
PO Box 2226
Norwood, MA 02062-2636
617-255-1766
Disability Served: all

This company manufactures electric ovens.

Gainor Medical USA Inc.

PO Box 93127
Long Beach, CA 90809-3127
800-825-8282
Disability Served: diabetes

This company manufactures a blood test puncture device for diabetics.

Gala Industries Inc.

181 Pauley Street
Eagle Rock, VA 24085
540-884-2589
http://gala-industries.com
Disability Served: all

This company makes underwater pelletizers, tempered water systems, and centrifugal pellet dryers for the plastics industry.

GAM Industries

PO Box 2226
Petersburg, VA 23804
804-733-4460, 800-342-4426
Disability Served: all

This company manufactures cervical collars, thermal wraps, hot packs, and ice packs.

Gambro Inc.

5000 Chestnut Avenue
Newport News, VA 23605
757-247-0105
Disability Served: all

Gambro manufactures a dialysis machine and individually packaged bloodline sets.

GameTime Inc.

PO Box 121
Ft Payne, AL 35967
205-845-5610
Disability Served: physically disabled

This company manufactures recreational equipment, including playground equipment, for children with disabilities.

GAR Hospital Equipment Inc.

PO Box 30271
Cleveland, OH 44130
216-546-1767
Disability Served: physically disabled

This company manufactures bed trays and a portable shower stretcher.

Garaventa (Canada) Ltd.

7505 134A Street
Surrey, BC V3W 7B3 Canada
604-594-0422, 800-663-6556
Disability Served: physically disabled

This company manufactures emergency evacuation carriers for persons with limited mobility as well as wheelchair lifts.

Garden Way's Troy Built Factory Store

102nd Street & 9th Avenue
Troy, NY 12180
800-833-6990
Disability Served: all

This store manufactures a garden cart.

Gardener's Supply Company

128 Intervale Road
Burlington, VT 05401
800-955-3370
http://www.gardeners.com
Disability Served: all

This company provides a catalog of gardening supplies, including gardening tools for physically challenged people.

Garon Products Inc.

1924 Highway 35 Cn 20
Wall, NJ 07719
800-631-5380
Disability Served: all

This company manufactures an anti-skid coating that can be applied to floors, ramps, and sidewalks like paint.

Gavrity Electronics

415 Cleveland Avenue
Highland Park, NJ 08904
908-937-4455
Disability Served: all

This company manufactures ChildFinder, a wireless signal transmitter designed so parents can locate children who have wandered off.

Gaymar Industries Inc.

10 Centre Drive
Orchard Park, NY 14127
716-662-2551, 800-828-7341
Disability Served: all

This company manufactures seat cushions and air flotation mattress surfaces.

Gendron Inc.

400 East Lugbill Road
PO Box 197
Archbold, OH 43502
419-445-6060, 800-537-2521
Disability Served: physically disabled

This company manufactures a variety of wheelchairs as well as wheelchair accessories.

General Electric

Housewares Division
1285 Boston Avenue
Bridgeport, CT 06602
203-382-2000
Disability Served: all

This company manufactures housewares that can be adapted for persons in wheelchairs and persons with other disabilities. Products include wall ovens, ranges, washers and dryers, portable cassette players, microwave ovens, and Braille controls for household appliances.

General Marine Company, Inc.

6001 192nd Street NE
Arlington, WA 98223
Disability Served: physically disabled

This company manufactures a boat that is wheelchair accessible.

General Partitions Manufacturing Corp.

1702 Peninsula Drive
PO Box 8370
Erie, PA 16505-0370
814-833-1154
http://www.genpartitions.com
Disability Served: all

This company manufactures accessible bathroom stall partitions for public facilities.

Genie Industries

18340 NE 76th Street
PO Box 69
Redmond, WA 98073-0069
425-881-1800, 800-536-1800
Disability Served: all

This company manufactures an elevating work platform that can be used as a ladder alternative.

Gentex Corporation

10985 Chicago Drive
Zeeland, MI 49464
616-392-7195, 800-436-8391
http://www.gentex.com
Disability Served: all

This company manufactures smoke detectors and signaling devices that meet ADA requirements.

Gentleman Door Company

PO Box 77
506 Dawson
Yorklyn, DE 19736
800-525-7078
http://www.coast-resources.com/gentlemandoorcompany
Disability Served: physically disabled

This company manufactures door and window operators for residential and light commercial use.

George H Snyder Enterprises

5809 NE 21st Avenue
Ft Lauderdale, FL 33308
954-491-2886
Disability Served: physically disabled

This company manufactures wheelchair accessories. Products include a bowling ball holder, wheel locks, key rings for wheelchairs, table attachments for wheelchairs, and a camera mount for wheelchairs.

Gerber Plumbing Fixtures Corp.

4656 West Touhy Avenue
Chicago, IL 60646
773-675-6570
Disability Served: all

This company produces bathroom and plumbing accessories, including lever faucets, tall toilets, and valves to control water temperature.

Geri Care Products

Division of Blessings Corp.
252 Wagner Street
Middlesex, NJ 08846
201-469-7722
Disability Served: all

This company manufactures incontinence aids and bibs.

Gestetner Corporation

599 West Putnam Avenue
PO Box 2656
Greenwich, CT 06836-2656
203-863-5506
Disability Served: physically disabled

This company manufactures a copy machine designed to be used by employees who are physically disabled.

Giant Lift Equipment Mfg. Co. Inc.

136 Lafayette Road
North Hampton, NH 03862
603-964-5127, 800-524-4268
Disability Served: physically disabled

This company manufactures a hydraulic wheelchair lift.

Ginco Medical Equipment

6804 Highway 6 South, Suite 353
Houston, TX 77083-3397
281-561-9033, 800-480-4514
http://www.ginco.com
Disability Served: physically disabled

Ginco manufactures a variety of lifts using the SureHands track system. Ginco makes swimming pool lifts, wall lifts, and mobile lifts on wheels.

Ginny, Inc.

1125 Satellite Boulevard, Suite 111
Suwanee, GA 30174
770-623-8998
Disability Served: all

Ginny, Inc. manufactures slings, supports, and orthoses.

Gintuzi

761 Fernhill Boulevard
Oshawa, ON L1J 5K2 Canada
416-571-1233
Disability Served: physically disabled

This company manufactures a permanent plastic bath seat that can be folded when not in use.

GKR Industries Inc.

12636-38 South Kroll Drive
Alsip, IL 60658
708-389-2003, 800-526-7879
Disability Served: physically disabled

This company produces a disposable urinal and vomit bag.

Glacier Cross Inc.

1694 Whalebone Drive
Kalispell, MT 59901
406-257-8822
http://www.glaciercross.com
Disability Served: physically disabled

This company manufactures cervical and lumbar traction equipment.

Gladys E Loeb Foundation, Inc.

2002 Forest Hill Drive
Silver Spring, MD 20903-1532
301-434-7748
Disability Served: vision

This all-volunteer organization provides assistive technology to people who are blind.

Global Assistive Devices, Inc.

4950 North Dixie Highway, Suite 121
Ft Lauderdale, FL 33334-3947
954-784-0035
TDD: 954-784-0035
http://www.globalassistive.com
Disability Served: hearing

This company manufactures assistive devices for the deaf and hard of hearing. Products include wake-up alarms (flashing and vibrating), door knock signalers, phone signalers, and vibrating watches.

Glynn Johnson

PO Box 6135
Indianapolis, IN 46206-6135
Disability Served: all

This company manufactures a door handle that can be manipulated by pushing or pulling.

GMR Labs

1030 East El Camino Real, #308
Sunnyvale, CA 94087
408-985-7200
Disability Served: communication

This company manufactures communication boards to accommodate persons with speech disabilities.

GN Netcom

7688 Executive Drive
Eden Prairie, MN 55344-3677
612-932-2992
Disability Served: hearing

This company manufactures hearing aids, telephone amplifiers, and telephone headsets.

Golden Fleece International Inc.

14240 60th Street North
Clearwater, FL 34620
813-531-5129, 800-562-7326
Disability Served: all

This company manufactures seat cushions, joint protectors, transfer aids, pressure relief pads, wheelchair cushions, and other home health aids.

Golden Technologies Inc.
159 Penn Avenue
Exeter, PA 18643
717-883-7423, 800-624-6374
Disability Served: all

This company manufactures powered scooters, motorized beds, seat lift chairs, arm chairs, and replacement seats for wheelchairs.

Good Health Inc.
405 Grand Avenue
PO Box 588
Dayton, OH 45405
937-226-3812, 800-426-3812
Disability Served: elderly

This company produces an exercise videotape designed for senior citizens.

Goodman Specialty Pillows Inc.
PO Box 29027
Dallas, TX 75229
214-243-3742, 800-423-1233
Disability Served: all

This company manufactures foam support pillows.

Goshen/Kind-in-Mind
PO Box 532
Fair Lawn, NJ 07410
800-286-8181
Disability Served: all

This company manufactures furniture, seating, school chairs, and desks for special needs children.

GPK Inc.
9380 Bond Avenue, Suite B
El Cajon, CA 92021
619-390-5884, 619-468-8679
Disability Served: physically disabled

This company manufactures exercise equipment called UPPERTONE for unassisted muscle strengthening and conditioning of the quadriceps.

Grab It Enterprizes
PO Box 703
Jackson, AL 36545
334-246-5116
http://www.grab-it-enterprises.com
Disability Served: all

This company makes reaching devices designed for picking up items without the need to bend over or reach high shelves unaided.

Grabber International
4600 Danvers SE
Grand Rapids, MI 49512
616-940-1914, 800-423-1233
Disability Served: all

This company manufactures disposable heating pads.

Graley Marketing
15935 El Soneto Drive
Whittier, CA 90603
562-947-7848
Disability Served: communication

This company makes a plastic direct-selection communication board.

Grand Traverse Technologies Inc.
1167 Hastings Street
Traverse City, MI 49684-4318
616-941-2041
Disability Served: physically disabled

This company manufactures an accessible whirlpool bathtub.

Grandmar Inc.
1311 63rd Street
Emeryville, CA 94608
510-428-0441
Disability Served: physically disabled

Grandmar manufactures wooden supports and rests for amputees, support cushions, lapboards, transfer boards, and solid seat supports.

Grant AirMass Corp.

986 Bedford Steet
PO Box 3456
Stamford, CT 06905
203-348-7779, 800-243-5237
Disability Served: physically disabled

This company manufactures alternating air pressure mattress and seat pads designed to stimulate circulation and thus reduce or prevent pressure sores, air flotation seat cushions, water-operated bath lifts, and shampoo basins for washing hair while lying in bed.

Grayline Housewares

373 Randy Road
Carol Stream, IL 60188
630-695-3900
Disability Served: all

Grayline manufactures wire cabinet organizers.

Great Wave Software

5353 Scotts Valley Drive
Scotts Valley, CA 95066
800-423-1144
http://www.greatwave.com
Disability Served: all

Great Wave Software publishes K-12 educational software, focusing on extensive customization to meet individual kids' special needs, core curriculum, nonviolence, and gender neutrality.

Greatest of Ease Company

2443 Fillmore Street, #345
San Francisco, CA 94115
415-441-6649, 800-845-1208
Disability Served: all

This company designs paging systems and emergency alert systems that are activated by pushing a button.

Greenwald Surgical Company

2688 De Kalb Street
Lake Station, IN 46405
219-962-1604
Disability Served: vision

This company manufactures male incontinence clamps.

Griffin Laboratories

27636 Ynez Road, Suite L7199
Temecula, CA 92591
800-330-5969
Disability Served: communication

This company manufactures augmentative communication aids for nonspeaking persons.

Grimm Scientific Industries

Box 2143
Marietta, OH 45750
614-374-3412, 800-223-5395
Disability Served: all

This company manufactures paraffin baths.

Grohe America Inc.

900 North Lively Boulevard
Wood Dale, IL 60191
630-350-2600
Disability Served: all

This company manufactures kitchen faucets, handshowers, and thermostats designed to control water temperature.

Guardian Angel Products

401-417 Fayette Avenue
Springfield, IL 62704
217-753-2505
Disability Served: hearing

This company manufactures a flashing baby monitor for parents with hearing impairments.

Guardian Products Inc.

A Sunrise Medical Company
4175 Guardian Street, #3190
Simi City, CA 93063-3382
818-504-2820, 800-255-5022
Disability Served: all

This company offers more than eighty daily living and health care aids. Products include grab bars, transfer benches, walkers, canes, commodes, shower and bathtub chairs, carrying accessories, and beds.

Guerdon Homes, Inc.
PO Box 657
982 Rundell Road
Gering, NE 69341
308-436-3131
Disability Served: all

This company manufactures accessible mobile homes.

Guidecraft Inc.
PO Box 324
Industrial Plaza
Garnerville, NY 10923-0324
914-947-3500, 800-544-6526
Disability Served: all

This company manufactures educational games and skill-building activities for children.

Guinta Associates
37 Terhune Avenue
Lodi, NJ 07644
212-594-4522, 800-631-0821
Disability Served: hearing

This company manufactures battery-operated auditory speech training devices.

Gunnell Inc.
8440 State Street
Millington, MI 48746
517-871-4529, 800-551-0055
Disability Served: physically disabled

This company manufactures recliners and chairs on wheeled bases, walkers, commodes, and seating systems for wheelchairs. Many of the company's products are made for children.

Gyro Tech Inc.
PO Box 906
South 82 West 18717 Gemini Drive
Muskego, WI 53150
414-679-0045
Disability Served: all

This company manufactures an electric door operator.

H & K Sales and Marketing, Inc.
13567 Y Street
Omaha, NE 68137
402-895-8643
Disability Served: physically disabled

This company distributes shower seats for the mobility impaired, including the Shower-A-Way Swivel Seat.

H. Weniger Inc.
70 12th Street
San Francisco, CA 94103
415-621-6876
Disability Served: physically disabled

This company manufactures splints and braces.

Hager Leather
Route 3, Box 145
Waseca, MN 56093
507-835-7785
Disability Served: all

This company makes a cordless telephone holder that can be attached to wheelchairs, walkers, crutches, belts, and more.

Hal Hen Company
35-53 24th Street
Long Island City, NY 11106
718-392-6020, 800-242-5436
Disability Served: hearing

This company offers a number of daily living aids, including bed vibrator alarm clocks, telephone accessories and amplifiers, stethoscopes, and doorbells.

Hallmark Orthopedic Co.
20 Laporte Street
PO Box 898
Arcadia, CA 91006
818-446-4882, 800-446-8668
Disability Served: orthopedic

This company manufactures pads, cushions, and supports, including arm slings, joint protectors, orthopedic shoes, neck pillows, and bed pads.

Halls Wheels
PO Box 784
Cambridge, MA 02238
617-628-7955
Disability Served: physically disabled

This company manufactures wheelchairs and wheelchair gloves.

Halsey Taylor/Thermos Co.
Route 75
Freeport, IL 61032
815-235-0066
Disability Served: physically disabled

This company manufactures accessible drinking fountains and water coolers.

Hamilton Scientific Inc.
1316 18th Street
Two Rivers, WI 54241
920-793-1121
Disability Served: physically disabled

This company manufactures a science laboratory chemical fume hood that is wheelchair accessible.

Han-D-Products Inc.
3999 Parkway Lane, Suite 1
Hilliard, OH 43026-1252
614-876-6625
Disability Served: physically disabled

This company manufactures a bathtub grab bar.

Hand In Hand, Catalogue Center
Route 26, RR 1
Box 1425
Oxford, ME 04270
800-872-3841
Disability Served: all

This company manufactures a number of educational items for children, including art supplies, puzzles, magnetic letters and numbers, blocks, balls, training cups, and more.

Handi Helps
PO Box 343
North Grafton, MA 01536
508-839-6170
Disability Served: all

This company offers numerous aids to daily living, including safety rails for bathrooms, crutch tips, on-screen keyboard programs, safety flags, tire sealant for wheelchair tires, crutch tips, and more.

Handi Medi Devices
PO Box 897
Plymouth, MA 02360
508-746-5861
Disability Served: all

This company makes an automatic leg bag emptier.

Handi Ramp Inc.
PO Box 745
1414 Armour Boulevard
Mundelein, IL 60060-0745
847-816-7525, 800-876-7267
Disability Served: physically disabled

This company manufactures metal ramps, portable metal tracks, and folding van ramps.

Handi-Patterns
5200 Quintilis Street
Spring Hill, FL 34608
904-688-2980, 800-676-2980
Disability Served: all

This company makes sewing patterns featuring adaptive clothing.

Handicaps Inc.
4335 South Santa Fe Drive
Englewood, CO 80110
303-781-2062, 800-782-4335
Disability Served: physically disabled

This company manufactures driving aids and accessories for persons with disabilities. Products include hand brakes, hand controls, motorhome lifts, left-foot accelerators, wheelchair restraints, and more.

Hands On Toys, Inc.

171 Merrimac Street
Woburn, MA 01801
617-932-8774
Disability Served: all

This company manufactures foam toys for children.

Happy Baby Products

719 Palermo Drive
Santa Barbara, CA 93105
805-687-9996, 800-549-8973
Disability Served: all

This company manufactures a seat and back support for children riding in grocery cart seats.

HARC Mercantile Ltd.
Hearing Aid Center of Kalamazoo

PO Box 3055
Kalamazoo, MI 49003
800-445-9968, 616-324-1615
http://www.harcmercantile.com
Disability Served: hearing

This company manufactures an electronic stethoscope that has an amplifier. HARC also specializes in a wide range of assistive listening devices for the hard of hearing and deaf. Products include alerting and signaling systems, personal and wide-area listening systems, wake-up systems, smoke/fire and security protection products for the automobile, and hearing aid maintenance products. ADA compliant.

HARD Manufacturing Co. Inc.

230 Grider Street
Buffalo, NY 14215
716-893-1800, 800-873-4273
Disability Served: all

This company manufactures beds and cribs, including manual adjustable beds, motorized beds, bed side rails, and safety cribs.

Harmony House, Inc.

111 West Maple Street, Suite 3002
Chicago, IL 60610
773-280-8334
Disability Served: hearing

This company makes a sign language training video.

Harriet Carter, Inc.

Department 34
North Wases, PA 19455
215-361-5151
Disability Served: physically disabled

This company manufactures a swivel seat for use in automobiles.

Hartwell Medical

6352 Corte Del Abeto, Suite J
Carlsbad, CA 92009-1408
760-438-5500, 800-633-5900
http://www.hartwellmedical.com
Disability Served: all

This company manufactures a waste/emesis collection bag.

Harvy Surgical Supply Co.

34-35 Collins Place
Flushing, NY 11354
718-939-1122, 800-221-0142
Disability Served: physically disabled

This company provides a safety frame for toilets, fixed-height commode chairs, and crutch handgrip cushions.

Hasten Help System

c/o AC Corp.
PO Box 16367
301 Creek Ridge Road
Greensboro, NC 27416
910-273-4472
Disability Served: all

This company offers a telephone emergency response unit, including special adapters.

Hatch Imports
1656 Walter Street, #B
Ventura, CA 93003-5600
805-642-0170, 800-767-1343
Disability Served: physically disabled

This company manufactures specialty gloves, including edema gloves and wheelchair gloves.

Hats with Heart, Inc.
10271 South 1300 East, Suite 166
Sandy, UT 84094
801-567-0066
Disability Served: all

This company manufactures turbans, scarves, and hats for women who have experienced hair loss.

Hausmann Industries Inc.
130 Union Street
Northvale, NJ 07647
888-428-7626
http://www.hausmann.com
Disability Served: all

This company manufactures physical therapy, occupational therapy, and rehabilitation equipment as well as treatment furniture.

Hausted
927 Lake Road
PO Box 710
Medina, OH 44256
216-723-3271, 800-428-7833
Disability Served: physically disabled

This company manufactures a stretcher wheelchair, a motorized bed, and a manual therapeutic bed.

Hawk Enterprises
PO Box 20490
San Jose, CA 95160
408-268-6466
Disability Served: physically disabled

This company manufactures a hanger with an extended hook and wheelchair gloves.

Haws Drinking Fountain Corp.
1435 Fourth Street
PO Box 1999
Berkeley, CA 94701-1499
510-525-5801
http://www.hawsco.com
Disability Served: physically disabled

This company manufactures accessible drinking fountains for outdoor and indoor use.

Health & Community Living Inc.
9833 Whetstone Drive
Gaithersburg, MD 20879
301-972-5129, 800-736-6617
Disability Served: physically disabled

This company manufactures a standing transfer aid, a commode seat lift, and a stair walker.

Health & Medical Techniques/Aquatherm
PO Box 2697
Smithtown, NY 11787
516-582-5900, 800-526-4296
Disability Served: physically disabled

This company manufactures mattresses, cushions, and pads.

Health Chair Enterprises Inc.
Route 3, Box 17
Calhoun City, MS 38916
601-637-2517
Disability Served: physically disabled

This company manufactures a recliner and seat lift chair.

Health Concepts, Inc.
279-B Great Valley Parkway
Malvern, PA 19355
610-889-7363, 800-673-7881
Disability Served: communication

This company makes speech and swallowing exercise devices for use by speech and language pathologists for therapy.

Health Equipment
PO Box 4887
San Diego, CA 92164-4887
619-283-9810
Disability Served: physically disabled

This company manufactures electronically adjustable exercise equipment for upper extremities.

Health Products Inc.
747 Kendrick, Suite 116
Houston, TX 77060
713-445-8341
Disability Served: physically disabled

This company manufactures air flotation mattresses.

Health Services R & D, Inc.
10470 Waterfowl Terrace
Columbia, MD 21044
410-964-9678, 800-4-KIMBRO
Disability Served: physically disabled

This company sells an inflatable lift and bedpan (Kimbro Comfort Lift) for easy toileting and personal hygiene care for persons with limited mobility.

Health Sonics Corp.
1056 Serpentine Lane
Pleasanton, CA 94566
510-462-4610
Disability Served: all

This company manufactures an electronic faucet with infrared sensors.

Healthdyne Inc.
1255 Kenneson
Marietta, GA 30066
770-499-1212
Disability Served: all

This company manufactures an infant monitor.

Healthguard
PO Box 60113
Chicago, IL 60626
312-973-1611
Disability Served: all

This company makes a toileting cleansing aid.

Healthscan Products Inc.
908 Pompton Avenue
Cedar Grove, NJ 07009
201-857-3414
Disability Served: all

This company manufactures a device designed to exercise inspiratory muscles.

Healthy Innovations
PO Box 391090
Cleveland, OH 44139
800-799-7436
Disability Served: all

This company produces exercise videos for persons with physical disabilities or low vision.

Hear You Are, Inc.
125 Main Street
Netcong, NJ 07857
973-347-7662, 973-347-0006
TDD: 973-691-0663
Disability Served: hearing

This education and communications skills center sells assistive listening devices, speech therapy products, and hearing supplies.

Hear-More, Inc.
PO Box 3413
Farmingdale, NY 11735
516-752-0738, 800-881-4327
Disability Served: hearing

This company manufactures alarm clocks with strobe lights for persons with limited or no hearing.

Hearing Services International (HSI)
10340 West 70th Street
Eden Prairie, MN 55344-3445
612-829-5757, 800-328-3832
Disability Served: hearing

This company manufactures hearing aids.

Heart Rate Inc.
3188-E Airway Avenue
Costa Mesa, CA 92626-6601
714-850-9716, 800-237-2271
Disability Served: all

This company manufactures a climbing and stepping exercise machine that allows the user to exercise just the arms, just the legs, or both the arms and legs.

HEAT
PO Box 1177
Calistoga, CA 94515
707-886-0893
Disability Served: all

This company manufactures warmers made of thermo-insulating wool. Products include gloves, socks, lower back warmers, shoulder warmers, and knee and elbow warmers.

Heelbo Inc.
5745 West Howard Street
Niles, IL 60648
800-323-5444
Disability Served: all

This company manufactures decubitus pads, joint protectors, and foot positioners.

Helluva Hunt
1562 Esterbrook Road
Douglas, WY 82633
307-358-6580
Disability Served: vision, mobility

This company coordinates an annual antelope hunt for sportsmen and sportswomen with disabilities.

Helm Distributing
911 Kings Point Road
Polson, MT 59860
406-883-2147
http://www.equalizerexercise.com
Disability Served: physically disabled

This company makes exercise machines for wheelchair users.

Help Me To Help Myself Communication Aid
324 Acre Avenue
Brownsburg, IN 46112-1318
317-852-4427
Disability Served: communication

This company offers communication boards and books for children.

Henley International
104 Industrial Boulevard
Sugar Land, TX 77478
713-240-2442, 800-237-8749
Disability Served: physically disabled

This company manufactures transcutaneous electrical stimulator (TENS) units and accessories.

Henry Lackey
PO Drawer T
Calhoun City, MS 38916
601-628-5131
Disability Served: physically disabled

This company manufactures a toilet seat lift.

Hens Nest
PO Box 531
Colby, KS 67701
913-833-5691
Disability Served: all

This company manufactures clothing.

Hepp Industries Inc.
687 Kildare Crescent
Seaford, NY 11783
516-735-0032
Disability Served: all

This company makes a toileting aid designed for anal cleansing and an oral hygiene aid.

Hermell Products, Inc.
Box 7345
522 Cottage Grove Road, Building G
Bloomfield, CT 06002
860-242-6550, 800-233-2342
Disability Served: physically disabled

This company manufactures orthopedic softgoods, such as wheelchair cushions, cervical and lumbar pillows, wedges, elastic supports, cervical collars, and podiatry products.

Hersh & Treadgold

6657 Camelia Drive
San Jose, CA 95120
408-997-7017
Disability Served: all

This company manufactures a reminder program designed to remind the user to perform tasks at certain times. The user wears a small pager that beeps and displays a text message.

Hitchcock Shoes Inc.

165 Beal Street
Hingham, MA 02043
617-749-3260
Disability Served: all

This company makes men's shoes in extra wide sizes.

HITEC Group International, Inc.

8160 Madison
Burr Ridge, IL 60521
630-654-9200, 800-288-8303
http://www.hitec.com
Disability Served: hearing, vision, physically disabled

This company distributes hundreds of assistive products for people who are deaf, hard of hearing, speech impaired, and visually and mobility impaired.

HJV Inc.

605B Country Club Drive
Bensenville, IL 60106
630-595-0860
Disability Served: all

HJV makes an emergency alert system. The user wears a transmitter that when activated calls for assistance through the telephone.

HK Eyecan Ltd.

36 Burland Street
Ottowa, ON K2B 6J8 Canada
800-356-3362, 613-860-0333
http://www.eyecan.ca
Disability Served: all

This company produces an alternative keyboard and communication aid that is controlled by eye movements. Users look through an eyepiece at a keychart and select letters, numbers, or commands, which are then transferred to a visual display. Users can type letters, play games, and surf the Web using only their eyes.

Hoffman Group

PO Box 728
Collierville, TN 38027
901-853-2781
Disability Served: all

This company manufactures a twin handle cup for persons with hand problems.

Holbrook

PO Box 447
Coldwater, MI 49036
517-278-2411
Disability Served: all

This company manufactures play equipment for children, including a balance beam set, a wooden boat, large foam shapes, and a balance board.

Hold-IT! Corporation

4500 College Boulevard, Suite 110
Overland Park, KS 66211
913-469-6458
Disability Served: all

This company manufactures a portable cup holder that attaches to the arm of a chair.

Hold-It, Inc.

PO Box 611391
Port Huron, MI 48061-1391
810-984-4213
Disability Served: physically disabled

This company manufactures and distributes thermoplastic materials that can be applied to a handle of any shape then custom molded to the user's hand.

Hollister Incorporated

2000 Hollister Drive
Libertyville, IL 60048
847-680-1000
Disability Served: all

This company manufactures incontinence aids and catheters.

Home Delivery Incontinent Supplies Co., Inc.

1215 Dielman Industrial Court
Olivette, MO 63132
800-269-4663
http://www.hdisnet.com
Disability Served: physically disabled

This company provides bladder control products.

Home Technology Center

352 Hungerford Drive
Rockville, MD 20850
301-738-1348
Disability Served: all

This company provides remote-controllable entry access, lighting devices, appliances, and motorized window drapes.

Homecare Products, Inc.

15824 SE 296th Street
Kent, WA 98042
206-631-4633, 800-451-1903
Disability Served: physically disabled

This company makes ramps, portable showers and baths to accommodate the bedridden, and air flotation mattresses.

HomeCare Suites, Inc.

805 East Maple Road, Suite 310
Birmingham, MI 48009
313-644-5757, 800-72-SUITE
Disability Served: physically disabled

This company manufactures a prefabricated house that can attach to an existing home. The house is wheelchair accessible.

Homedics Inc.

6841 North Rochester Road, Building H
Rochester Hills, MI 48306
810-650-9400, 800-333-8282
Disability Served: all

This company manufactures cushions, support pillows, and massage pillows.

Honeywell Residential Controls

1985 Douglas Drive North
Golden Valley, MN 55422-3992
612-542-7500
Disability Served: vision

This company provides a tactile thermostat designed with large numbers for the visually impaired.

HOPE Inc.

PO Box 6044
Athens, GA 30604
706-769-7935, 800-241-7046
Disability Served: all

This company manufactures a commode with a powered elevating seat lift.

Horton Automatics

Division of Overhead Door Corp.
4242 Baldwin Boulevard
Corpus Christi, TX 78405
512-888-5591, 800-531-3111
Disability Served: all

This company manufactures powered door openers.

Hosmer Dorrance Corp.

561 Division Street
PO Box 37
Campbell, CA 95008-6905
408-379-5151, 800-827-0070
Disability Served: physically disabled

This company manufactures prosthetic devices, including a baseball glove attachment, a bowling attachment, button hooks to facilitate dressing, a steering wheel spinner ring, a prosthetic elbow, and more.

Hospitak Inc.

1144 Route 109
Lindenhurst, NY 11757
516-957-5300
Disability Served: all

This company makes a hyperbaric oxygen cushion for healing wounds.

Hotpoint WCE

Division of GE
Appliance Park
Louisville, KY 40225
Disability Served: physically disabled

This company manufactures a wall oven that can be adjusted to accommodate wheelchair users and a microwave oven.

Housing Devices Inc.

407 R Mystic Avenue
Medford, MA 02155
617-395-5200, 800-392-5200
Disability Served: vision

This company produces intercom-based call signal systems.

Howbrite Solutions, Inc.

12254 25th Street SW
PO Box 880
Cokato, MN 55321
320-286-2597, 800-505-MATH
Disability Served: physically disabled

This company manufactures and sells a math tool to help people learn basic arithmetic. Math Line is manipulative and is made in large print, Braille, and for the physically disabled.

Howda Designz, Inc.

PO Box 451
Newburyport, MA 01950
508-462-6260, 800-348-3884
Disability Served: back injury

This company manufactures a posture chair designed to provide support for persons with lower back problems.

Howe Press of Perkins School for the Blind

175 North Beacon Street
Watertown, MA 02172
617-924-3490
Disability Served: vision

This company manufactures items for persons with visual impairments. Products include Braille paper, Braille styluses, Braillers, erasers, rulers, copy holders, and more.

Howell Design, Inc.

192 Thomas Lane
Stowe, VT 05672
802-253-4468, 800-867-7869
http://www.readerswindow.com
Disability Served: physically disabled

This company manufactures a bookholder, Reader's Window, for people who have difficulty positioning themselves comfortably while reading or who have difficulty holding books while reading. Normal finger dexterity is required.

Hoyle Products Inc.

302 Orange Grove
Fillmore, CA 93015
805-524-1211, 800-345-1950
Disability Served: all

This company manufactures lap desks, bookholders, and grips for pens.

Hudson Photographic Industries

Division of Kamar Products Inc.
PO Box 227
Irvington on Hudson, NY 10533
914-591-8700
Disability Served: all

This company manufactures physical therapy mirrors.

Huey Co.

10100 Franklin Avenue
Franklin Park, IL 60131
847-671-6150, 800-333-4839
Disability Served: physically disabled

This company makes a drafting table that can be adjusted to accommodate wheelchair users.

Huggie Aids

837 NW 10th Street
Oklahoma City, OK 73106
405-232-7848
Disability Served: hearing

This company manufactures hearing aid retainers.

Hugh Macmillan Rehabilitation Centre

350 Rumsey Road
Toronto, ON M4G 1R8 Canada
416-425-6220, 800-363-2440
Disability Served: all

This company manufactures switches, standing aids, keyboard modification programs, bath seats, and more.

Hughes Lighting Technologies

Yacht Club Drive
Lake Hopatcong, NJ 07849
201-663-1214
Disability Served: all

This company designs lights for the treatment of seasonal affective disorder.

Hughes Toy Company

24675 Glenwood Drive
Los Gatos, CA 95033-8541
408-353-2137
Disability Served: all

This company manufactures a swimming aid to help persons stay afloat.

Human Performance Measurement Inc.

PO Box 1996
Arlington, TX 76004-1996
817-640-7178
Disability Served: physically disabled

This company makes measurement tools that evaluate motor control and strength.

Humanicare International Inc.

1471 Jersey Avenue
North Brunswick, NJ 08902-1622
908-214-0660
Disability Served: vision

This company manufactures incontinence garments for men and women.

Humphrey Inc.

9212 Balboa Avenue
San Diego, CA 92123
619-565-6631
Disability Served: all

This company manufactures a hand dryer.

Huntleigh Technology Inc.

227 Route 33 East
Manalapan, NJ 07726
908-446-2500, 800-223-1218
Disability Served: physically disabled

This company manufactures mattress surfaces and hyperbaric sleeves to stimulate blood flow.

Hy-Ko Products Company

7370 Northfield Road
Walton Hills, OH 44146
800-292-0550
Disability Served: all

This company manufactures access signs, parking signs, and a long-handled sponge.

Hydra Fitness Industries

2121 Industrial
Belton, TX 76513
800-433-3111
Disability Served: physically disabled

This company makes exercise equipment, including a rowing machine and a hydraulic exercise machine for the upper extremities.

Hygenic Corporation (The)

1245 Home Avenue
Akron, OH 44310
330-633-8460, 800-321-2135
http://www.thera-band.com
Disability Served: all

This company manufactures a resistive exercise band designed to strengthen and stretch upper and lower extremities.

Hygienics Industries, Inc.

PO Box 427
Wayne, PA 19087-0427
610-397-0788
Disability Served: all

This company makes incontinence aids such as pads and panty shields.

I.C.E. Down

9870 Marconi Drive, Suite F
San Diego, CA 92173
800-482-0302
Disability Served: all

This company manufactures cold packs.

IDC Tectonics Ltd.

PO Box 2104, Station B
St Catherines, ON L2M 6P5 Canada
905-646-6335
Disability Served: physically disabled

This company manufactures plastic lapboards, prone standers, and hardware for wheelchair accessories.

IM Inc.

Health Care Division
PO Box 658
Fairfield, NJ 07006
201-227-3740, 800-962-1292
Disability Served: all

This company manufactures male incontinence garments, urinary drainage bags, urinary leg bags, and catheter straps.

Imaginart International, Inc.

307 Arizona Street
Bisbee, AZ 85603
520-432-5741, 800-828-1376
http://www.imaginart.com
Disability Served: all

This company publishes and distributes materials for speech and occupational therapy.

Inclinator Company of America

2200 Paxton Street
PO Box 1557
Harrisburg, PA 17105-1557
717-234-8065
Disability Served: physically disabled

This company manufactures residential lifts, elevators, and dumbwaiters.

Independent Living Aids, Inc.

27 East Mall
Plainview, NY 11803
516-752-8080, 800-537-2118
http://www.independentliving.com
Disability Served: vision

This company sells aids to the blind and visually impaired, primarily through mail order.

Independent Specialty Co.

PO Box 39
Middle Haddam, CT 06456
203-267-9792
Disability Served: physically disabled

This company manufactures lapboards.

Independent Transfer Equipment Co.

5482 Business Drive, Unit C
Huntington Beach, CA 92649
714-898-9005, 800-622-4832
Disability Served: physically disabled

This company manufactures an overhead transfer lift.

Indepth Sock Company

92 Candy Lane
Syosset, NY 11791
516-921-6789
http://www.widehealthsocks.com
Disability Served: all

This company provides oversized socks for those who require socks that do not bind.

Indiana Ramps, Inc.

PO Box 504
Goshen, IN 46526
219-534-2451
Disability Served: physically disabled

This company manufactures indoor and outdoor aluminum portable ramps.

Industrial Research and Engineering Inc.

2409 North Kerby
Portland, OR 97227
503-288-5817
Disability Served: all

This company manufactures handrails.

Infinite Access Corporation

PO Box 942
Mt Vernon, IL 62864
618-244-7823
Disability Served: physically disabled

This company builds modular ramps to provide wheelchair access.

Infra-Link Inc.

16260 SW Upper Boones Ferry Road
PO Box 1008
Portland, OR 97224-7220
503-598-7531, 800-395-3596
Disability Served: all

This company distributes environmental control systems that use infrared signals and are wireless.

Infusaid Corporation

1400 Providence Highway
Norwood, MA 02062
617-769-8330, 800-451-1050
Disability Served: diabetes

This company manufactures a syringe infuser that allows for a continuous flow of medication.

Innerface Architectural Signage Inc.

5320 Webb Parkway
Liburn, GA 30247
404-921-5566, 800-445-4796
Disability Served: all

This company manufactures access and parking area signs that are ADA compliant.

Innovatex Research & Development Inc.

Klick Products Sales Corp.
34 Boston Street
Lynn, MA 01904
617-599-4620
Disability Served: physically disabled

This company manufactures a telescopic cane and telescopic crutches that come with programmable memory.

Innovative Care Systems

PO Box 401
Fruitport, MI 49415
616-847-3623
Disability Served: all

This company develops a control switch that allows the user to manipulate the telephone with just one switch.

Innovative Control Systems Inc.

2325 Parklawn Drive, Building N
Waukesha, WI 53186
414-785-0645
Disability Served: all

This company makes a wandering patient detection system.

Innovative Products Unlimited Inc.

4351 West College Avenue, Suite 505
Appleton, WI 54914
920-738-9090, 800-833-2826
Disability Served: physically disabled

This company manufactures shower chairs, commodes, walkers, transfer chairs, and shower stretchers.

Innoventions, Inc.

5921 South Middlefield Road, Suite 102
Littleton, CO 80123-2877
303-797-6554, 800-854-6554
http://www.magnicam.com/magnicam
Disability Served: vision

This company manufactures a portable electronic magnification system which utilizes the television set to magnify printed materials.

Instant Replay, Inc.

2601 South Bayshore Drive, Suite 1050
Coconut Grove, FL 33133
305-854-8777, 800-749-8779
Disability Served: hearing

This company manufactures a telecaption video recorder.

Interior Mediquip Ltd.

3401 33rd Avenue
Vernon, BC V1T 2P2 Canada
250-542-1363, 800-561-8998
http://www.intermedd.com
Disability Served: physically disabled

This company manufactures the Aquatic Wheelchair for use in chlorinated pools, the Shower Wheelchair for shower use, and the Sand Wheelchair for beach use.

Interkal Inc.

PO Box 2107
Kalamazoo, MI 49003-2107
616-349-1521
Disability Served: all

This company manufactures a portable stage.

Intermatic Inc.

Intermatic Plaza
Spring Grove, IL 60081-9698
815-675-2321
http://www.intermatic.com
Disability Served: all

Intermatic manufactures a timing switch that automatically activates appliances and lights.

International Cushioned Products, Inc.

#202-8360 Bridgeport Road
Richmond, BC V6X 3C7 Canada
604-244-7638, 800-TUB-SOFT
Disability Served: all

This company manufactures cushioned bathtubs.

International Healthcare Products

4222 South Pulaski Road
Chicago, IL 60632
800-423-7886
http://www.fabricoinfo.com/bathomatic
Disability Served: all

This company manufactures Bath-O-Matic products, which are designed to assist disabled individuals with bathing.

International Krown Technologies

605 Hindry Avenue
Inglewood, CA 90301
310-64-KROWN
Disability Served: hearing

This company manufactures devices for the hearing impaired, including text telephone devices.

International Steel Company

PO Box 3442
401 West Tennessee Street
Evansville, IN 47733
812-425-3311
Disability Served: physically disabled

This company manufactures a revolving door large enough for wheelchairs.

Intromark Inc.

701 Smithfield Street
Pittsburgh, PA 15222-3906
412-288-1331
Disability Served: physically disabled

This company manufactures therapeutic mattresses and carrying accessories for walkers or wheelchairs.

Invacare Canada Inc.

5970 Chedworth Way
Mississauga, ON L5R 3T9 Canada
905-890-8300, 800-668-5324
http://www.invacare.com
Disability Served: physically disabled

This company manufactures durable medical equipment such as power wheelchairs; custom, standard, and rehabilitation manual chairs; seating and positioning products; patient aids; respiratory products; and homecare beds.

Invacare Corporation
One Invacare Way
Elyria, OH 44035
216-329-6000, 800-333-6900
http://www.invacare.com
Disability Served: all

This company manufactures and distributes home health care products and mobility products for people with disabilities.

Inventronic Inc.
Richard Martin Friedmar
2823 Kenwood Boulevard
Toledo, OH 43606
419-536-7777
Disability Served: vision

This company manufactures a music reading aid that magnifies musical scores onto a screen.

Invisible Structures, Inc.
20100 East 35th Drive
Aurora, CO 80011-8160
800-233-1510
http://www.invisiblestructures.com
Disability Served: physically disabled

This company manufactures paving products to increase accessibility.

Iron-A-Way, Inc.
220 West Jackson
Morton, IL 61550
309-266-7232
Disability Served: physically disabled

This company manufactures a wheelchair accessible ironing board.

ITT
7635 Plantation Road
PO Box 7065
Roanoke, VA 24019
540-563-0371
Disability Served: vision, hearing

This company manufactures a large-button Braille flashing telephone for persons with low vision or limited hearing.

J & B Foam Fabricators Inc.
PO Box 144
Ludington, MI 49431
616-843-2448, 800-621-3626
Disability Served: all

This company makes float swimming aids and swim belts.

J. E. Burke Co.
PO Box 549
Fond du Lac, WI 54935
920-921-9220
Disability Served: physically disabled

This company makes basketball backstops, funnel ball games, wheelchair swings, and accessible picnic tables.

J. T. Posey Company
5635 Peck Road
Arcadia, CA 91006
818-443-3143, 800-447-6739
Disability Served: all

This company manufactures more than fifty kinds of restraints.

Jack Harvey, Rehabilitation Engineer
8728 Arnold Road, Route 3
Manton, MI 49663-9004
616-824-3430
Disability Served: physically disabled

Jack Harvey manufactures a motorized artist's easel designed to accommodate persons with physical disabilities.

Jaclo Inc.
162 Carlton Avenue
Brooklyn, NY 11205
800-852-3906
Disability Served: all

This company manufactures a variety of hand showers.

JACO Enterprises Inc.
PO Box 22084
Phoenix, AZ 85028
800-678-0078
Disability Served: all

This company makes a neoprene ear protector for swimmers with ear tubes or those who are prone to swimmer's ear. It also produces extra-soft silicone ear plugs in a variety of colors for water protection.

Jaeco Orthopedic Specialties

214 Drexel
PO Box 75
Hot Springs, AR 71901
501-623-5944
Disability Served: orthopedic

This company manufactures a number of orthotics and supports.

James Leckey Design, Inc.

360 Merrimack Street
Riverwalk, Building 9
Lawrence, MA 01843
978-691-5220, 800-532-5390
http://www.leckey.com
Disability Served: all

This company manufactures and supplies positioning equipment for children and adults with special needs.

James Stanfield Co., Inc.

PO Box 41058
Santa Barbara, CA 93140
800-421-6534
http://www.stanfield.com
Disabilities Served: learning disabled, developmentally disabled

This company produces and distributes video programs and curricula for persons with mild to moderate learning or developmental disabilities.

Janice Invalid Security Alert Systems Inc.

7218 Lanai
Long Beach, CA 90808
562-421-3367
Disability Served: all

This company manufactures a portable emergency alert system that can be attached to wheelchairs, carried by hand, or fastened to a belt.

Jay L. Warren, Inc.

PO Box 25413
Chicago, IL 60625
312-275-1525
Disability Served: hearing

This company manufactures a speech amplification system to facilitate persons with hearing impairments.

Jay Medical, Ltd.

PO Box 18656
Boulder, CO 80308-8656
303-442-5529, 800-648-8282
Disability Served: all

This company manufactures cushions, supports, and pads.

Jayfro Corp.

976 Hartford
Waterford, CT 06385
203-447-3001
Disability Served: all

This company manufactures chin-up exercise bars, parallel handrail bars for swimming pools, floor ladders for scooter boards, bean bag games for children, and scooter boards.

JC Penney Company Inc.

Catalog Distribution Center
Atlanta, GA 30390-0370
800-222-6161
Disability Served: all

This company manufactures clothing.

JE Medical Ltd. (dba MOPAC Ltd.)

PO Box 3094
Eau Claire, WI 54702
715-834-2710, 800-944-8589
Disability Served: physically disabled

This company manufactures and distributes the Swivel Walker, which enables para and quadriplegic patients to ambulate without crutches.

Jean Rose
369 East Van Koevering
Rialto, CA 92376-5143
714-875-0285
Disability Served: hearing

This company produces a lip-reading tutorial videotape.

Jefferson Industries Inc.
1985 Rutgers University Boulevard
Lakewood, NJ 08701
908-905-9001, 800-257-5145
Disability Served: physically disabled

This company manufactures flotation mattresses and flotation cushions.

Jetta Products Inc.
500-A Centennial Boulevard
Edmond, OK 73013
405-340-6661, 800-288-7771
Disability Served: all

This company manufactures a hydrotherapy whirlpool.

JH Industries
8901 East Pleasant Valley Road
PO Box 31267
Cleveland, OH 44131
216-524-7520
Disability Served: physically disabled

This company makes ramps.

Jimmy Systems Inc.
PO Box 2715
Country Club Hills, IL 60478
800-779-0926
Disability Served: physically disabled

This company manufactures a nonslip writing board.

Jobst Institute
Box 653
Toledo, OH 43694
419-698-1611, 800-537-1063
Disability Served: all

This company manufactures therapeutic stockings and a water flotation pad.

John Deere
1400 Third Avenue
Moline, IL 61265
800-544-2122
Disability Served: all

This company manufactures a long-handled edging shear and a garden cart.

John Van Note, Specially Customized Bicycles
9352 New Martinsville Avenue
Englewood, FL 34224
813-475-6646
Disability Served: all

This company performs custom modifications of bicycles for children.

Jokari US Inc.
1205 Venture Court
Dallas, TX 75006
214-416-5202
Disability Served: all

This company offers the Bottle Grabber, a pouring handle that fits over two-liter bottles.

Jordan Medical Enterprises
12555 Garden Grove Boulevard, Suite 507
Garden Grove, CA 92643
714-530-5123, 800-541-1193
Disability Served: vision

This company manufactures a syringe filling device to assist persons with limited vision and an insulin syringe injector.

Joy Enterprises Inc.
3800 North Fairfax Drive, #1301
Arlington, VA 22203
703-528-4220
Disability Served: hearing

This company offers a videotape of the *Joy of Signing Dictionary.*

JSR Enterprises Inc.
12275 Greenleaf Avenue
Potomac, MD 20854
301-279-2994
Disability Served: physically disabled

This company develops exercise workouts for wheelchair users. Workouts include audiocassettes and instruction manuals.

Julius Blum & Co. Inc.

PO Box 816
Carlstadt, NJ 07072
800-526-6293
Disability Served: all

This company manufactures handrails.

Just For You Fashions

810 Busch Court
Columbus, OH 43229
614-846-6133, 800-445-8474
Disability Served: all

This company provides clothing for people with special needs.

Just Manufacturing Company

9233 King Street
Franklin Park, IL 60131
847-678-5150
Disability Served: all

This company manufactures stainless steel plumbing fixtures, faucets, and related accessory products.

Just Two Bikes, Inc.

4821 Washington Avenue
White Bear Lake, MN 55110
800-499-1548
http://www.justtwobikes.com
Disability Served: physically disabled

This company manufactures dual recumbent cycles for the disabled.

K & L Resources Inc.

PO Box 2612
Springfield, VA 22152
703-455-1503
Disability Served: all

This company manufactures a slantboard designed for reading, writing, and drawing. The company also makes therapy putty for therapeutic hand exercise.

K'NEX Industries

2990 Bergey Road
PO Box 700
Hatfield, PA 19440-0700
215-997-7722, 800-KID-KNEX
Disability Served: all

This company manufactures a toy construction set with pieces that snap together into cars. The toy is designed to stimulate and enhance cognitive skills and eye-hand coordination.

K.Bow Med, Inc.

1201 School Street, Suite E
Wilkesboro, NC 28697
800-755-KBOW
Disability Served: all

K.Bow manufactures a pediatric reflux positioner and an infant positioning wedge designed to prevent reflux problems.

Kadco USA

9 Granger Avenue
Saratoga Springs, NY 12866
518-587-2224
Disability Served: all

This company manufactures a garden cart.

Kamenstein Inc.

565 Taxter Road, #500
Elmsford, NY 10523-2300
Disability Served: all

This company manufactures a revolving utensil organizer and a revolving spice rack.

Kapable Kids Inc.

227-4 Knickerbocker Avenue
Bohemia, NY 11716
800-356-1564
Disability Served: all

This company manufactures toys, puzzles, and assistive switches for the developing and special needs child.

Kardex Systems, Inc.

Route 7 North
Marietta, OH 45750
614-374-9300, 800-234-3654
http://kardex.com
Disability Served: physically disabled

This company makes a powered filing cabinet, shelving, and file folders.

Kay Elemetrics Corp.

12 Maple Avenue
PO Box 2025
Pine Brook, NJ 07058-2025
201-227-2000
Disability Served: communication

This company manufactures computer-based speech instruction programs and sound spectrographs to assist persons with speech disorders.

Kaye Products Inc.

535 Dimmocks Mill Road
Hillsborough, NC 27278
919-732-6444
Disability Served: all

This company distributes a number of daily living aids for children, including child toilet seats, walkers, therapy mats, positioning chairs, incontinence garments, and adjustable benches.

Keane Monroe Corporation

PO Box 5016
Monroe, NC 28111-5016
704-289-5581, 800-438-1937
Disability Served: physically disabled

This company manufactures a powered door operator.

Kees Goebel/Medical Specialties Inc.

9663 Glades Drive
Hamilton, OH 45011
513-874-2201, 800-354-0445
Disability Served: all

This company manufactures foam mattresses, foam wheelchair cushions, and foam hand exercisers.

Keitzer Check Writing Guide

K Enterprises
PO Box 491440
Leesburg, FL 34749-1440
904-326-3437
Disability Served: vision

This company manufactures a plastic check-writing guide to assist persons with limited vision.

Kel Tech Inc.

9285 North 32nd Street
Richland, MI 49083-0405
616-629-4814, 800-999-4320
Disability Served: physically disabled

This company manufactures an instant hot water heater for persons whose skin is not sensitive to temperature.

Kelco Building Products

PO Box 216
Scituate, MA 02066
617-545-9255
Disability Served: physically disabled

This company manufactures fiberglass ramps.

Keller Enterprises

930 East Lake Street
Aurora, IL 60506
630-859-2864
Disability Served: physically disabled

This company makes a long-handled stocking and trouser aid.

Kelvinator International Company

3 Parkway Center
Pittsburgh, PA 15220
412-928-8555
http://www.kelvinator-intl.com
Disability Served: physically disabled

This company sells accessible drinking fountains and water coolers internationally.

Ken McRight Supplies, Inc.

7456 South Oswego
Tulsa, OK 74136
918-492-9657
Disability Served: physically disabled

This company manufactures and distributes the Bye-Bye Decubiti inflatable wheelchair cushions and the BBD hospital bed mattress products for the prevention of decubiti.

Kimberly Clark Corp.

PO Box 2001
Neenah, WI 54956
800-242-6463
Disability Served: physically disabled

This company manufactures Depend incontinence garments and pads.

Kinetic Concepts

3417 Steen Drive
San Antonio, TX 78219
800-531-5396
Disability Served: physically disabled

This company manufactures a support bed designed to prevent pressure sores and a rotating bed.

Kinetic Diversified Industries, Inc.

7746 Arjons Drive
San Diego, CA 92126
619-566-4850, 800-451-6206
Disability Served: all

This company manufactures gel flotation seat cushions and foam seat cushions.

Kinetic Rehabilitation Instruments, Inc.

155-J Webster Street
Hanover, MA 02339
617-871-5200, 800-244-8882
Disability Served: physically disabled

This company makes a reaching device that can be switch activated and attached to wheelchairs.

Kinetic Resource Corporation

17 Elizabeth Place
Armonk, NY 10504
914-273-5320
Disability Served: all

This company manufactures a window opening aid for double-hung windows. The aid is a crank handle that is rotated to open and close windows.

Kingstar International America Inc.

1443 North Dearborn
Chicago, IL 60610
312-951-1115, 800-336-6550
Disability Served: all

This company manufactures a lumbar and back support cushion.

Kiwi Brands Inc.

Healthcare Products Division
Route 622 North
Douglassville, PA 19518
800-523-1210
Disability Served: physically disabled

This company manufactures incontinence aids, including a chair pad and waterproof sheets.

Kiwi Connection

82 Shelburne Center Road
Shelburne, MA 01370
413-625-9506
Disability Served: physically disabled

This company manufactures a door control system that provides easier access for persons with physical disabilities.

Kloz Ez

1065-D Shary Circle
Concord, CA 94518
510-689-1316, 800-848-5540 (CA)
Disability Served: physically disabled

This company makes incontinence garments.

Knight Protective Industries

7345 Varna Avenue
North Hollywood, CA 91605-4009
818-765-0600, 800-356-4448
Disability Served: physically disabled

This company manufactures a portable emergency alert system that plugs into a telephone jack.

Kohler Company

444 Highland Drive
Kohler, WI 53044
414-457-4441
Disability Served: all

This company makes plumbing items, including hand showers, baths, whirlpools, countertops, faucets, toilets, and drinking fountains.

Kojis Accessibility Products

509 East Main Street
Waterford, WI 53185
414-534-3935, 800-750-3935
Disability Served: physically disabled

This company makes a drinking glass with a lid and spout to accommodate persons with physical disabilities.

Kopptronix Co.

Box 361
Stanhope, NJ 07874
201-543-6819
http://kopptronix.com
Disability Served: hearing

This company manufactures sign-language games.

Koregon Enterprises Inc.

9735 Southwest Sunshine Court, Suite 100
Beaverton, OR 97005
800-544-4240
http://www.nitetrain-r.com
Disability Served: vision

This company manufactures an incontinence alarm designed for use at night to prevent bed-wetting.

Krissie Products Inc.

232 Taylor Road
Portsmouth, RI 02871
401-846-1701, 401-846-1702, 800-846-1701
Disability Served: physically disabled

This company offers a machine-washable poly/terrycloth bib for persons with arthritis or physical disabilities.

Kryger Enterprises

7253 Viar Avenue
San Diego, CA 92120
619-582-3451
Disability Served: physically disabled

This company manufactures a timed signal device designed to remind wheelchair users to shift their weight to prevent and reduce pressure sores.

Kuschall of America Inc.

708 Via Alondra
Camarillo, CA 93012-8713
805-484-3595, 800-654-4768
Disability Served: physically disabled

This company manufactures a variety of lightweight wheelchairs, including the Champion and Kusch'Kin series.

Kustom Built Athletic Equipment Inc.

North 409 Dyer Road
Spokane, WA 99212
509-534-4680, 800-537-5539
Disability Served: physically disabled

This company manufactures exercise equipment for wheelchair users.

KVM Rehabilitation, Inc.

9431 West Belt South
Houston, TX 77099-9998
713-271-0852
Disability Served: all

This company manufactures a continuous passive motion device designed for temporomandibular joints (TMJ).

Kwik Kut Manufacturing Co.
125 Columbia Street
PO Box 116
Mohawk, NY 13407-0116
315-866-2741
Disability Served: all

This company manufactures a food chopper and a device designed to cool hot liquids quickly.

L & L Manufacturing Company
1222 North Fancher Avenue
Fresno, CA 93727
209-255-2078
Disability Served: physically disabled

This company manufactures a portable, wheelchair accessible restroom.

L'Nard Associates Inc.
11236 47th North Street
Clearwater, FL 34622
813-573-1595, 800-627-1595
Disability Served: all

This company manufactures a knee stabilizer and splint systems for feet.

La Z Boy Inc.
1284 North Telegraph
Monroe, MI 48162
313-242-1444
http://www.lazboy.com
Disability Served: physically disabled

This company manufactures recliner chairs and power-lift chairs.

Labac Systems Inc.
3535 S. Kipling Street
Lakewood, CO 80235
303-791-6000, 800-445-4402
Disability Served: physically disabled

This company manufactures recliner seating systems for wheelchairs as well as switches to activate the powered recliner seating systems and headrests and arm supports.

LaCome Inc.
PO Box 77
Taos, NM 87571
505-758-5816
Disability Served: physically disabled

This company manufactures ski equipment for persons with disabilities. Products include a crutch-style outrigger for standing skiers with disabilities or seated skiers and a forearm crutch that can be used as an outrigger.

Lafayette Instrument
Box 5729
3700 Sagamore Place
Lafayette, IN 47903
765-423-1505
Disability Served: all

This company manufactures a goniometer, a muscle evaluation system that measures isometric strength, a dynamometer to measure grip strength, and a battery-operated muscle tester.

Lakeshore Learning Materials
2695 East Dominguez Street
PO Box 6261
Carson, CA 90749
310-537-8600, 800-421-5354
http://www.lakeshorelearning.com
Disability Served: learning disabled

This company supplies teachers, parents, and children with learning materials. Developmentally appropriate educational supplies, from block play to science and outdoor play to arts and crafts, are offered.

Lamson & Goodnow Manufacturing Company
PO Box 128
Shelburne Falls, MA 01370
413-625-6331, 800-872-6564
Disability Served: physically disabled

This company manufactures kitchen cutlery.

Landscape Structures Inc.
601 7th Street South
Delano, MN 55328
612-479-2546, 800-328-0035
Disability Served: physically disabled

This company manufactures playground equipment, including an adjustable basketball backstop, an infant maze, playground systems with wheelchair accessibility, and rubber mats for playground surfaces.

Lane Bryant
2300 Southeastern Avenue
Indianapolis, IN 46201
317-266-3300
Disability Served: all

This company manufactures large-size clothing for women.

Larkotex Company
1002 Olive Street
PO Box 449
Texarkana, TX 75501
903-793-4647, 800-972-3037
Disability Served: physically disabled

This company manufactures aids to daily living, including safety grab bars, commodes, walkers, shower chairs, restraint systems, orthotics, pads, and cushions.

Larry G. Fox Group, Inc.
2500 Sahler Street
Omaha, NE 68111
800-528-8628
Disability Served: physically disabled

This company manufactures handicap-adjustable cabinets, kitchens, baths, bedrooms, and offices.

Lasco Bathware
3255 East Miraloma Avenue
Anaheim, CA 92806
714-572-8686, 800-877-0464
Disability Served: physically disabled

This company manufactures bathroom aids and equipment, including a variety of tubs and showers.

Laszlo Corporation
PO Box 1182
Florissant, MO 63031
314-830-3222
Disability Served: physically disabled

This company manufactures a number of items, including swing-away lapboards for wheelchairs; back rests that allow upright sitting while in bed; bed chairs; and the Ziggy Medi-Chair, a multifunctional lift and transfer system.

Laurel Designs
98 Main Street, Suite 537
Tiburon, CA 94920
415-435-1891
http://www.laureldesigns.com
Disability Served: physically disabled

This company sells products for people with disabilities, including wheelchair and walker bags, wheelchair rain ponchos, videos, and cookbooks.

Lauri
PO Box F
Phillips-Avon, ME 04966
207-639-2000, 800-451-0520
Disability Served: physically disabled

This company manufactures and distributes learning toys for use by teachers of the learning disabled, physical therapists, occupational therapists, and vision therapists. Lauri toys assist in building fine motor skills and are suitable for the physically challenged and visually impaired.

LCN Closers
Division of Schlage Lock Co.
PO Box 100
Princeton, IL 61356
815-875-3311
Disability Served: physically disabled

This company manufactures powered door operators and spring-powered door closers.

Learning Pillows
PO Box 345
Greenfield, NH 03047
603-827-3859
Disability Served: all

This company manufactures multisensory educational products and tapes and provides programs and activities for children that are geared toward literacy.

Learning Products Inc.
700 Fee Fee Road
St Louis, MO 63043-3210
314-997-6400
Disability Served: all

This company develops large plastic blocks, a round plastic scooter board, and a plastic rocking boat used for balance.

Leisure-Lift, Inc.
1800 Merriam Lane
Kansas City, KS 66106
800-255-0285
http://www.pacesaver.com
Disability Served: physically disabled

This company manufactures three-wheeled wheelchair alternatives and seat-lift chairs in recliner, rocker, or contemporary styles.

Les Equipements Adaptes Physipro Inc.
783 rue Longpre
Sherebrooke, QC J1G 4S8 Canada
819-823-2252
Disability Served: physically disabled

This company manufactures a seating simulator used to evaluate custom seating needs and a prone stander.

Levenger
420 Commerce Drive
Delray Beach, FL 33445-4696
407-276-4141, 800-544-0080
Disability Served: physically disabled

This company provides reading and writing aids, including bookstands, lap desks, reader's pillows, and foot rests.

LGS Health Products
PO Box 12335
Sioux Falls, SD 57101-1235
605-321-0356
Disability Served: physically disabled

This company offers a pill crusher and a pill splitter.

Lidbuster Inc.
19527 Bay View Road
Boca Raton, FL 33434
561-483-9178
Disability Served: physically disabled

This company manufactures a jar opener designed to accommodate persons with little or no hand strength.

Life Essentials
345 Burnett Road
West Lafayette, IN 47906
765-742-6707, 800-543-3740
Disability Served: physically disabled

This company manufactures a door opener and closer and an exterior seat lift for automobiles.

Life Like Laboratory
Division of Marmich Inc.
2718 Hollandale Lane, Suite 400
Dallas, TX 75234
214-620-0203
Disability Served: physically disabled

This company manufactures custom hand and foot prostheses.

Lifecall Medical Alert Systems Inc.
1300 Admiral Wilson Boulevard
Camden, NJ 08101
609-665-9500
Disability Served: all

This company manufactures a personal emergency call system.

Lifecare
655 Aspen Ridge Drive
Lafayette, CO 80026
303-666-9234
Disability Served: physically disabled

This company manufactures health care aids, including ventilators and nebulizers.

Lifeguard Lift Inc.

95 Monument Plaza
Pleasant Hill, CA 94523
510-686-4664
Disability Served: physically disabled

This company manufactures a hydraulic hot tub lift and a hydraulic pool lift.

Lifeline International, Inc.

1421 South Park Street
Madison, WI 53715
608-251-4778, 800-553-6633
Disability Served: all

This company manufactures the Lifeline Wall Pulley System, a pulley exerciser for those in physical rehabilitation.

Lifeline Systems Inc.

640 Memorial Drive
Cambridge, MA 02138-4851
617-923-4141, 800-451-0525
Disability Served: all

This company provides an emergency call system that sends a signal to the Lifeline Emergency Response Center when the system is activated.

Lifescan Inc.

1051 South Milpitas Boulevard
Milpitas, CA 95035
800-227-8862
Disability Served: all

This company manufactures numerous blood glucose monitoring systems.

Lifestyle Innovations

PO Box 2643
Zanesville, OH 43702-2643
614-455-3419
Disability Served: physically disabled

This company manufactures a bed shower so bedridden patients can bathe.

Lifetek Co.

PO Box 1505
Stowe, VT 05672
802-253-4173
Disability Served: vision

This company manufactures vibrating canes used to alert the user of changes in ground surface.

Lift & Storage Systems, Inc.

3582 Hoffman Road East
White Bear Lake, MN 55110
612-777-1554
Disability Served: physically disabled

This company offers an elevating platform as an alternative to ramps and lifts.

Lift Aid

38281 Schoolcraft, Suite A
Livonia, MI 48150
800-951-4243
http://www.liftaid.com
Disability Served: physically disabled

This company manufactures patient lifts with a capacity of up to 500 pounds.

Light Bright Books

2930 East Fourth Avenue
Durango, CO 81301
970-259-0563
Disability Served: vision

This company manufactures Light Bright Illuminated Story Books for children with low vision and the Discovery Light Box, designed to illuminate the Light Bright Books.

Lindsay Russell

100 Memorial Drive, Apartment 5-18-C
Cambridge, MA 02142
617-547-0819
Disability Served: vision

This manufacturer provides an electronic mobility aid that uses ultrasonic sound to investigate the upcoming path.

Lindustries Inc.
21 Shady Hill Road
Weston, MA 02193
508-237-8177
Disability Served: physically disabled

This company manufactures a door handle lever to accommodate persons with limited hand strength.

Linear Electronics
PO Box 9003
Carlsbad, CA 92008
800-421-1587
Disability Served: hearing

This company manufactures a wireless signal transmitter.

Lite Walker Inc.
7715 Lacorn Court
St Louis, MO 63121
314-383-4968
Disability Served: physically disabled

This company manufactures a height-adjustable wheeled walker.

LiteTouch Inc.
3550 South 700 West
Salt Lake City, UT 84119-4120
Disability Served: all

This company manufactures lighting control systems.

Little Tikes Company
2180 Barlow Road
PO Box 2277
Hudson, OH 44236-0877
800-321-0183
Disability Served: all

This company makes a teaching clock for children.

Living Wall Garden Company
2044 Chili Avenue
Rochester, NY 14624
716-374-2340
Disability Served: all

This company manufactures a gardening container.

Lloyd Matheson Inc.
PO Box L
Charlestown, NH 03603
603-826-5777
Disability Served: physically disabled

This company manufactures door handles and security chains for doors.

LMB Hand Rehab Products Inc.
PO Box 1181
San Luis Obispo, CA 93406
800-541-3992
Disability Served: all

This company manufactures rehabilitative and therapeutic products, including wrist supports, exercise putty for hand strengthening activities, foam hand orthoses, work station pads, and more.

Logan Inc.
3041 South Shannon Street
Santa Ana, CA 92704
714-556-6441
Disability Served: all

This company manufactures whirlpool chairs.

Logan Powell Company
1225 Thomas Road
Wayne, PA 19087
610-995-0973
Disability Served: physically disabled

This company manufactures a heat protection device that automatically turns off electric ranges after a specified amount of time.

Longstreet Pharmacal Corp.
1224 50th Street
Brooklyn, NY 11219
718-436-9200, 800-633-7878
Disability Served: physically disabled

This company manufactures an incontinence garment for men.

Lossing Orthopedic
777 Harding Street NE, Suite M-4
PO Box 18298
Minneapolis, MN 55418
612-331-3985
Disability Served: physically disabled

This company develops traction systems.

Lott Company
PO Box 1107
Santa Monica, CA 90406
310-397-4217, 800-359-4554
Disability Served: all

This company makes an emergency alert speakerphone and emergency alert systems activated by pendant transmitters.

Lotus Health Care Products
31 Sheriden Drive
Naugatuck, CT 06770
203-723-1494
Disability Served: physically disabled

This company manufactures cushions, mattresses, and pressure evaluation systems.

Love Electronics Inc.
395 Vosberg Lane
Goldendale, WA 98620-3415
509-773-5958
Disability Served: vision

This company manufactures access signs for persons with low vision and a voice output screen access system for computers.

Love Lift
PO Box 2158
1274 Industrial Avenue
Holland, MI 49423-2158
616-393-8941, 800-456-8826
Disability Served: physically disabled

This company manufactures a transfer aid to assist persons in wheelchairs.

LPB, Inc.
28 Bacton Hill Road
Frazer, PA 19355
610-644-1123
http://www.lpbinc.com
Disability Served: hearing

This company manufactures hearing-assistive transmission systems.

LS & S Group, Inc.
PO Box 673
Northbrook, IL 60065
847-498-9777, 800-468-4789
TTY/TDD: 800-317-8533
http://www.lssgroup.com/
Disability Served: vision, hearing

This company distributes aids and appliances for the visually and hearing impaired via a yearly catalog.

Luba Medical Supplies Inc.
6187 NW 167th Street, #H24
Miami, FL 33015
305-556-5559
Disability Served: all

This company manufactures and distributes aids to daily living as well as therapeutic aids. Products include toilet seats, walkers, support cushions, bath and shower benches, crutches, orthoses, and more.

Lubidet USA Inc.
950 South Cherry Street, Suite 506
Denver, CO 80222-2664
303-757-3031, 800-582-4338
Disability Served: all

This company manufactures a toilet bidet.

Lumex
Division of Lumex, Inc.
100 Spence Street
Bay Shore, NY 11706-2290
516-273-2200, 800-645-5272
Disability Served: all

This company manufactures and distributes numerous aids for daily living. Products range from crutch covers to kitchen tongs to mattresses.

Luminaud, Inc.
8688 Tyler Boulevard
Mentor, OH 44060
440-255-9082, 800-255-3408
Disability Served: all

This company manufactures, sells, and services artificial larynges, voice amplifiers, small communications boards, switches for limited motion capability, and other specialized products for people in need of assistance in communication.

Lutron Electronics Co., Inc.
7200 Suter Road
Coopersburg, PA 18036-1299
215-282-3800
http://www.lutron.com
Disability Served: all

This company manufactures lighting control systems and controls for persons with disabilities.

Luxury Liners
14545 Ballyview Avenue
Santa Fe Springs, CA 90670
800-247-4203
Disability Served: physically disabled

This company manufactures a number of items for persons with disabilities, including wheelchair seatbelts, support systems, foam cushions and supports, footboards, lap trays, and harness systems.

M+IND Corporation
Seattle Medical Systems Group
861 Poplar Place South
Seattle, WA 98144
206-325-0715, 800-248-MIND
Disability Served: physically disabled

This company manufactures prosthetics.

M.E.S.A. Inc.
9807 Fredericksburg Road
San Antonio, TX 78240
210-699-6911, 800-383-6437
Disability Served: all

This company manufactures a lumbar support belt designed to protect against strain and injury when lifting objects.

MA Rallis Corporation
2031 Highway 130
Building 1F
Mammoth Junction, NJ 08852
908-940-0456, 800-852-8898
Disability Served: vision

This company manufactures an electric metronome with flashing lights.

Mac's Lift Gate Inc.
2801 South Street
Long Beach, CA 90805
562-634-5962
Disability Served: physically disabled

This company manufactures van lifts and home wheelchair lifts.

Mada Medical Products Inc.
60 Commerce Road
Carlstadt, NJ 07072
201-460-0454, 800-526-6370
Disability Served: all

This company manufactures oxygen carts and portable oxygen systems.

Maddak Inc.
6 Industrial Road
Pequannock, NJ 07440
973-628-7600, 800-443-4926
http://www.maddak.com
Disability Served: all

This company is manufacturer of Ableware self-help products for daily-living needs. Ableware products are designed to increase mobility and facilitate everyday activities such as dressing, bathing, grooming, and eating. The catalog features more than 500 products that enable people to remain active and maximize their independence at home and work.

Magic Box Inc.
PO Box 65233
Lubbock, TX 79464
806-799-1462
Disability Served: all

This company manufactures exercise equipment based on push-pull action.

Magic Industries
PO Box 30333
Portland, OR 97230
503-252-4760
Disability Served: physically disabled

This company manufactures an exercise machine designed for wheelchair users to exercise their upper extremities.

Magnisight, Inc.
3360 Adobe Court
Colorado Springs, CO 80907
719-578-8893, 800-753-4767
http://www.magnisight.com
Disability Served: vision

This company manufactures electronic low-vision aids.

Magnistitch Inc.
3756 Rockhill Road
Birmingham, AL 35201
205-967-8326
http://magnistitch.com
Disability Served: vision

This company manufactures various magnifying lenses, including a magnifier for use with sewing machines.

Maico Hearing Instruments Inc.
7375 Bush Lake Road
Minneapolis, MN 55439-2029
612-835-4400, 800-328-6366
Disability Served: hearing

This company develops hearing aids.

Mailhawk Manufacturing Co.
PO Box 445
5292 Whitehouse Parkway
Warm Springs, GA 31830
706-655-3849
http://www.mailhawkmfg.com
Disability Served: all

This company manufactures a reaching device for health care and municipal, state, home, and industry trash pickup.

Major-Lab Manufacturing
4408 North Sewell
Oklahoma City, OK 73118
Disability Served: all

This company manufactures a fixed height commode, canes, a home traction unit, shower chairs, a powered door opener, and safety grab bars.

Makit Products, Inc.
4659 Mint Way
Dallas, TX 75236
214-330-6667
Disability Served: all

This company manufactures Make-A-Plate, a kit that allows children to draw and design a plate. The drawing is sent to the company and imposed on a plastic plate.

Makita USA, Inc.
14930 Northam Street
La Mirada, CA 90638
562-522-8088, 800-851-0537
Disability Served: all

Makita makes an environmental control unit designed to automatically open and close draperies.

Manhelp of San Antonio
3110 Wroxton Road
San Antonio, TX 78217-3952
210-653-6512
Disability Served: vision

This company produces, markets, and sells playground equipment for the visually impaired. Products include soccer balls and basketballs.

Mankind Research Foundation Inc.
1315 Apple Avenue
Silver Spring, MD 20910
301-587-8686
Disability Served: all

This company manufactures electrical stimulators, crib monitors, biofeedback relaxation units, transfer mats for transferring patients from beds to tables or stretchers, and thermometers.

Maple Leaf Chapter Bell Telephone of Canada
483 Bay Street
Toronto, ON M5S 2E1 Canada
Disability Served: hearing

This company manufactures a voice amplifier headset telephone.

Maramed Orthopedic Systems
2480 West 82nd Street
Hialeah, FL 33016
305-823-8300
http://maramed.com
Disability Served: all

This company manufactures orthoses and braces, including leg splints, hand immobilizers, and leg braces.

Marc Us Inc.
639 South Washington Street
Naperville, IL 60546
630-357-3828
Disability Served: physically disabled

This company produces a chair with a seat lift to assist those who have difficulty getting in and out of chairs.

Marlen Manufacturing & Development Co.
5150 Richmond Road
Cleveland, OH 44146
216-292-7060
Disability Served: all

This company develops personal care wound products, including colostomy pouches, colostomy irrigating systems, cleaning brushes, and ostomy supplies.

Mart Cart/Assembled Products Corp.
115 East Linden Street
Rogers, AR 72756
501-636-5776
http://assembledproducts.com
Disability Served: physically disabled

This company manufactures shopping carts and a home-use cart.

Marusya, Inc.
PO Box 13925
Albany, NY 12212
518-274-1745
Disability Served: all

This company manufactures and sells ceramic and plastic tableware designed for those with any disability affecting hand function.

Mary-Jane Goodrich
c/o Mies Van Der Roh's Home School
2971 53rd Street SE
Auburn, WA 98092-8310
253-735-6350
Disability Served: communication

This company makes tactile symbols to aid persons with communication and/or visual disabilities.

Mason Medical Products
Division of MRC Industries, Inc.
8000 Cooper Avenue, Building 28
Glendale, NY 11385
718-326-3100
Disability Served: physically disabled

This company manufactures a motorized bed that comes with an electric hand control to adjust the head and foot sections. The company also produces foam seat cushions.

Mat Factory, Inc.
760 West 16th Street, Building E
Costa Mesa, CA 92627
949-645-3122, 800-628-7626
http://www.matfactoryinc.com
Disability Served: physically disabled

This company manufactures Safety Deck II, an interlocking tile system that installs directly on the ground, providing wheelchair access over grass.

Maxi-Aids

42 Executive Boulevard
Farmingdale, NY 11735
800-522-6294
http://www.maxiaids.com
Disability Served: all

This company sells products to enable independent living.

Maxi-Signal Products

Division of Mill Specialties, Inc.
5 East 49th Street
PO Box 398
La Grange, IL 60525
708-354-4730, 800-227-9636
Disability Served: hearing

This company manufactures signals and alarms that use flashing lights to accommodate persons with hearing impairments.

Maximum Performance Technologies

13765 Alton Parkway, Suite E
Irvine, CA 92718
714-707-2728
Disability Served: all

This company manufactures electrical stimulators for pain management.

Mayline/Hamilton

619 North Commerce Street
Sheboygon, WI 53082-2728
414-457-5537, 800-822-8037
Disability Served: physically disabled

This company produces a height-adjustable, electrically powered drafting table.

McCarty's

3329 Industrial Avenue
Coeur d'Alene, ID 83815
208-765-8408, 800-635-3557
Disability Served: all

This company manufactures pillows, cushions, and back supports.

McDavid Knee Guard Inc.

5420 West Roosevelt Road
Chicago, IL 60650
800-237-8254
Disability Served: all

This company manufactures ankle guards, knee guards, and stability braces.

McKay's Inc.

1421 Hamilton Avenue
Janesville, WI 53545
608-756-4600, 800-227-0679
Disability Served: all

This company manufactures a key holder that offers leverage to facilitate key turning as well as a light switch aid.

McKinney Electronics

Division of Overhead Door Corp.
1315 East Saint Andrew Place #6
Santa Ana, CA 92705-4919
714-432-9922
Disability Served: physically disabled

This company manufactures a residential vertical lift carrier called Dumb Waiter.

MD Products Inc.

4720 SE Fort King Street
Ocala, FL 32671
800-255-5493
Disability Served: all

This company manufactures a portable transcutaneous electrical neuromuscular stimulator (TENS) designed to alleviate chronic pain.

Med Covers Inc.

1103 Transport Drive
Raleigh, NC 27603
800-327-4571
Disability Served: physically disabled

This company manufactures carrying aids for wheelchairs, covers for wheelchairs and scooters, and oxygen cylinder carrying cases.

Med Lift & Mobility Inc.
PO Box 1249
Calhoun City, MS 38916
601-682-7533, 800-748-9438
Disability Served: physically disabled

This company manufactures lift chairs and a motorized bed for residential use.

Med/West
Division of Western Manufacturing Corp.
702 South 3rd Avenue
PO Box 130
Marshalltown, IA 50158
515-752-5446, 800-247-7594
Disability Served: physically disabled

This company makes a powered, elevating toilet seat lift to assist persons with limited mobility.

MedCare Apparel
6573 Cochran Road
Solon, OH 44139
216-248-8400, 800-633-0929
Disability Served: all

This company manufactures men's and women's clothing.

Medco
Division of KKC Inc.
1421 Champion Drive, Suite 311
Carrollton, TX 75006
214-241-7240
Disability Served: physically disabled

This company manufactures a body support pad designed to prevent pressure sores and a wedge-shaped pillow that can be used as a back rest.

MedDev Corporation
2468 Embarcadero Way
Palo Alto, CA 94303-3313
650-494-1153
http://www.meddev-corp.com
Disability Served: physically disabled

This company manufactures hand therapy equipment used for the rehabilitation of patients suffering from hand injuries. Products include the Hand Helper, a resistance exerciser, the Iso Hand Helper, an isometric exerciser, specialized exercisers for the thumb and individual fingers, and the FiddLink, a digital-dexterity developer also useful for children with ADHD.

MedFlex
19046 Emory Road
Pal, TN 37849
800-925-2294
Disability Served: all

MedFlex manufactures elastic back supports and wrist splints.

Medi Athleti-K Inc.
2175 Place Thimens
St Laurent, QC H4R 1K8 Canada
514-331-7214, 800-361-6857
Disability Served: physically disabled

This company manufactures orthoses, support stockings, mattresses, pillows, and cushions.

Medi Crush Company
PO Box 16237
4801 West Fourth Street, Suite L-10
Hattiesburg, MS 39402-6237
800-262-6334
Disability Served: all

This company manufactures a pill splitter, a pill crusher, a pill case, and a shampoo basin.

Medi Sports Health Homecare Corp.
75 York Avenue
PO Box 302
Randolph, MA 02368
617-961-1232, 800-225-8634
Disability Served: all

This company makes leg bags, breathing exercisers, sitz baths, catheters, and ice packs.

Medic ID's International
18730 Oxnard Street, Suite 210
Tarzana, CA 91356
818-705-0595, 800-926-3342
http://medicid.com
Disability Served: all

This company makes medical identification tags.

Medic-Air Corp. of America

1963 Palmer Avenue
Larchmont, NY 10538
800-247-7455
http://www.novicom.com/ptpmedicair.htm
Disability Served: all

This company manufactures back pillows and supports.

Medical Devices International (MDI)

3849 Swanson Court
Gurnee, IL 60031
847-336-6611, 800-323-9035
Disability Served: all

This company makes a urinary drainage bag, ice bags, inflatable ring cushions, and leg bags.

Medical Disposables/INBRAND

1169 Canton Road
Marietta, GA 30066
770-422-3036, 800-241-8205
Disability Served: physically disabled

This company manufactures incontinence aids for men and women.

Medical Flotation Systems

3229 Flagler Avenue, Suite 107
Key West, FL 33040-4687
800-336-0332
Disability Served: all

This company manufactures adjustable water flotation mattresses.

Medical Line Warehouse

6130 Clark Center Avenue, #103
Sarasota, FL 34238
941-924-2058, 800-247-2256
Disability Served: all

This company offers numerous aids for daily living and health care products. Some of the products include catheters, eating utensils, toilet seats, flotation cushions, and crutch pads.

Medical Monitoring Systems Inc.

3802 Hackers Avenue
Madison, WI 53704
608-241-1234
Disability Served: all

This company manufactures a passive emergency alert system. If the timer is set, the system requires the user to check in at various intervals. If there is no response, the monitoring center will be alerted.

Medical Products of America

704 Dolphin Drive West
Highland, IL 62249
800-633-7374
Disability Served: all

This company makes a small, liquid crystal thermometer that is applied to the skin and does not have to be removed for several days.

Medical Technology Inc.

2601 Pinewood Street
Grand Prairie, TX 75051
214-647-0884, 800-527-3666
Disability Served: physically disabled

This company makes a passive motion exerciser.

Medical Technology, Inc.

1710 Adams Street
Cedar Falls, IA 50613
800-277-1710
Disability Served: vision

This company manufactures a specialized camera that detects vision problems in children.

Medicool Inc.

23761 Madison Street
Torrance, CA 90505
800-654-1565
Disability Served: diabetes

This company makes a portable cooler to carry insulin.

Medinorm Ergonomic Kitchens

Division of Twin Oaks Management
48525 Yale Road East
Chilliwack, BC V2P 6H4 Canada
604-792-1450
Disability Served: physically disabled

This company designs and manufactures height-adjustable and adaptable kitchens and vanities. Three electric height-adjustable systems are available, as are shallow sinks with single or double bowls, shallow sinks with two sloped sides, and long-handled faucets.

MediUSA

76 West Seegers Road
Arlington Heights, IL 60005
847-640-8400, 800-633-6334
Disability Served: all

This company makes therapeutic stockings and pressure wraps.

Medmart Inc.

PO Box 724
Glendora, CA 91740
626-963-0620, 800-724-1414
Disability Served: all

This company manufactures and sells products to laryngectomees, including stoma covers and shower shields.

Medmax Inc.

5105 East 39th Avenue
Denver, CO 80207-1108
Disability Served: all

This company manufactures an electronic stethoscope that is equipped with an amplifier to increase volume output.

Medpro Inc.

275 Highway 18
East Brunswick, NJ 08816
908-238-1444, 800-257-5145
Disability Served: all

This company manufactures mattress surfaces, seat cushions, and bed underpads.

Medtek Resources, Inc.

204 A North Clay
St Louis, MO 63122
314-966-0221, 800-397-0222
Disability Served: physically disabled

This company manufactures bathroom safety devices, including grab bars, flip-up safety bars, toilet roll accessories, and back rests.

Medx Corporation

1401 NE 77th Street
Ocala, FL 34479
352-622-2112
http://www.medxonline.com
Disability Served: back injury, neck injury, knee injury

This company makes computerized exercise machines designed by medical professionals for rehabilitation.

Memry Corporation

57 Commerce Drive
Brookfield, CT 06804
203-740-7311, 800-582-5454
Disability Served: all

This company manufactures a water temperature control unit for showers.

Mentor Corporation

5425 Hollister Avenue
Santa Barbara, CA 93111
805-681-6000, 800-235-5731
Disability Served: physically disabled

This company makes an incontinence garment for men.

Mentor O & O, Inc.

3000 Longwater Drive
Norwell, MA 02061
617-871-6950
Disability Served: all

This company manufactures nerve stimulators, catheters, magnifiers, and urinary bags.

Merillat Industries Inc.

PO Box 1946
Adrian, MI 49221
517-263-0771
Disability Served: physically disabled

This company manufactures accessible kitchen cabinet accessories.

Meroni Locks of America, Inc.

2121 West 60th Street
Hialeah, FL 33016
305-557-7050, 800-749-5625
Disability Served: physically disabled

This company makes door knobs designed for hands-free opening of doors.

Merry Walker Corporation

1357 Northmoor Court
Northbrook, IL 60062
847-498-9028, 800-827-8318
Disability Served: physically disabled

This company manufactures a wheeled walker.

Metavox Inc.

8375 Leesburg Pike, PMB #421
Vienna, VA 22182
703-698-0802
Disability Served: hearing

This company makes a tactile assistive device.

Metpar Steel Products Corp.

95 State Street
Westbury, NY 11590
516-333-2600
Disability Served: all

This company manufactures accessible restroom stall partitions.

Mettler Electronics Corporation

1333 South Claudina Street
Anaheim, CA 92805-9844
800-854-9305
Disability Served: physically disabled

This company manufactures an electrode garment, ultrasound units used for pain relief, and electrical stimulators.

Meyra Inc.

59 Wedgewood Road
Newark, DE 19711-2055
302-324-4400, 800-833-9962
Disability Served: physically disabled

This company manufactures wheelchairs, hydraulic lifts for transferring patients, and commode wheelchairs.

MG Equipment Co.

6990 Blaine Avenue
Inner Grove Heights, MN 55076
612-227-9298
Disability Served: all

This company manufactures head supports and headrests.

Micro Audiometrics Corp.

2200 South Ridgewood Avenue, US #1
South Daytona, FL 32119-3018
904-788-9331, 800-729-9509
Disability Served: hearing

This company makes audiometers designed to test hearing.

Midwest Contracting & Manufacturing Co. Inc.

East Highway 40
PO Box 175
WaKeeney, KS 67672
913-743-5460
Disability Served: physically disabled

This company manufactures wheelchair lifts and wheelchair headrests.

MIG

800 Hearst Avenue
Berkeley, CA 94710
510-845-7549
Disability Served: all

This company produces texts that provide technical and design information related to the ADA and universal design.

Mila Engineering Corp.
11554 Encino Avenue
Granada Hills, CA 91344
818-363-1908
Disability Served: physically disabled

This company manufactures a mechanical feeder.

Mill-Tech Enterprises Inc.
PO Box 2614
Northbrook, IL 60065
800-726-5438
Disability Served: all

This company makes an elevating toilet seat lift that can be used with a standard toilet or with a bedside commode.

Miller Building Systems Inc.
58120 County Road #3 South
Elkhart, IN 46517
219-295-1214
Disability Served: physically disabled

This company builds a wheelchair accessible mobile home.

Miller's Adaptive Technologies
2023 Romig Road
Akron, OH 44320-3819
800-837-4544
Disability Served: physically disabled

This company manufactures wheelchair support systems and accessories.

Milwaukee Machine & Engineering Corporation
2550 South 170th Street
New Berlin, WI 53151
414-782-3510
Disability Served: physically disabled

This company manufactures a manual wheelchair that converts to a commode chair.

Mirac
542 Route 62
Winchester, OH 45697
513-442-2401
Disability Served: hearing

This company manufactures smoke alarms, TDD phone enclosures, and alarm clocks for persons with hearing disabilities.

Misty Mate
162 West Boxelder, #2
Chandler, AZ 85224
602-892-1226, 800-233-6478
Disability Served: all

This company makes the Misty Mate Personal Cooling System, a device that sprays a water mist in order to cool the user.

MITEC Controls, Inc.
3040 F Business Park Drive
Norcross, GA 30071
770-662-0094
Disability Served: physically disabled

This company makes a fire alarm extension handle so wheelchair users can trigger fire alarms.

MNO Medical Products
441 Cedar Haven Way
Anaheim, CA 92807
714-637-8501
Disability Served: physically disabled

This company manufactures a urinary drainage system for use with wheelchairs.

Mobility Limited
475 Arbutus Avenue
Morro Bay, CA 93442
805-772-9253, 800-366-6038
http://www.mobilityltd.com/index.html
Disability Served: physically disabled

This company produces and distributes exercise videos for people with physical disabilities.

Mobility Systems
1125 Hastings Street
Traverse City, MI 49684-4318
616-941-4626
Disability Served: physically disabled

This company manufactures restraints and positioners.

Mobility Transfer Systems, Inc.

19 Lafayette Street
PO Box 922
Randolph, MA 02368-0922
617-963-4564, 800-854-4687
http://www.bed-mobility.com
Disability Served: all

This company makes transfer aids for getting in and out of beds.

Modern Healthcare Concepts

2303 First Street
Holiday Garden Estate
New Port Richey, FL 34652
813-846-0194
Disability Served: physically disabled

This company manufactures a geriatric chair and a reclining wheeled chair.

Modern Transfer Industries Inc.

PO Box 78290
Shreveport, LA 71107
318-222-3436, 800-356-1572
Disability Served: physically disabled

This company manufactures a transfer aid.

Modu-Tray

9 Orlando Drive
Chattanooga, TN 37415
423-870-3245
Disability Served: physically disabled

This company manufactures a lapboard with a bookholder that can be used as a tray or as a writing board for wheelchair users.

Modular Medical Corp.

1513 Olmsted Avenue
Bronx, NY 10462
718-829-2626
Disability Served: physically disabled

This company provides belt restraints, foam for creating seating devices, protective helmets, and folding bath seats.

Modulex Signs, Inc.

204 West Newberry Road
Bloomfield, CT 06002
860-726-1910, 800-742-6543
Disability Served: vision

This company manufactures ADA compliance signs to assist persons with low vision.

Moen Incorporated

25300 Al Moen Drive
North Olmsted, OH 44070
216-962-2000, 800-321-8809
http://moen.com
Disability Served: physically disabled

This company manufactures kitchen sinks, faucets, and hand showers.

Monadnock Lifetime Products

PO Box B
Fitzwilliam, NH 03447
603-585-6810
Disability Served: physically disabled

This company provides an attachment for canes and crutches designed to provide gripping and prevent skidding on snow and ice.

Monmouth Vans, Access & Mobility Equipment

5105 Route 33/34
Farmingdale, NJ 07727
732-919-1444, 800-221-0034
http://www.monmouth.com
Disability Served: physically disabled

This company provides complete modifications to vans and cars, stairway or vertical lifts, automatic door openers, modular ramp systems, and patient transfer systems.

Monoject

1831 Olive Street
St Louis, MO 63103
314-621-7788
Disability Served: all

This company manufactures a puncture device used for self-monitoring blood sugar levels.

Moore and Moore Inc.

1202 South 17th Avenue
Maywood, IL 60153
708-343-8710
Disability Served: physically disabled

This company manufactures an arm exerciser for paralyzed arms and an arm sling.

Morfam Inc.

3002 North Home Street
PO Box 113
Mishawaka, IN 46545
219-259-4581, 800-338-7014
Disability Served: all

This company manufactures a portable electric massager.

Motion Analysis Corporation

3617 Westwind Boulevard
Santa Rosa, CA 95403-1067
707-579-6500
Disability Served: all

This company develops computer-based motion evaluation systems for use by research laboratories, physical education departments, and sports facilities.

Motor Development Corp.

9340 Buell Street
Downey, CA 90241
562-862-6741
Disability Served: all

This company manufactures a board designed to provide standing support, balance boards, support chairs, a vest that maintains body temperature, and positioning wedges.

Mount Sinai Medical Center

Patient Representative Department
1 Gustave Levy Place
PO Box 1161
New York, NY 10029-6574
212-659-8990
Disability Served: communication

The Center manufactures a portable communication board.

Mountain Man

720 Front Street
Bozeman, MT 59715
406-587-0310
Disability Served: physically disabled

This company manufactures skis and accessories for persons with disabilities.

Mountain Medical Equipment, Inc.

10488 West Centennial Road
Littleton, CO 80127
303-973-1200
Disability Served: physically disabled

This company manufactures an ultrasonic nebulizer.

Mountainsmith

18301 West Colfax Avenue
Heritage Square, Building P
Golden, CO 80401
303-279-5930
Disability Served: physically disabled

This company makes sleds.

Mr. America Manufacturing Inc.

PO Box 587
Ooltewah, TN 37363
615-238-5388, 800-251-6040
Disability Served: physically disabled

This company manufactures supports, including low back orthoses and wrist splints.

Mueller Magnum Orthopedic

One Quench Drive
Prairie du Sac, WI 53578
608-643-8530, 800-356-9522
Disability Served: orthopedic

This company manufactures a number of braces and supports, including ankle braces, elbow supports, knee supports, and more.

Multiple Sclerosis Foundation, Inc.

6350 North Andrews Avenue
Ft Lauderdale, FL 33309
954-776-6805, 800-441-7055
http://www.msfacts.org
Disability Served: multiple sclerosis

The Multiple Sclerosis Foundation, Inc. is a nonprofit organization that provides traditional and alternative health care options and home care assisted programs. It also publishes a newsletter and provides phone support, in-house library information and referrals, and networking with regional support groups. The Foundation awards grants to universities for research of the cause, cure, prevention, and treatment of MS. Temporary custodial home care, home renovations, used medical equipment, and summer camp programs are also offered.

Murials Comfort Clothing

21 Harvey Street
Kingston, ON K7K 5C1 Canada
910-996-3370
Disability Served: physically disabled

This company manufactures clothing for men and women.

Murphey Door Bed Co.

42 Central Avenue
Farmingdale, NY 11735
516-543-0234
Disability Served: physically disabled

This company manufactures an accessible kitchen unit.

Murphys Products Corp.

PO Box 1826
Murphys, CA 95247
209-728-2075, 800-334-4896
Disability Served: physically disabled

This company manufactures a curb ramp.

N-K Products Company Inc.

2500 Rosedale Avenue
Soquel, CA 95073
408-462-6509, 800-462-6509
Disability Served: physically disabled

This company manufactures exercise equipment and therapeutic aids used for physical rehabilitation.

Naace Industries Inc.

5032 North Royal Atlanta Drive
Tucker, GA 30084
770-938-6500, 800-438-1900
Disability Served: physically disabled

This company manufactures a portable shampoo tray and a shampoo basin. Both are designed for washing the bedridden individual's hair.

Nada-Chair

783 Haroing Street NE
Minneapolis, MN 55413-2813
800-722-2587
Disability Served: physically disabled

This company makes the Nada Chair, an adjustable posture chair that provides extra support for the lower back.

Nady Systems Inc.

6701 Shellmound Street
Emeryville, CA 94608-1023
510-652-2411
http://www.nady.wireless.com
Disability Served: hearing

This company makes a television amplification system for the hard of hearing and large-area RF and IR assistive listening systems.

Nancy V Becker

22 Grove Place
Unit 27, White Horse Common
Winchester, MA 01890
617-437-3064
Disability Served: hearing

This company manufactures an address book for the hearing impaired. The book has sections for TDD numbers and features American Sign Language symbols.

National Association for Visually Handicapped

22 West 21st Street, 6th Floor
New York, NY 10010
212-889-3141
Disability Served: vision

The Association offers numerous items to accommodate persons with limited vision.

Products include magnifiers, telephone accessories, watches, and playing cards.

National Captioning Institute

1900 Gallows Road, Suite 3000
Vienna, VA 22182
800-533-9673
http://www.us.net/nci/
Disability Served: hearing

NCI, a nonprofit corporation founded in 1979, is the nation's largest provider of closed-captioned television services for the broadcast, cable, and home video industries.

National Guard Products Inc.

540 North Parkway
PO Box 7853
Memphis, TN 38107
800-647-7874
Disability Served: physically disabled

This company makes an accessible door threshold.

National Hearing Aid Distributors, Inc.

145 Tremont Street
Boston, MA 02111
617-426-9845, 800-627-9930
Disability Served: hearing

This company manufactures a personal amplification system.

National Identification Co.

11531 Rupp Drive
Burnsville, MN 55337-1248
303-295-1453
Disability Served: all

This company makes medical alert tags.

National Invention Services Inc.

4133 Highway 17 North
Pawleys Island, SC 29585
803-237-7755
Disability Served: all

This company makes a timing device that acts as a reminder for persons with cognitive disabilities.

National Medical Industries Inc.

PO Box 3268
1440 West Bannock Street
Boise, ID 83703
208-343-3639
Disability Served: physically disabled

This company manufactures a portable ramp for wheelchair users, a three-wheeled motorcycle, and a powered tricycle.

National Patient Care Systems Inc.

23 Poplar Street
East Rutherford, NJ 07073
800-876-BEDS
Disability Served: all

This company manufactures an air flotation mattress.

National Presto Industries

3925 North Hastings Way
Eau Claire, WI 54703
Disability Served: all

This company manufactures a food processor.

National Wheel-O-Vator Co., Inc.

509 West Front Street
Roanoke, IL 61561
800-551-9095
http://www.wheelovator.com
Disability Served: physically disabled

This company manufactures stairway chairlifts, vertical platform lifts, and private residence elevators.

Nationwide Emergency Alert Systems

PO Box 61331
Potomac, MD 20859
301-469-9564
Disability Served: all

This company makes a personal emergency call system.

Navitar
Division of DO Industries Inc.
200 Commerce Drive
Rochester, NY 14623-3589
716-359-4000
Disability Served: vision

Navitar manufactures a low-vision projection screen that allows the user to view greatly magnified images.

Nearly Me
PO Box 2501
Waco, TX 76702-2501
817-330-7500, 800-421-2322
Disability Served: physically disabled

This company designs bathing suits for women who have had mastectomies.

Nemectron Medical
28069 Diaz Road, Unit A
Temecula, CA 92390
800-428-4010
Disability Served: physically disabled

This company manufactures stimulators for pain management and muscle stimulation as well as a traction system.

Neurodyne Medical
51 Winchester Street
Newton, MA 02161
800-328-4266
Disability Served: physically disabled

This company manufactures an EMG feedback unit.

Neuropedic
120 North Abington Road
Clarks Summit, PA 18411
717-586-1323
Disability Served: physically disabled

This company manufactures motorized beds and orthopedic mattresses.

New Abilities Now, Inc.
PO Box 208
Excelsior, MN 55331
612-930-5216, 800-876-2300
Disability Served: physically disabled

This company manufactures carrying aids for wheelchairs and a commercial stand for wheelchairs.

New Dimensions Design
90127 West Demming Road
Elmira, OR 97437
541-935-3162
Disability Served: physically disabled

This company manufactures a hand-propelled cycle.

New Freedom Inc.
Clawur Rocker Shoe Company
PO Box 428
Rexburg, ID 83440
208-356-0061
Disability Served: all

This company manufactures wooden shoes designed to allow the wearer to walk without lifting his/her legs.

New York Telephone Co. Western Frontier Co.
65 Franklin Street, 1st Floor
Buffalo, NY 14202
716-824-7258
Disability Served: vision

This company manufactures a signal beacon used to locate buildings.

Next Page
394 Craigleith Drive
Waterloo, ON N2L 5T2 Canada
519-747-9444
Disability Served: all

This company manufactures the Next Page page turner, which is designed for any level of disability.

NFSS Communications

8120 Fenton Street
Silver Spring, MD 20910
888-589-6671
http://www.nfss.com
Disability Served: hearing

This company distributes and services assistive devices for the deaf and hard of hearing.

NIKKEN Inc.

10866 Wilshire Boulevard, #250
Los Angeles, CA 90024
Disability Served: all

This company manufactures therapeutic aids, including foam mattresses, massagers, support pillows, massaging shoe inserts, and support wraps.

NILFISK-Advance America Inc.

300 Technology Drive
Malvern, PA 19355
610-647-6420
http://www.pa.nilfisk-advance.com
Disability Served: all

This company manufactures a vacuum cleaner designed for persons with allergies.

NK and Associates, Inc.

3506 Clearwater Drive
Fayetteville, NC 28311
919-822-4747
Disability Served: physically disabled

This company makes a wide-angle-view peephole.

No Rinse Labs, LLC

900 East Franklin Street
Centerville, OH 45459
800-223-9348
http://www.NoRinse.com
Disability Served: all

This company makes no-rinse hair-care and body-care products, including shampoo, hair conditioner, and lotion.

Noir

6155 Pontiac Trail
PO Box 159
South Lyon, MI 48178
313-769-5565, 800-521-9746
Disability Served: vision

This company offers sunglasses that absorb ultraviolet and near infrared rays.

Nor-Am Patient Care Products Inc.

PO Box 543
Lewiston, NY 14092
716-285-7548
Disability Served: physically disabled

This company manufactures a hydraulic transfer lift that can be operated by one person.

Noraxon USA, Inc.

13430 North Scottsdale Road, #104
Scottsdale, AZ 85254-4057
800-848-4912
Disability Served: physically disabled

This company makes an EMG feedback unit.

North Coast Medical, Inc.

187 Stauffer Boulevard
San Jose, CA 95125-1042
408-283-1900, 800-821-9319
Disability Served: all

This company offers a wide array of daily living aids and health care products. Items range from back supports to jar openers to pantyhose aids.

Northern Electric Company

1501 East Woodfield Road, Suite 400N
Schaumburg, IL 60173-5402
847-267-5100
Disability Served: all

This company makes a variety of heating pads.

Northern Industrial Tool Co.

PO Box 49601
Blaine, MN 55449
612-786-6155
Disability Served: physically disabled

This company manufactures a carrying caddy for wheelchairs.

Northland Aluminum Products Inc.
5005 Highway 7
Minneapolis, MN 55416
612-920-2888
Disability Served: physically disabled

This company manufactures the Nordicware Microwave Micro Max, a cooking tool designed for persons with limited hand dexterity.

Northport, Inc.
3701 South Cedar Drive
Excelsior, MN 55331
612-474-7996
Disability Served: physically disabled

This company manufactures height-adjustable desks and work stations.

Norton Company Inc.
4910 West Linebaugh Avenue
Tampa, FL 33624
813-962-4012
Disability Served: physically disabled

This company makes a bowling game similar to skee ball and Stomper, a game in which lighted panels flash under the player and the player stomps on the panel that is lit. Stomper comes in a wheelchair version and a stand-up version.

Norton Door Controls
Yale Security Inc.
PO Box 25288
Charlotte, NC 28212
704-283-2101, 800-438-1951
Disability Served: physically disabled

This company manufactures door closers.

Nova Health Systems Inc.
409 VPR Commerce Center
Blackwood, NJ 08012
609-228-8833, 800-225-6682
Disability Served: physically disabled

This company manufactures an air pressure flotation mattress designed to prevent pressure sores.

Nova Technologies, Inc.
89 Cabot Court, Unit L
Hauppauge, NY 11788
516-434-8811
Disability Served: physically disabled

This company manufactures a motorized bed designed to transfer persons from bed to wheelchair.

Novo Nordisk Pharmaceuticals Inc.
100 Overlook Center, Suite 200
Princeton, NJ 08540-6213
609-987-5800
Disability Served: diabetes

This company makes an insulin injection aid that looks like a pen and uses insulin cartridges.

NTRON
104 Industrial Boulevard
Sugarland, TX 77478
915-472-4600, 800-777-8367
Disability Served: physically disabled

This company manufactures electrical nerve and muscle stimulators.

Nu Hope Laboratories Inc.
12640 Branford Street
Pacoima, CA 91331
818-899-7711
Disability Served: all

This company manufactures catheters, colostomy pouches, skin care products designed to protect the stoma area, and urinary pouches.

Nurion
Station Square, Building 2
Paoli, PA 19301
610-640-2345
Disability Served: vision

This company manufactures electronic guiding devices for the blind, deaf-blind, and visually impaired persons. Products include the Laser Cane and Polaron, which are both hand-held units. They also produce Pathfinders, which are devices for mounting on wheelchairs, scooters, or walkers.

Nytone, Inc.—Medical Division
2424 South 900 West
Salt Lake City, UT 84119
801-973-4090
http://www.stopbedwetting.net
Disability Served: all

This company manufactures an enuretic alarm for children with night-time enuresis. It is also used as a moisture detector for incontinence.

Oak Hill Industries Ltd.
6200 McKay Avenue, Suite 145-934
Burnaby, BC V5H 4M9 Canada
604-250-7859
Disability Served: physically disabled

This company manufactures powered transfer lifts.

Oakworks
PO Box 99
34 Main Street
Glen Rock, PA 17327-0099
717-235-6807, 800-558-8850
Disability Served: all

This company manufactures a variety of treatment tables and chairs for therapists.

Oberon Terrazzo Products
4260 Kearney Street
Denver, CO 80216
303-331-0304
Disability Served: physically disabled

This company manufactures shower basins that can be rolled in and out of bath areas.

OBUS Forme, Ltd.
550 Hopewell Avenue
Toronto, ON M6E 2S6 Canada
416-785-1386, 800-361-1378
Disability Served: back injury

This company manufactures back support cushions and therapeutic seat panels.

Ohio Medical Instrument Company Inc.
3924 Virginia Avenue
Cincinnati, OH 45227
513-561-2241
Disability Served: all

This company manufactures a support pillow designed for premature infants.

Olympic Fiberglass Industries Inc.
PO Box 920
East 4th Street
Rochester, IN 46975
219-223-3101
Disability Served: physically disabled

This company manufactures a wheelchair accessible portable toilet.

Olympic Medical
5900 First Avenue South
Seattle, WA 98108-3249
206-767-3500, 800-426-0353
http://olymed.com
Disability Served: all

This company manufactures a seating and positioning system that molds to the patient's figure.

Omni Group Inc.
PO Box 398
Timonium, MD 21094
410-296-5404
Disability Served: all

This company manufactures wireless emergency alert systems and closed circuit security/monitoring systems.

Omni Hearing Systems
3418 Midcourt, Suite 105
Carrollton, TX 75006
214-934-2961, 800-527-0872
Disability Served: hearing

This company manufactures hearing aids.

Omni Manufacturing Inc.

4355 International Boulevard
Norcross, GA 30093
800-554-9215
Disability Served: all

This company manufactures walkers, shower and tub benches and chairs, commodes, canes, recliners with seat lifts, motorized beds, and more.

Omni Scientific, Inc.

179 Mason Circle
Concord, CA 94520
510-682-1155, 800-448-6664
Disability Served: orthopedic

This company manufactures a knee brace.

Omron Healthcare, Inc.

300 Lakeview Parkway
Vernon Hills, IL 60061-1800
847-680-6200
Disability Served: all

This company manufactures an electronic thermometer, a harness restraint for strollers, and an electronic sphygmomanometer that provides a digital readout of blood pressure.

On The Wall

Teddi Kessie
13061 Hartsook Street
Sherman Oaks, CA 91423
818-784-1572
Disability Served: all

This company manufactures a wall-mounted, folding ironing board.

Ondine from Interbath Inc.

665 North Baldwin Park Boulevard
City of Industry, CA 91746-1502
626-369-1841, 800-423-9485
http://www.interbath.com
Disability Served: all

This company manufactures hand showers and accessories.

One Hand Stethoscope

PO Box 1406
4444 East Avenue R, Unit 127
Palmdale, CA 93550
805-947-0025
Disability Served: all

This company manufactures a one-hand stethoscope.

One Shoe Crew

86 Clavela Avenue
Sacramento, CA 95828-4647
916-634-SHOE
Disability Served: physically disabled

This company provides a shoe-sharing service for persons who need only one shoe. The company matches persons with the same shoe sizes.

One Step Closer

PO Box 691
Weston, MA 02193
508-653-6272
Disability Served: physically disabled

This company makes carrying accessories for wheelchairs.

One To One Communicators

1714 Penrose
Olathe, KS 66062
913-764-4072
Disability Served: hearing

This company develops a personal amplification system for persons with hearing impairments.

Open Sesame

1933 Davis Street, Suite 279
San Leandro, CA 94577
800-673-6911
http://www.opensesamedoor.com
Disability Served: physically disabled

This company manufactures remote control door systems primarily for quadriplegic individuals.

Optelec US, Inc.

6 Lyberty Way
Westford, MA 01886
800-828-1056
http://www.optelec.com
Disability Served: vision

This company manufactures video magnifiers and hand-held magnifiers for people with low vision.

Ora Genics

6409 SE Monroe
Milwaukie, OR 97222
503-224-2316
Disability Served: all

This company manufactures a toothbrush with suction control.

Oralgiene USA, Inc.

10920 Wilshire Boulevard, Suite 330
Los Angeles, CA 90024
213-824-6363, 800-368-6725
Disability Served: all

This company manufactures a battery-powered toothbrush.

Organization for Enhanced Capability, Inc.

502 Bedford Street, Suite 16
Fall River, MA 02720
800-733-4334
Disability Served: all

OEC offers services that monitor users' health and safety. Access911 Response Service provides a twenty-four-hour connection to friends, neighbors, health and safety needs, or even emergency response with the push of a button. CompuMed, an automated medication/vitamin dispenser, dispenses the proper amount of medication at the proper time, alerting the user with an alarm. It is monitored for any noncompliance issues. WanderWatch, a home-based wandering management system, creates a safety zone for anyone with a tendency to wander.

Ortho Concepts

285 Alpha Park
Highland Heights, OH 44143
216-449-8222
Disability Served: all

This company offers a modular seating system that can be fit to wheelchairs.

Ortho Mold Bracing Systems

646 Brookline Avenue
Brookline, MA 02146
617-232-1201, 800-344-1012
Disability Served: all

This company manufactures custom-molded back and arm orthoses.

Ortho Support Wraps

PO Box 816
Norco, CA 91760
714-737-5649, 800-854-5149
Disability Served: all

This company manufactures support wraps for ankles, backs, elbows, knees, wrists, thighs, and more.

Ortho-Kinetics Inc.

West 220 North 507 Springdale Road
PO Box 1647
Waukesha, WI 53187-1647
414-542-6060, 800-558-7786
Disability Served: all

This company offers aids to daily living, including shower and bath chairs, seat-lift recliners and chairs, walkers, commodes, and standers.

Orthomedics Inc.

2950 East Imperial Highway
Brea, CA 92621
714-996-9500, 800-854-3259
Disability Served: all

This company manufactures orthotics, including cervical supports, hip abduction splints, and adjustable sockets for prosthetic devices.

Orthopedic Physical Therapy Products

PO Box 47009
Minneapolis, MN 55447-0009
800-367-7393
http://www.optp.com
Disability Served: all

This company distributes physical therapy products including lumbar rolls, swiss balls, exercise devices, and stretching products.

Orthopedic Products Corp.

10381 Jefferson Boulevard
Culver City, CA 90232-3511
310-202-7766
Disability Served: all

This company manufactures back and seat supports and foot stools.

OrthoPro, Inc.

PO Box 10628
Reno, NV 89510
702-826-1866
Disability Served: physically disabled

This company manufactures a mono-ski for downhill skiing.

Orthotic Systems Inc.

PO Box 20262
Houston, TX 77025
713-666-7928
Disability Served: all

This company manufactures orthotics, including powered orthotics.

Osbon Medical Systems

PO Box 1478
Augusta, GA 30903-1478
706-821-6850, 800-438-8592
Disability Served: all

This company manufactures an erection aid for impotence.

Ostergaard Enterprises

3228 West Olive
Fresno, CA 93722
209-275-4695
Disability Served: physically disabled

This company makes a drink holder for wheelchairs, a camera mount for wheelchairs, tilting lapboards for wheelchairs, and canes.

Oticon, Inc.

29 Schoolhouse Road
PO Box 6724
Somerset, NJ 08875-6724
800-526-3921
http://www.oticonus.com
Disability Served: hearing

This company manufactures advanced hearing instruments and accessories, including 100 percent digital hearing instruments.

OtoSonic, Inc.

4200 West Bryn Mawr Avenue
Chicago, IL 60646
773-463-9173, 800-837-6642
Disability Served: hearing

This company manufactures hearing aids.

Otto Bock

3000 Xenium Lane North
Minneapolis, MN 55441
612-553-9464, 800-328-4058
http://www.ottobockus.com
Disability Served: all

This company offers both adult and pediatric seating systems as well as positioning support, mounting hardware, power and manual wheelchairs, bath and safety products, and pediatric mobility bases.

Oval Window Audio

33 Wildflower Court
Nederland, CO 80466
303-447-3607
http://www.ovalwindowaudio.com
Disability Served: hearing

This company manufactures hearing-assistance technologies and multisensory sound systems for hearing-impaired children and adults.

Overcast Cover Co.
1655 Middlefield Road
PO Box 122
Palo Alto, CA 94301
650-327-2188, 800-321-4467
Disability Served: all

This company manufactures and sells cast and dressings protectors for bathing and showering.

Overseer Electronic Visual Aids
6826 Logan Avenue South
Richfield, MN 55423
612-866-7606
Disability Served: vision

This company manufactures a low-vision reading system that magnifies the reading material by using a video monitor or television monitor.

OXO International
1536 Beech Street
Terre Haute, IN 47804
800-545-4411
Disability Served: all

This company manufactures kitchen utensils with rubber grips.

Pac All Carriers Inc.
2321 Carolton Road
Maitland, FL 32751
407-830-6604, 800-628-6672
Disability Served: physically disabled

This company makes carrying accessories for wheelchairs.

Pacific Lotus Technology, Inc.
411 108th Avenue NE, Suite 235
Bellevue, WA 98004
425-454-7374, 800-243-2710
TDD: 425-646-3085
Disability Served: hearing

This company manufactures telecaption decoders for persons with hearing impairments.

Page Net
1121 Industrial Road
San Carlos, CA 94070-4106
650-591-7900
Disability Served: hearing

This company manufactures a vibrating paging system for persons with hearing impairments.

Palco Laboratories
8030 Soquel Avenue
Santa Cruz, CA 95062
408-476-3151
Disability Served: all

This company manufactures medical aids, including puncture devices for blood tests, syringe injection aids, insulated coolers for carrying medication, and pediatric incontinence alarms.

Palmetto Technologies Inc.
PO Box 498
Duncan, SC 29334
803-576-2886
Disability Served: hearing

This company manufactures a telephone device that decodes touch-tone phone messages.

Panasonic Company
1 Panasonic Way
Mail Stop 2F3
Secaucus, NJ 07094
201-348-7000, 800-447-4700
Disability Served: all

Panasonic manufactures cassette recorders and players designed for the visually impaired, vibrating alarm clocks, a massage recliner, and hearing aids.

Paper Pak Products Inc.
1941 White Avenue
PO Box 1060
La Verne, CA 91750
909-392-1200
Disability Served: vision

This company makes a waterproof bed pad.

Papworth Industries Inc.
278 SW 33rd Court
Ft Lauderdale, FL 33315
954-525-7411
Disability Served: physically disabled

This company manufactures a wheelchair console that has storage shelves.

Para Medical Distributors
2020 Grand Avenue
PO Box 19777
Kansas City, MO 64141
800-245-3278
Disability Served: all

This company manufactures braces and supports, including cast boots, body socks, fracture socks, and elastic bandages.

Paradigm Enterprises Inc.
PO Box 339
Hixson, TN 37343-0339
615-877-7097
Disability Served: all

This company makes pill organizers as well as a smoke alarm for persons with hearing impairments.

ParaMed Exercise Equipment, Inc.
PO Box 6469
Jackson, MS 39282
601-354-2211, 800-844-4480
Disability Served: physically disabled

This company manufactures Nautilus weight and exercise machines for wheelchair users.

Parent's Helper, Inc.
RR 2, Box 1600
Campton, NH 03223
800-413-7446
http://www.childsafety.com
Disability Served: all

This company manufactures and markets the Be Alert—Children driveway warning signs to help protect playing children.

Parisi Enterprises, Inc.
23 Southward Avenue
Congers, NY 10920
914-268-5983
Disability Served: physically disabled

This company manufactures a powered door operator that is activated by the touch of a button.

Parity Inc.
PO Box 3593
Oak Park, IL 60303
800-848-3585
Disability Served: all

This company manufactures a child's swing.

Park Surgical Co. Inc.
5001 New Utrecht Avenue
Brooklyn, NY 11219
718-436-9200
Disability Served: communication

This company makes speech amplifiers and speech aids.

Parker Bath Developments Inc.
Village Green Business Center
805 Tela Drive
Gallatin, TN 37066
800-457-8827
Disability Served: all

This company manufactures a reclining whirlpool unit.

Passy-Muir, Inc.
4521 Campus Drive, PMB 273
Irvine, CA 92612
800-634-5397 (CA)
http://www.passy-muir.com
Disability Served: communication

This company manufactures the patented closed-position "no-leak" Passy-Muir Tracheostomy and Ventilator Speaking Valves.

Patient Care Corporation
PO Box 3716
Carson City, NV 89702
702-882-0300, 800-829-6006
Disability Served: physically disabled

This company makes an attendant-operated body positioner for bedridden patients.

Patient's Personal Needs Inc.
275 Centre Street
Holbrook, MA 02343
617-767-5776, 800-289-4776
Disability Served: physically disabled

This company manufactures a geriatric chair with a reclining back on a wheelchair frame.

PatientGuard Products, Inc.
4407 Old William Penn Highway
Murrysville, PA 15668
800-748-8273
Disability Served: vision

This company manufactures a waterproof bed underpad.

Patroni Armcycles
9005 Amherst Avenue
Margate, NJ 08402
609-823-8121
Disability Served: physically disabled, elderly

This company manufactures and sells arm-powered tricycles.

Patton Enterprise
PO Box 7100
Jacksonville, FL 32210
904-388-1182
Disability Served: physically disabled

This company manufactures the Active Life Glove for those with little or no hand dexterity. The glove can be used for exercise equipment and sport.

Pawling Corporation
Standard Products Division
PO Box 200
Wassaic, NY 12592
914-373-9300, 800-431-3456
Disability Served: all

This company develops hand rails and cushioned rubber mats that can be used as play surfaces.

PCP Champion
PO Box 125
Ripley, OH 45167-0125
513-392-4301, 800-888-0867
Disability Served: all

This company manufactures a number of items for people with disabilities. Products include canes, adjustable commodes, slings and supports, shoes, cushions, crutches, toilets, side rails, bath and shower benches, and walkers.

Peachtree Medical Systems
5002 North Royal Atlanta Drive, Suite P
Tucker, GA 30084
770-939-1122
Disability Served: physically disabled

This company makes a powered wheelchair controller that allows wheelchair control through head movement.

PECO Inc.
4707 SE 17th Avenue
PO Box 82189
Portland, OR 97282-0189
503-233-6401
Disability Served: all

This company manufactures a rolling cart with a wire basket ideal for shopping purposes.

Pedicraft
4134 St. Augustine Road
Jacksonville, FL 32207
904-396-9627, 800-223-7649
http://www.pedicraft.com
Disability Served: all

This company manufactures pediatric aids, including cribs, mesh-enclosed beds, infant slings, and therapeutic foam wedges.

Pelton Shepherd Industries

PO Box 30218
Stockton, CA 95213-0218
209-983-0893, 800-258-3423
Disability Served: all

This company manufactures hot and cold therapy packs and heating pads.

Penox Technologies Inc.

One Penox Plaza, Commerce Road
PO Box 785
Pittston, PA 18640
717-655-1421, 800-233-3029
Disability Served: all

This company manufactures an oxygen concentrator and container.

PEP Inc.

HC 06 Box 17
Park Rapids, MN 56470
218-732-1407
Disability Served: all

This company manufactures a vaporizer tent and a reflex positioner for infants.

Phillips & Brooks/Gladwin, Inc.

1485 Redi Road
PO Box 267
Cumming, GA 30130
404-887-9901
Disability Served: all

This company manufactures enclosures for pay telephones that meet ADA standards.

Phoenix Management, Inc.

5195 Fontaine Boulevard
Fountain, CO 80817
719-392-1442
Disability Served: hearing

This company provides a telecommunication device for the deaf that works with hearing aids.

Phoenix Poke Boats, Inc.

207 North Broadway
PO Box 109
Berea, KY 40403
606-986-2336
http://www.pokeboat.com
Disability Served: all

This company produces lightweight kayaks and poke boats used primarily for paddling, fishing, hunting, and photography.

Phonak, Inc.

850 East Diehl Road
PO Box 3017
Naperville, IL 60566
877-887-9905
Disability Served: hearing

This organization is a leading manufacturer of high-quality, high-performance hearing aids, including programmable and digital units as well as the world's smallest FM receiver for special communication needs.

Phonetics Inc.

901 Tryens Road
Aston, PA 19014
215-558-2700
Disability Served: all

This company makes an emergency alert system that is triggered by changes in the environment.

Phonics Phun

PO Box 716
Bryn Mawr, PA 19010
800-869-8336
http://www.learningdifferences.com
Disability Served: all

Phonics Phun teaches letter recognition, phonics, and words.

Physical Research Corporation

Box 189, Route 20
Charlton, MA 01507
617-248-5244
Disability Served: all

This company manufactures a suspension traction system and a thoracic bench designed to extend the thoracic and cervical vertebrae.

PI Professional Therapy Products

PO Box 1067
Athens, TN 37303
615-744-1395
http://www.pi-inc.com
Disability Served: all

This company manufactures a cold pack with an inflatable sleeve to provide pressure.

Pick A Lift Inc.

2051 East Edgewood Drive
Lakeland, FL 33803
941-665-5355, 800-328-5438
Disability Served: physically disabled

This company performs van modifications and manufactures van lifts and wheelchair carriers.

Pillow Place

1940 Moores Mill Road NW
Atlanta, GA 30318
800-832-2022
Disability Served: all

This company manufactures support cushions for the lower back and neck.

Pillow Talk Inc.

348 Pond Road
Freehold, NJ 07728
732-780-9483
Disability Served: all

This company makes allergy-proof waterproof mattress pads, total light-control drapes, and bed pillows.

Pilot Luggage

4670 Old Pike Road
Pilot, VA 24138
703-382-1056
Disability Served: physically disabled

This company manufactures wheelchair carrying accessories.

Pin Dot Products

6001 Gross Point Road
Niles, IL 60648-4027
847-774-1700, 800-451-3553
Disability Served: all

This company makes hardware, cushions, straps, shower chairs, and other aids to daily living and health care.

Pitts Corporation

4260 North 650 East
Provo, UT 84604
801-225-6441
Disability Served: communication

This company manufactures Eye-Com, a portable communication aid.

Plantronics

345 Encinal Street
Santa Cruz, CA 95060
800-544-4660
Disability Served: hearing

This company makes a microphone telephone headset and a phone amplifier.

Playground Environments Inc.

PO Box 578
22 Old Country Road
Quogue, NY 11959
516-653-5465, ext. 133
http://playgroundenvironments.com
Disability Served: all

This company designs and manufactures playground equipment.

Playskool
PO Box 200
Pawtucket, RI 02862
401-431-8697, 800-752-9755
Disability Served: all

Playskool develops toys and activities for children, including the 4-in-1 Busy Activity Center, which is designed to teach motor and mobility skills, and Kids of Color Dress-Me-Up Pal, a toy that helps children practice dressing activities.

Playskool Baby
108 Fairway Court
Northvale, NJ 07647
201-767-0900, 800-777-0371
Disability Served: all

This company makes pediatric aids, including travel cups, medicine spoons, bowls, bottle grippers, and the Tommee Tippee cup.

Plow & Hearth
301 Madison Road
Box 830
Orange, VA 22960
800-527-5247
Disability Served: all

This company makes a gardening container mounted on casters and a wheeled thatcher.

Plum Enterprises Inc.
9 Clyston Circle
PO Box 283
Worcester, PA 19490
215-584-5003
Disability Served: all

This company makes protective helmets.

Ply Gems Barrier Free
6948 Frankford Avenue
Philadelphia, PA 19135
215-331-3434
Disability Served: physically disabled

This company manufactures door hinges to widen the width of doors for wheelchair accessibility.

Polar Ware Co.
2806 North 15th Street
PO Box 211
Sheboygan, WI 53082-0211
920-458-3561
http://www.polarware.com
Disability Served: all

This company manufactures bedpans, sitz baths, and male urinals.

Poppin and Company Communication Materials
PO Box 176
Unity, ME 04988
207-437-2746
Disability Served: all

This company specializes in AAC, articulation, and language materials that use DynaSyms, the symbols on DynaVox devices.

Porta Ramps
Division of Young Enterprises
5592 East La Palma Avenue
Anaheim, CA 92807
714-970-0683, 800-654-7267
Disability Served: physically disabled

This company manufactures portable fiberglass ramps, van ramps, and ramp hand rails for wheelchair use.

Portable Isokinetics Inc.
3522 Lousma Drive SE
Grand Rapids, MI 49548
616-243-5105
Disability Served: all

This company manufactures exercise equipment for isometric exercise.

Porter Shower of America Inc.
3 Dunham Road
Billerica, MA 01821-5728
800-422-0098
Disability Served: physically disabled

This company manufactures a portable shower with ramp.

Porto Lift Corporation
PO Box 5
Higgins Lake, MI 48627
517-821-6688
Disability Served: physically disabled

This company makes a hydraulic patient lift and accessories.

Pos-T-Vac, Inc.
1701 North 14th Avenue
PO Box 1436
Dodge City, KS 67801
800-279-7434
Disability Served: all

This company makes an erection aid for impotency.

Positive Image Orthotics, Inc.
1002 Commons Way
Toms River, NJ 08755
732-286-0690
Disability Served: all

This company provides cosmetic enhancement for orthotic and prosthetic devices.

Positron Industries
5101 Buchan Street
Montreal, QC H4P 2K9 Canada
514-345-2200
TDD: 514-731-8690
Disability Served: hearing

This company manufactures a text telephone for the deaf that can be connected to a home computer.

Postcraft Company
625 West Rillito Street
Tucson, AZ 85705
800-528-4844
http://www.postcraft.com
Disability Served: all

This company manufactures mattress and pillow protectors as well as shower curtains.

Posture Comfort Cushion Co.
59-29 174th Street
Fresh Meadows, NY 11365
718-631-1734
Disability Served: all

This company makes foam seat cushions.

PosturMate Inc.
139 Burke Lane
Kneeland, CA 95549
707-445-4841
Disability Served: physically disabled

This company manufactures a height-adjustable desk.

Power Access Corporation
106 Powder Mill Road
42 Bridge Street
Collinsville, CT 06022
860-693-0751, 800-344-0088
http://www.power-access.com
Disability Served: physically disabled

This company makes a powered door opener.

PPP Enterprises: 'Lastic Laces
2027 Pheasant Creek Drive
Martinez, GA 30907
706-855-7059
http://webehave.com
Disability Served: physically disabled

This company manufactures 'Lastic Laces—a curly, spring elastic lace available in many colors. Once inserted, shoes never have to be tied again. PPP Enterprises also manufactures incentives for children for use with toilet training and general behavior.

Practical Answers
2616 D Philadelphia Pike, Suite 102 D
Claymont, DE 19703
800-553-6748
Disability Served: all

This company makes a toilet seat cleaner ideal for cleaning public toilet seats before use.

Pre Vocational Training Systems
PO Box 183
Sparta, MI 49345
616-887-1685
Disability Served: developmentally disabled

This company develops a work simulator used for vocational training of persons with mental disabilities.

Pre-Cast Reddi-Ramp, Inc.
PO Box 2288
Lenox, MA 01240
413-637-2644
Disability Served: physically disabled

This company manufactures a modular, concrete ramp to accommodate wheelchairs.

Precious Bundles
7882 South Valentia Way
Englewood, CO 80112
303-220-5572
Disability Served: all

This company manufactures a horseshoe-shaped support pillow that can be used for back support, reading, nursing, and more.

Precision Acoustics
501 Fifth Avenue, Suite 704
New York, NY 10017
212-986-6470
Disability Served: hearing

This company manufactures auditory and speech trainers for persons with hearing disabilities.

PRECO Products
8019 Flood Road
Baltimore, MD 21222
410-285-1135, 800-426-6503
Disability Served: physically disabled

This company manufactures walkers, crutches, bath aids such as toilet seats and commodes, and handgrip cushions.

PrePak Products
4055 Oceanside Boulevard, Suite K
Department M/D-1A
Oceanside, CA 92056
760-643-0390
http://www.prepak.com
Disability Served: all

This company manufactures exercise and therapeutic equipment, including shoulder pulleys and weight bags. The company also offers arm slings and massage creams.

Preso Matic Lock Co. Inc.
3048 Industrial 33rd Street
Ft Pierce, FL 34946
305-465-7400
Disability Served: all

This company manufactures keyless locks for doors.

Prevent Care Products Inc.
1006 Arnold Avenue
Point Pleasant, NJ 08742
732-295-8092
http://improvetoothbrush.com
Disability Served: all

This company makes the Improve toothbrush, which makes it possible to brush at a 45-degree angle for effective plaque reduction at the gumline.

Pride Health Care, Inc.
71 South Main Street
Pittston, PA 18640
717-655-5574, 800-800-8586
Disability Served: physically disabled

This company manufactures lift chairs, recliner chairs, and scooters.

Primak Educational Foundation
PO Box 701
Devon, PA 19333
610-644-6435, 800-444-5729
Disability Served: developmentally disabled

This company provides curricula and training for teachers of children who are developmentally three through six years old. Programs exist in perceptual development, oral language, early math, and science.

Principle Business Enterprises, Inc.

PO Box 129
Pine Lake Industrial Park
Dunbridge, OH 43414-0129
419-352-1551, 800-467-3224
http://www.gopeach.com
Disability Served: physically disabled

This company manufactures incontinence garments and pads.

Priva Inc.

PO Box 448
Champlain, NY 12919-0448
800-761-8881
http://www.priva-inc.com
Disability Served: all

This company manufactures and distributes reusable incontinence care products and aids to daily living.

Pro Massage Co.

PO Box 9220
Denver, CO 80209
303-722-2225, 800-947-1470
Disability Served: all

This company manufactures a neuromuscular stimulator to relieve and treat pain.

PRO MAX

2200 NE 65th Avenue, #C
Vancouver, WA 98661
360-694-7722, 800-654-3539
Disability Served: all

This company makes a resistive arm exerciser.

Pro Orthopedic Devices, Inc.

PO Box 31401
Tucson, AZ 85751
520-294-4401, 800-523-5611
http://www.proorthopedic.com
Disability Served: all

This company manufactures braces for ankles, knees, elbows, lower backs, wrists, and more.

Procter and Gamble Co.

PO Box 599
Cincinnati, OH 45201
800-543-0480
Disability Served: vision

This company makes Attends disposable diapers for adults.

Prodyne

PO Box 212
Montclair, CA 91763
714-628-1316
Disability Served: all

This company manufactures a cheese slicer that is a cutting board with a wire cutting arm.

Professional Medical Products

PO Box 3288
Greenwood, SC 29648
803-223-4281, 800-845-4571
Disability Served: physically disabled

This company manufactures incontinence garments and pads.

Profex Medical Products

8013 Maryland Avenue
PO Box 16043
St Louis, MO 63105
314-727-2996, 800-325-0196
Disability Served: all

This company makes a foam mattress.

Promenade Inc.

1004 East Jefferson Street
Charlottesville, VA 22901
804-296-3980
Disability Served: physically disabled

This company manufactures carrying bags that attach to crutches.

Prospect Designs

11 Prospect Street
New Hartford, CT 06057
203-379-7858
Disability Served: all

This company manufactures adjustable chairs for children.

Prospect Marketing
60 East Main
PO Box 479
Stockbridge, MA 01262
413-298-4371
Disability Served: all

This company develops a book that attaches to refrigerators and is designed to teach the alphabet.

Pure Flite Gear
4321 NE 16th Avenue
Pompano Beach, FL 33064
954-784-0800
Disability Served: physically disabled

This company manufactures carrying bags for persons with physical disabilities.

PW Minor & Sons
3 Treadeasy Avenue
Batavia, NY 14020
716-343-1500
Disability Served: all

This company manufactures women's shoes.

Qualitone
Hearing Aids & Audiometers
4931 West 35th Street
Minneapolis, MN 55416
612-927-7161, 800-328-3897
Disability Served: hearing

This company manufactures hearing aids.

Quality Lifestyles
PO Box 1365
Carrollton, GA 30117
270-834-2013, 800-466-4675
Disability Served: physically disabled

This company manufactures a seating and standing lift cushion that helps people get up or down from any chair.

Quest Electronics
510 South Worthington Street
Oconomowoc, WI 53066
414-567-9157, 800-245-0779
Disability Served: hearing

This company manufactures paging systems for persons with hearing impairments.

Quick Deck Inc.
PO Box 607
Livermore, CA 94550
510-449-8686
Disability Served: physically disabled

This company manufactures a modular ramp.

Quick Q Industry
PO Box 684
Duncansville, PA 16635
814-695-6897, 800-852-8750
Disability Served: all

This company manufactures a spring-activated pool cue.

R & H Adaptive Equipment Co.
PO Box 175
Thompson, IA 50478
515-584-2025, 800-255-6956
Disability Served: physically disabled

This company manufactures support frames and seating systems for persons with physical disabilities.

R. C. Musson Rubber Co.
1320 Archwood Avenue
PO Box 7038
Akron, OH 44306
330-773-7651
Disability Served: all

This company manufactures a nonslip stair tread covering made of rubber.

R. G. Abernethy Inc.
PO Box 11733
Winston-Salem, NC 27116
919-768-6544, 800-334-0128
Disability Served: all

This company makes custom orthopedic shoes.

R. Smith Company
PO Box 5175
Emerald Isle, NC 28594-5175
Disability Served: all

This company manufactures magnification mirrors on stands.

R.E.A.L. Design Inc.
187 South Main Street
Dolgeville, NY 13329
315-429-3071, 800-696-2041
http://www.disabilitymall.com/REAL/
Disability Served: cerebral palsy

This company manufactures pediatric rehabilitation products, including seating systems and wheelchair tables.

Radventure, Inc.
20755 SW 238th Place
Sherwood, OR 97140
503-628-2895
Disability Served: all

This company manufactures and distributes Yetti mono-skis and outriggers for adults and children who enjoy snow skiing.

Railnet
PO Box 9077
Missoula, MT 59807-9077
800-221-3584
Disability Served: all

This company manufactures netting designed to be attached to railings to provide barriers for infants and toddlers.

Rainshine Co.
PO Box 5615
Madison, WI 53705-0615
608-257-9330
Disability Served: vision

This company manufactures white canes for persons with visual impairments.

RAM Marketing Inc.
1641 Broad Street
Greensburg, PA 15601-5403
412-837-5811, 800-833-9002
Disability Served: physically disabled

This company manufactures a canvas sling that can be used as a manual transfer device or as an emergency evacuation carrier.

Rampus Inc.
PO Box 37
Coldwater, MI 49036
800-876-9498
Disability Served: physically disabled

This company manufactures a variety of ramps.

Rand-Scot Incorporated
401 Linden Center Drive
Ft Collins, CO 80524
970-484-7967, 800-467-7967
http://www.easypivot.com
Disability Served: physically disabled

This company manufactures the EasyPivot Patient Lifting system for strain-free lifting and toileting of the disabled individual.

Ransberg
PO Box 1727
Columbus, IN 47202-1727
812-372-2284
Disability Served: all

This company manufactures an acrylic bathroom caddy.

RAR Enterprises
PO Box 126
Round Mountain, TX 78663
512-825-3242, 800-231-3553
Disability Served: all

This company manufactures bath aids and fixtures, including grab bars, faucets and handles, towel dispensers, and accessible lavatories.

Raychem Corp.
300 Constitution Drive
Menlo Park, CA 94025
650-361-3333
Disability Served: all

This company develops a snow melting and anti-icing system for use on concrete pavement.

RCA Rubber Company
1833 East Market Street
PO Box 9240
Akron, OH 44305-0240
330-784-1291, 800-321-2340
Disability Served: vision

This company manufactures the Glo Strip, a nonslip stair tread covering that glows in the dark to accommodate persons with visual impairments.

RD Equipment, Inc.
230 Percival Drive
West Barnstable, MA 02668
508-362-7498
http://www.capecod.net/rdequip
Disability Served: all

This company produces the Electric Leg Bag Emptier and the Tub Slide Shower Chair.

RDM Sales
PO Box 95
North Hollywood, CA 91603
818-851-2786
Disability Served: hearing

This company manufactures a telephone cutoff switch and a voice amplifier for telephones.

Re Heater Inc.
15828 South Broadway, Suite C
Gardena, CA 90248
310-719-9582, 800-331-7066
Disability Served: all

This company manufactures a reusable heat pack.

RE TEC—Rehabilitation Technologies
121 Haven Ridge
Peachtree City, GA 30269
404-351-4486
Disability Served: physically disabled

This company manufactures carrying bags for wheelchairs, restraints, lapboards, push gloves, and wheels.

Reach Paging System, Inc.
PO Box 30193
Bethesda, MD 20824
301-601-8733, 800-875-2724
Disability Served: hearing

This company manufactures an emergency paging system for the hearing impaired.

Reb Manufacturing, Inc.
PO Box 276
Carey, OH 43316
419-396-7651
Disability Served: physically disabled

This company manufactures electrohydraulic lifts and gravity lifts for vans and building exteriors.

Red Line Supply Inc.
15020 63rd Street, Court E
Sumner, WA 98390
206-474-1145
Disability Served: all

This company makes a plastic headset attachment for telephones.

REDCO
1055 36th Street
Grand Rapids, MI 49501-2994
616-248-3000
Disability Served: physically disabled

This company manufactures height-adjustable work tables for wheelchair users.

REDD Team Manufacturing, Inc./Universal Ramp Systems

6587 State Route 21
Keystone Heights, FL 32656
352-473-7246, 800-648-3696
http://www.reddteam.com
Disability Served: all

This company builds prefabricated modular aluminum access ramps designed to accommodate everyone, regardless of means of mobility. Custom and standard applications are available.

Reese Enterprises Inc.

PO Box 459
Rosemount, MN 55068
612-423-1126, 800-334-8823
Disability Served: physically disabled

This company manufactures aluminum ramps and thresholds.

Regency Elevator Products Corp.

870 Mount Prospect Avenue
Newark, NJ 07104
201-481-1400
Disability Served: physically disabled

This company manufactures an elevator call button designed to accommodate wheelchair users.

Rehab Centre for Children

633 Wellington Crest
Winnipeg, MB R3M 0A8 Canada
204-452-4311
Disability Served: all

This community-based company provides a broad range of specialty clinics, physiotherapy and occupational therapy, a preschool Developmental Day Program, assessment and fabrication of special aids, and a communication program.

Rehab Plus Therapeutic Products Inc.

6104 45th Street, #D
Lubbock, TX 79407-3742
806-791-2288, 800-288-8059
Disability Served: all

This company makes ankle and wrist weights.

Rehabilicare Inc.

1811 Old Highway 8
New Brighton, MN 55112-1828
612-631-0590, 800-551-7939
http://www.rehabilicare.com
Disability Served: physically disabled

This company makes an electrical stimulator for home or clinical use and a transcutaneous electrical nerve stimulator (TENS) unit.

Rehabilitation Technical Components, Inc.

PO Box 784
1256 Liberty Avenue
Hillside, NJ 07205
908-687-8275
Disability Served: all

This company manufactures orthotics, aluminum holders designed to hold utensils, and wheelchair hardware.

Rehabilitative Health Products

3950 Atlantic Avenue, Suite 59
Long Beach, CA 90807
562-423-2750
Disability Served: physically disabled

This company manufactures a passive motion exerciser designed for wheelchair users.

Rehrig International

901 North Lombardy Street
Richmond, VA 23220
804-656-5876, 800-446-2729
Disability Served: physically disabled

This company makes a shopping cart for wheelchairs.

Relaxo Bak Inc.

PO Box 812
319 East California Street
Gainesville, TX 76240
800-752-8889
Disability Served: back injury

This company manufactures a plastic back support.

Reliable Fire Equipment Co.
12845 South Cicero Avenue
Alsip, IL 60658
708-597-4600
Disability Served: hearing

This company manufactures a flashing smoke alarm.

Remston Electronics Corporation
PO Box 31
Itasca, IL 60143
800-797-6565
Disability Served: physically disabled

This company makes a paging system so individuals needing wheelchair service into a building can notify attendants inside the building to provide wheelchair service.

REON
7486 La Jolla Boulevard, #555
La Jolla, CA 92037
619-450-1325, 800-776-7366
Disability Served: all

This company makes showerheads and soap dispensers for home use.

Repetitive Motion Trauma Corporation
810 Arlington Heights Road
Itasca, IL 60143
847-285-8900, 800-860-RMTC
Disability Served: all

This company makes a hand exerciser designed for persons overcoming Carpal Tunnel Syndrome.

ReSound Corporation
220 Saginaw Drive
Seaport Centre
Redwood City, CA 94063
800-582-4327
Disability Served: hearing

This company manufactures hearing aids.

Resources for Industry
RD 3, Box 12
Prospect Avenue
Walton, NY 13856-9711
607-865-7184
Disability Served: all

This company makes a height-adjustable work table.

Respironics Inc.
1001 Murry Ridge Drive
Murrysville, PA 15668-8517
412-733-0200
Disability Served: all

This company manufactures an apnea respiration monitor.

Rhamdec, Inc.
476 Ellis Street
Mountain View, CA 94043-2240
650-965-3251, 800-428-0620
Disability Served: physically disabled

This company manufactures various lapboards and mounting hardware.

RHM Enterprises
PO Box 19948
Houston, TX 77024
713-493-3353, 800-669-3353
Disability Served: all

This company manufactures adjustable foam positioning cushions called Sta-On-Pads.

Richer Life of Iowa
Box 12
Boyden, IA 51234
712-725-2334
Disability Served: physically disabled

This company manufactures an exercise machine designed for persons with physical disabilities.

Ricon Corporation
12450 Montague Street
Pacoima, CA 91331
818-899-7588, 800-322-2884
Disability Served: physically disabled

This company makes powered driver seat bases and van lifts.

Ridgley Enterprises

16161 Ventura Boulevard, Suite 744
Encino, CA 91436
818-788-7322
Disability Served: all

This company makes a battery-operated spice dispenser that is operated by pushing a button.

Ridon Group Inc.

PO Box 31042
Palm Beach Gardens, FL 33418
561-627-9647, 800-628-7812
Disability Served: physically disabled

This company manufactures a shower cabinet.

Rifton Equipment

Route 213
Rifton, NY 12471-0901
800-777-4244
http://www.rifton.com
Disability Served: physically disabled

This company works with teachers and therapists to develop products for positioning and mobilizing children with disabilities for functional activity.

RIKO Medical & Scientific Instrument Corp.

600 Sylvan Avenue
Englewood Cliffs, NJ 07632-3101
516-354-3080, 800-222-7456
Disability Served: all

This company manufactures Pocket Potty, a disposable urinal.

Rimball Inc.

PO Box 5785
Peoria, IL 61601
309-688-7515
Disability Served: all

This company makes basketball backstops.

Rinz LO Pillow Company

340 West Maplehurst
Ferndale, MI 48220
248-548-3993
Disability Served: all

This company manufactures support cushions and pillows.

Rival Manufacturing Co.

36th and Bennington
Kansas City, KS 64129
913-861-1000
Disability Served: all

This company manufactures a slow cooker.

Rixson Firemark

Division of Conrac Corporation
9100 West Belmont Avenue
Franklin Park, IL 60131
847-671-5670
Disability Served: all

This company manufactures an automatic door closer.

Rock N' Roll Marketing

PO Box 1558
Levelland, TX 79336
806-894-5700, 800-654-9664
http://www.rocknrollcycles.com
Disability Served: physically disabled

This company provides therapy cycles for those from age two to adult.

Rogers Engineering Corporation

4805B Eisenhower Avenue
Alexandria, VA 22304
703-370-5628
Disability Served: all

This company manufactures a remote control security system for persons with hearing and physical disabilities.

ROHO, Inc.

100 North Florida Avenue
PO Box 658
Belleville, IL 62221
618-277-9150, 800-851-3449
http://www.roho.inc
Disability Served: all

This company manufactures assorted therapeutic cushions and accessories.

Rol Fol Table Inc.

30916 Broadbeach Road
Malibu, CA 90265-2664
Disability Served: all

This company manufactures height-adjustable drafting tables and work tables.

Rollins Protective Services Co.

2170 Piedmont Road
Atlanta, GA 30324
404-252-4440
Disability Served: all

This company manufactures a computerized security system.

Roloke Company

5760 Hannum Avenue
Culver City, CA 90230
310-649-1807, 800-533-8212
Disability Served: all

This company manufactures support cushions, cervical pillows, heating pads, and furniture leg extenders.

Romet, Inc.

PO Box 31
Chester, VA 23831
800-758-8255
Disability Served: communication

This company manufactures augmentative and alternative communication aids for the nonspeaking population.

Rouse Communicator

2140 Woodbury Place
Escondido, CA 92026
760-743-5145
Disability Served: communication

This one-man shop makes the Rouse Communicator as a hobby. The owner does not sell them but gives them away to nonvocal persons to facilitate communication.

Royal Doulton

700 Cottontail Lane
Somerset, NJ 08873
201-356-7880
Disability Served: all

This company manufactures ceramic plates and other housewares.

Royalcare Systems/Royal Industries International

Route 14, Box 230
Highway 64 West
Morganton, NC 28655
704-433-5909, 800-843-9750
Disability Served: physically disabled

This company manufactures a shopping basket that attaches to wheelchairs.

Royce Medical Products

PO Box 1368
Culver City, CA 90232-0601
800-521-0601
http://www.roycemedical.com
Disability Served: all

This company manufactures splints, supports, and immobilizers.

Rugg Manufacturing Company

105 Newton Street
Greenfield, MA 01301
413-773-5471
http://www.rugg.com
Disability Served: back injury

This company manufactures snow shovels, push brooms, and lawn rakes designed to lessen stress on the back.

Rystan Company, Inc.
47 Center Avenue
PO Box 214
Little Falls, NJ 07424-0214
201-256-3737
Disability Served: all

This company makes an odor control tablet taken by patients to control bowel odor that can result from incontinence, colostomy, or ileostomy.

S & S Worldwide
PO Box 513
Colchester, CT 06415-0513
800-243-9232
Disability Served: all

This company manufactures cross stitch patterns for persons with low vision, magnifying lenses, large crayons, self-opening scissors, and training scissors.

S & W Enterprises, Inc.
10044 Goodhue Street NE
Blaine, MN 55449
800-328-1281, 612-786-2808
Disability Served: all

This company manufactures wooden products for medical and physical therapy needs.

S&S Adaptability
75 Mill Street
Colchester, CT 06415-0513
800-243-9232
Disability Served: all

This company makes furniture, games, workstations, cabinets, and other products to help people with disabilities.

S&S Manufacturing Import/Export Co.
PO Box 2485
York, PA 17405
717-843-2745
Disability Served: all

This company makes a lapboard that attaches to wheelchairs, hospital beds, and upholstered chairs.

S. A. Richards, Inc.
PO Box 1037
Ft Lee, NJ 07024
201-947-3850, 800-722-6403
Disability Served: all

This company makes a bookholder for hands-free reading.

S. Walters Inc.
30423 Canwood Street, Suite 115
Agoura Hills, CA 91301
818-706-2202, 800-992-5837
http://ourworld.compuserve.com/homepages/walters_low_vision
Disability Served: vision

This company provides low-vision optics and manufactures and distributes the Seewell Reading Enhancer.

Safe Care Products Inc.
60525 Decatur Road
Cassopolis, MI 49031
616-445-2413
Disability Served: all

This company manufactures child proof appliance plug locks, electrical outlet plates, cabinets, and extension cord covers. The company also makes inflatable bathtub cushions.

Safe Guard Surfacing Corp.
PO Box 801
St James, NY 11780
516-862-1276, 800-899-8703
Disability Served: all

This company makes a rubber mat and ground retention grid designed to prevent injuries and falls on playgrounds and other surfaces.

Safe T Bath
185 Millbury Avenue
Millbury, MA 01527
508-865-2361
Disability Served: all

This company manufactures a fiberglass, elevated bathtub.

Safe T Spin Inc.
21380 Lorain Road
Fairview Park, OH 44126
216-333-2323
Disability Served: physically disabled

This company manufactures a car emergency sign designed for drivers with disabilities to call for help.

Safe-Stride of Iowa
305 West Montgomery Street
Knoxville, IA 50138
515-842-2442, 800-682-5159
Disability Served: all

This company manufactures a nonslip floor coating that can be used on a bathtub surface.

Safeline Children's Products Co.
5335 West 48th Avenue, #300
Denver, CO 80212-2709
303-455-8335
Disability Served: all

This company manufactures a child car seat that can be converted into a stroller unit with one hand.

SafeTek International Inc.
PO Box 23
Melbourne, FL 32902
407-952-1300
Disability Served: physically disabled

This company manufactures bath aids, including bars, shower and tub benches and seats, and whirlpools.

Safety Operating Systems
415 North State Street, Suite 120
Lake Oswego, OR 97034
503-697-7267
Disability Served: all

This company manufactures a posture switch that alerts the wearer of the switch when he/she bends up to a ninety-degree angle.

Salco Toys, Inc.
11445 150th Street East
Nerstrand, MN 55053
507-645-8720
Disability Served: all

This company manufactures toys designed for active stimulation, including large-handled, wooden puzzles and form boards with one to nine pieces. They also produce magnetic manipulators, trackers, and puzzle switches.

Salk Co.
119 Braintree Street
PO Box 452
Boston, MA 02134
617-782-4030
Disability Served: physically disabled

This company manufactures incontinence garments and aids for men and women.

Sammons Preston
4 Sammons Court
Bolingbrook, IL 60440
630-226-1300, 800-323-5547
TDD: 800-325-1745
http://www.sammonspreston.com
Disability Served: physically disabled

This company provides products that help disabled people manage physical challenges and achieve the highest level of independence.

Samson Dynamics
43 Niguel Pointe
Laguna Niguel, CA 92677
714-363-1627, 800-728-2278
Disability Served: all

This company manufactures an arm and leg exerciser that can be used in both active and passive modes.

Sani Fem Corp.
PO Box 4117
Downey, CA 90241
800-542-5580
http://www.freshette.com
Disability Served: all

This company manufactures a portable urinal that can be used by men or women.

Sani Med
PO Box 1367
1 Tuffy Lane
Columbus, MS 39703
662-328-4000
Disability Served: physically disabled

This company manufactures elevated toilet seats and support arms for toilets.

Sanlex International Corp.
PO Box 14717
Dayton, OH 45414
937-297-3011, 800-424-1224
Disability Served: all

This company manufactures a bidet.

Saratoga Access & Fitness, Inc.
PO Box 1427
Ft Collins, CO 80522-1427
970-484-4010, 800-474-4010
http://www.saratoga-intl.com/fitness
Disability Served: physically disabled

This company manufactures and distributes exercise equipment for people with disabilities.

Sargent and Co.
100 Sargent Drive
New Haven, CT 06509
203-562-2151
Disability Served: all

This company makes panic bars for doors.

SASCO Products, Inc.
25972 Novi Road, #201
Novi, MI 48375
248-449-6684, 800-660-1002
Disability Served: all

This company manufactures self-adhesive products such as the Invisible Corner Guard, a flexible tape that is abrasion-resistant and intended to protect painted and wallpapered corners.

Savaria Inc.
1011 Highway #13
Chomedey Laval, QC H7W 4V3 Canada
514-681-5655
Disability Served: physically disabled

This company makes wheelchair platform lifts and residential elevators.

Scale-Tronix
200 East Post Road
White Plains, NY 10601
914-948-8117
Disability Served: all

This company manufactures scales, including chair, floor, ramp, and wheelchair scales.

Schindler Elevator Corp.
20 Whippany Road
PO Box 1935
Morristown, NJ 07962-1935
973-397-6500
http://www.us.schindler.com
Disability Served: physically disabled

This company offers an elevator call button for persons with disabilities. All elevators manufactured by this company meet or exceed ADA requirements.

Schlage Lock Co.
2401 Bayshore Boulevard
San Francisco, CA 94134
415-541-8881
Disability Served: all

This company manufactures security systems and door locks, including keyless door locks.

Schuco Inc.
1419 Expressway Drive North
Toledo, OH 43608
419-726-9000, 800-645-2500
Disability Served: all

This company manufactures portable nebulizers and aspirators.

Schukra of North America Ltd.
310 Carlingview Drive
Etobicoke, ON M9W 5G1 Canada
800-663-7248
Disability Served: all

This company designs back support cushions.

Schwinn Bicycle Co.
1690 38th Street
Boulder, CO 80301-2602
303-454-7400
Disability Served: all

This company manufactures an exercise ergometer.

Scott Designs
2169 Las Positas Court, Suite C
Livermore, CA 94550
510-294-1700
Disability Served: physically disabled

This company manufactures supports, pads, straps, wheelchairs, and hardware.

Scott Health Care Products
Scott Plaza
Philadelphia, PA 19113
800-992-9939
Disability Served: vision

This company manufactures incontinence aids and garments.

Scott Orthopedics Inc.
PO Box 12207
5300 West 44th Avenue
Denver, CO 80212
303-423-8510, 800-821-5795
Disability Served: all

This company manufactures orthoses.

Scott Sign Systems, Inc.
PO Box 1047
Tallevast, FL 34270-1047
800-237-9447
http://www.scottsigns.com
Disability Served: vision

This company manufactures and supplies signs, architectural systems, and component parts produced from a variety of materials, including plastic, acrylic, foam, vinyl, and wood. Standard and custom offerings include signs to comply with ADA.

Scott Specialties
PO Box 129
Belleville, KS 66935
913-527-5627, 800-255-7136
Disability Served: all

This company manufactures a number of restraints, pads, orthopedic shoes, and supports.

SCU Marketing Inc.
Shepherd Care Unit
PO Box 190
Ashland, KY 41105-0190
606-324-9713
Disability Served: physically disabled

This company makes a wheelchair-accessible shower unit.

Second Chance Manufacturing Co.
14335 Sherman Way, #125
Van Nuys, CA 91405
818-901-7595
Disability Served: physically disabled

This company manufactures a wire basket that attaches to wheelchairs.

Secure Care Products Inc.
104 High Street
Boscawen, NH 03303-2602
603-225-7838, 800-451-7917
Disability Served: all

This company manufactures a wandering patient detection system.

Security Components
17880 Sky Park Circle, Unit 101
Irvine, CA 92714
714-250-8753
Disability Served: all

This company manufactures an electronic safe that has keypad access.

Security Engineering Inc.
560 Birch Street
PO Box 9337
Forestville, CT 06010
203-584-9158
Disability Served: all

This company manufactures a remote control deadbolt lock.

Security Tag Systems
1615 118th Avenue North
St Petersburg, FL 33716-2302
813-576-6399, 800-451-6610
Disability Served: all

This company manufactures a wandering patient detection system.

See A Need
8864 Kalmar Drive
Colorado Springs, CO 80920
719-282-0141
Disability Served: vision

This company manufactures the RedLite, an optical pointer to use with communication boards.

Seeing Technologies Inc.
7074 Brooklyn Boulevard
Minneapolis, MN 55429
612-560-8080, 800-462-3738
Disability Served: vision

This company manufactures a magnification reading system for persons with visual impairments.

Seiko Corporation of America
1111 MacArthur Boulevard
Mahawah, NJ 07430
201-529-5730
Disability Served: vision

Seiko manufactures talking watches and clocks for persons with limited vision.

Selcom Inc.
21654 Melrose
Southfield, MI 48075
248-355-5900
Disability Served: all

This company manufactures an electronic motion evaluation system.

SEMCO
N9096 Dairyland Drive
PO Box 451
Cleveland, WI 53015
877-736-2663, 920-693-2824
http://www.quadjoy.com
Disability Served: all

This company manufactures a computer mouse for quadriplegics. The mouse can be mounted on a computer workstation and activated through sip and puff maneuvers.

SENCO Inc.
PO Box 306
Marquette, MI 49855
906-225-0274
Disability Served: all

This company manufactures a wheelchair accessible camouflage blind for rifle or bow hunting.

Senior Technologies/WanderGuard
1620 North 20th Street
PO Box 80238
Lincoln, NE 68501-0238
402-475-4002, 800-824-2996
http://www.seniortechnologies.com
Disability Served: all

This company manufactures a departure alert system mobility monitors, a wireless communications system, and delayed-egress magnetic locks.

Sennheiser Electronic Corporation
PO Box 987
6 Vista Drive
Old Lyme, CT 06371
203-434-9190
Disability Served: hearing

This company manufactures personal amplification systems.

Sentry S Division

8181 North Stadium Drive
Houston, TX 77054
713-799-8585
http://www.sleepsentry.com
Disability Served: diabetes

This company manufactures an insulin reaction monitor that can be worn on the wrist while sleeping.

Service Associates

PO Box 953
Cedar Falls, IA 50613
319-268-1915
Disability Served: physically disabled

This company manufactures an exercise bar designed to work the upper body and a swing-away lapboard for wheelchairs.

Seton Name Plate Company

PO Box 1331
New Haven, CT 06505
203-488-8059, 800-243-6624
TTY/TDD: 800-824-7259
Disability Served: all

This company manufactures a large variety of access signs.

SFH Products Inc.

1801 East Medlock Drive
Phoenix, AZ 85016
602-265-7370
Disability Served: physically disabled

This company manufactures a platform van lift and a mobile home lift.

SH Industries Inc.

1315 61st Avenue East
Bradenton, FL 34203
813-756-8297
Disability Served: all

This company manufactures a bathroom spray hose that is used to clean or rinse items in the bathroom.

Shamrock Medical Inc.

3620 SE Powell Boulevard
Portland, OR 97202-1880
503-233-5055, 800-231-2225
Disability Served: all

This company manufactures traction systems.

Sharn, Inc.

4801 George Road
Tampa, FL 33634
813-889-9614, 800-325-3671
http://www.sharn.com
Disability Served: all

This company makes a skin response biofeedback unit that measures skin temperature.

Sharp Electronics

10 Sharp Plaza
Paramus, NJ 07652
Disability Served: vision

This company manufactures a chime clock and a wide-angle light probe to assist persons with limited vision.

Shircliffe Enterprises

5002 Greenwood Road
Louisville, KY 40258
502-935-9931
Disability Served: physically disabled

This company manufactures mouthsticks.

Shower Aide, Inc.

444 Woodville Road
PO Box 339
Pelzer, SC 29669-0339
864-243-4187, 800-680-4187
http://www.showeraide.com
Disability Served: physically disabled

This company manufactures the Shower Aide, a bath chair that allows the disabled to enter outside the bathtub or shower, bathe, then exit on the outside without leaving the chair. The chair swivels 360 degrees and has folding arms.

Showerwall Industries Inc.
130 West Gore Street
Thunder Bay, ON P7E 3V9 Canada
807-577-6636
Disability Served: physically disabled

This company manufactures an accessible bathtub.

Siemens Hearing Instruments Inc.
10 Constitution Avenue
PO Box 1397
Piscataway, NJ 08855-1397
908-562-6600, 800-766-4500
Disability Served: hearing

This company manufactures aids for the hearing impaired, including hearing aids, personal amplification systems, amplification systems for televisions, infrared amplification systems, and speech amplifiers.

Sierra Laboratories Incorporated
PO Box 27005
Tucson, AZ 85726
520-324-0580
Disability Served: physically disabled

This company manufactures leg bags, urinals, catheters, and a cleaner designed to clean and deodorize urinary and ostomy products.

Sigvaris Inc.
PO Box 570
Branford, CT 06405
203-481-5588, 800-322-7744
Disability Served: all

This company manufactures therapeutic hosiery.

Silcraft Corp.
528 Hughes Drive
Traverse City, MI 49684
616-946-4221, 800-678-7100
Disability Served: physically disabled

This company manufactures bath aids, including shower seats, bathtubs with whirlpools, and showers with built-in grab bars and seats.

Silent Call Communications Corporation
PO Box 868
Clarkston, MI 48347-0868
248-673-0221, 800-572-5227
TTY/TDD: 800-572-5227
http://www.silent-call.com
Disability Served: hearing

This company manufactures and distributes assistive alerting devices for persons who are hearing impaired or deaf-blind.

Silver Creek Industries
1909 Silver Creek Road
PO Box 1988
Manitowoc, WI 54221-1988
920-684-1225, 800-533-3277
http://www.silvercreekindustries.com
Disability Served: hearing

This company makes personal amplification systems in headset form and a hand-held unit with separate headphones.

Silver Ring Splint Co.
PO Box 2856
Charlottesville, VA 22902
804-971-4052
Disability Served: all

This company manufactures a finger splint.

Simpson Timber Company
Third and Franklin
Shelton, WA 98584
206-426-3381
Disability Served: all

This company manufactures nonslip floor coverings of plywood.

Sintaur Corporation
123 Old Carriage Road
Ponce Inlet, FL 32019
904-432-1939
Disability Served: physically disabled

This company manufactures a bicycle exercise device that replaces standard wheelchair footrests.

Sinties Scientific, Inc.

5616-A South 122nd East Avenue
Tulsa, OK 74146
918-254-7395, 800-852-6869
Disability Served: all

This company serves the commercial rehabilitation and fitness markets as well as the home medical market. Sinties started in home medical with its Power Trainer line of wheelchair-accessible fitness equipment.

SIS Human Factor Technologies, Inc.

55C Harvey Road
Londonderry, NH 03053-7414
603-432-4495
Disability Served: physically disabled

This company manufactures adjustable-height tables from sit to stand for computer application. Other features include bilevel and single-surface design, forearm supports, monitor arms, printer stands, and copy holders.

Siskiyou Medical Systems

PO Box 3156
Central Point, OR 97502
541-664-5262
Disability Served: back injury

This company manufactures a gravity-assisted traction system that focuses traction to the lumbar spine.

Ski Eze USA Inc.

4401 Devonshire Avenue
Lansing, MI 48910
517-882-4608
Disability Served: physically disabled

This company manufactures ski stabilizers for skiers with disabilities.

Sleeper Lounge

701 East Kings Hill Place
Carson, CA 90746
800-437-3636
Disability Served: physically disabled

This company manufactures a motorized bed for the home.

SLM Inc.

PO Box 1070
Gloversville, NY 12078
518-725-8101
Disability Served: all

SLM manufactures a hand exerciser designed to strengthen hand grip.

SMART DOT

2655 West Central Avenue
Toledo, OH 43606
800-984-1137
Disability Served: all

This company manufactures a blood sugar test strip for persons with visual impairments or upper extremity disabilities.

Smith & Davis Manufacturing Co.

1100 Corporate Square Drive
St Louis, MO 63132-2908
314-569-3515, 800-788-3633
Disability Served: physically disabled

This company manufactures aids to daily living, including side rails, raised toilet seats, motorized and manual beds, patient chairs, canes, bath benches, commodes, and much more.

Smith & Hawken

25 Corte Madera
Mill Valley, CA 94941
415-383-4050
Disability Served: all

This company manufactures gardening tools and accessories.

Smith & Nephew Richards

1450 Brooks Road
Memphis, TN 38116
800-238-7538
Disability Served: all

This company manufactures a wide variety of support systems, slings, and immobilizers.

Smith & Nephew, Inc.
DonJoy Division
5966 La Place
Carlsbad, CA 92008
619-438-9091, 800-336-6569
http://www.donjoy.com
Disability Served: all

This company manufactures orthopedic devices, including knee braces, foot & ankle braces, and products for the upper extremities and back.

Smith & Nephew, Inc.
Rehabilitation Division
North 104 West 13400 Donges Bay Road
PO Box 1005
Germantown, WI 53022-8205
414-251-7840, 800-558-8633
http://www.smithnephew.com/
Disability Served: all

Snug Seat, Inc.
PO Box 1739
12801 East Independence Boulevard
Matthews, NC 28106-1739
704-847-0772, 800-336-SNUG
http://ww.snugseat.com
Disability Served: all

This company manufactures and distributes pediatric and adult wheelchairs, walkers, shower and commode products, aids for daily living, gait trainers, standers, strollers, and car seats for children with special needs.

So Cal Orthopedics Inc.
1717 East Lincoln Avenue
Anaheim, CA 92805
714-556-2663
Disability Served: orthopedic

This company manufactures flotation support systems, including cervical pillows, lumbar supports, neck supports, knee supports, and posture supports.

Solar World
2807 North Prospect
Colorado Springs, CO 80907
719-635-5125
Disability Served: hearing

This company makes a button battery tester and a solar-powered hearing aid battery charger.

Solutions for Accessibility
167 Union Avenue
Framingham, MA 01701
Disability Served: all

This company makes a bottle holder that holds a one-liter soda bottle.

Sonic Alert Inc.
1750 West Hamlin Road
Rochester Hills, MI 48309
810-656-3110
Disability Served: hearing

This company manufactures daily living aids for persons with hearing impairments. Products include doorbell signalers, alert systems, alarm clocks, sound monitors, and various sound signalers.

Sony Industries
Business Products Division
9 West 57th Street
New York, NY 10019
212-368-5000
Disability Served: vision

This company manufactures cassette recorders for persons with limited vision.

Sorbothane Inc.
2144 State Route 59
PO Box 178
Kent, OH 44240
216-678-9444
Disability Served: all

This company makes a foam material often used as shoe inserts.

SOS Rehabilitation Products

136 Merizzi Street
St Laurent, QC H4T 1S4 Canada
514-737-3422, 800-667-3422
Disability Served: physically disabled

This company manufactures a child car seat base that can serve as a custom seating insert for children with physical or mobility disabilities.

Sound Resources Inc.

201 East Ogden Avenue
Hinsdale, IL 60521
630-323-7970
Disability Served: hearing

This company manufactures telephone accessories for persons with hearing impairments. Products include amplified telephone handsets, telephone amplifiers, ring signalers and flashers, and more.

SOUNDBEAM Project (The)

3850 Sedgwick Avenue
Bronx, NY 10463
718-543-9481
http://www.soundbeam.co.uk
Disability Served: all

This company produces and distributes SOUNDBEAM, SOUNDBOX, and SOUNDBED for music therapy and vibro-acoustic therapy.

Southpaw Enterprises, Inc.

109 Webb Street
Dayton, OH 45403
937-252-7676, 800-228-1698
http://www.southpawenterprises.com
Disability Served: all

This company manufactures and distributes equipment for people with special needs in the area of sensory integration and developmental delay.

Southwest Technologies Inc.

2018 Baltimore
Kansas City, MO 64108
816-221-2442, 800-247-9951
Disability Served: all

This company makes the Elasto-Gel supports, pillows, and wraps.

Space Tables Inc.

8035 Ranchers Road NE
PO Box 32082
Minneapolis, MN 55432-0082
612-786-9301, 800-328-2580
Disability Served: physically disabled

This company manufactures height-adjustable, accessible tables and work stations.

Span America Inc.

PO Box 5231
Greenville, SC 29606
803-288-8877, 800-888-6752
Disability Served: all

This company makes support pillows, cushions, and splints.

Spanners

17671 Metzler A-9/10
Huntington Beach, CA 92647
714-841-6292, 800-878-7726
Disability Served: physically disabled

This company manufactures carrying bags for wheelchairs and a safety belt for wheelchairs.

Sparta, Inc.

9455 Towne Centre Drive
San Diego, CA 92121-1964
619-455-1650
Disability Served: orthopedic

This company makes lightweight leg braces.

Special Ballooning Adventures, Inc.

202 Ironwood
PO Box 282
Correctionville, IA 51016
712-372-4373, 712-372-4421
Disability Served: physically disabled

This company flies a wheelchair-accessible hot air balloon.

Special Clothes
PO Box 333
East Harwich, MA 02645
508-896-7939
http://www.special-clothes.com
Disability Served: all

This company manufactures clothing for children and adults.

Special Health Systems Ltd.
5970 Chedworth Way
Missassauga, ON L5R 3T9 Canada
416-841-1032, 800-263-2223
Disability Served: physically disabled

This company manufactures seat cushions and a swing-away lapboard.

Specially for You, LLC
PO Box 272
Willow Lake, SD 57278
605-625-3765, 605-625-5270
http://www.dailypost.com/speciallyforyou
Disability Served: all

This company designs and sews adaptive clothing for the physically challenged with special needs.

Spectrum Disposable Medical Products
8430 Santa Monica Boulevard
Los Angeles, CA 90069
Disability Served: all

This company manufactures a heel or elbow protector and a hot and cold pack.

Spectrum Pool Products
7100 Spectrum Lane
Missoula, MT 59802
406-543-5309, 800-776-5309
http://www.spectrumproducts.com
Disability Served: physically disabled

This company manufactures swimming pool access products for people with disabilities, including lifts, ramps, railings, and ladders, as well as stainless steel hydrotherapy tanks for the swimming pool and medical therapy markets.

Spenco Medical Corp.
PO Box 2501
Waco, TX 76702
817-772-6000, 800-433-3334
Disability Served: all

Spenco makes support pillows, pads, and hot and cold packs.

Sperzel Industries Inc.
PO Box 411
1010 North Osage
Nevada, MO 64772
417-667-6073, 800-326-4803
Disability Served: physically disabled

This company manufactures elevated toilet seats and support arms for toilet seats.

SPF Distributors
715 North Central Avenue, #213
Glendale, CA 91203-1225
626-242-7546
Disability Served: all

This company makes the Headache Ice Pillow, a cervical cold pack.

Sports Health Products
527 West Windsor Road
Glendale, CA 91204
800-289-7889
Disability Served: physically disabled

This company manufactures Power Putty, hand therapy putty in four color-coded resistances. This putty is used for hand rehabilitation and carpal tunnel prevention and treatment.

Sports Supports Inc.
400 Union Bower Court
Erving, TX 75061
214-554-1174, 800-527-5273
Disability Served: all

This company manufactures supports designed primarily for athletics. Products include ankle supports, elbow supports, lumbar supports, thigh supports, knee supports, and wrist supports.

Sportsplay Equipment Inc.

5642 Natural Bridge
St Louis, MO 63120
314-389-4140, 800-727-8180
http://www.sportsplayinc.com
Disability Served: all

This company manufactures playground and recreational equipment, such as swings, basketball backstops, wheelchair accessible jungle gyms, modular play structures, and picnic tables.

SR 77 Enterprises Inc.

363 Maple Street
Chadron, NE 69337
308-432-2894
Disability Served: physically disabled

This company manufactures a rifle mount for wheelchairs.

St. Joseph Hospital

220 Overton Avenue
Memphis, TN 38105
901-577-2772, 800-955-2668
Disability Served: physically disabled

This company manufactures boot orthotics that immobilize the ankles and feet. They are designed for the rehabilitation of spinal cord injury patients.

Sta Products, Inc.

PO Box 1438
Arvada, CO 80001-1438
303-420-5688, 800-782-6288
Disability Served: all

This company manufactures nonslip matting that can be used for placemats or shelves.

Stall and Dean

95 Church Street
Brockton, MA 02403
508-586-2414
Disability Served: all

This company manufactures protective helmets.

Stand Aid of Iowa Inc.

1009 Second Avenue
Sheldon, IA 51201
712-324-2153, 800-831-8580
http://www.stand-aid.com
Disability Served: physically disabled

This company makes a wheelchair scale, hydraulic standing aids, exercise machines, and a power adapter for wheelchairs.

Stanley Magic-Door

Attn: Rich Reed
Route 6 at Hyde Road
Farmington, CT 06032
203-677-2861, 800-232-3663
Disability Served: all

This company manufactures powered door operators for sliding doors and swinging doors.

Stanley Works

PO Box 1800
New Britain, CT 06050
203-225-5111, 800-232-3663
Disability Served: all

This company manufactures door hinges that allow greater access width.

Stanton Magnetics LLC

2821 Evans Street
Hollywood, FL 33020
954-929-8999
http://www.stantonmagnetics.com
Disability Served: communication

This company manufactures bone conduction microphone/speaker systems, and button receivers for hearing aids.

Staodynamics Inc.

1225 Florida Avenue
Longmont, CO 80501
303-772-3631
Disability Served: back injury

This company manufactures a portable traction system to treat cervical and lower back problems.

Staplex Company
777 Fifth Avenue
Brooklyn, NY 11232
718-768-3333, 800-221-0822
http://www.staplex.com
Disability Served: all

This company makes an electric mail opener and electric staplers, including a hand-held, battery-powered stapler.

Starkey Labs Inc.
6700 Washington Avenue South
PO Box 9457
Minneapolis, MN 55440
612-941-6401, 800-328-8602
Disability Served: hearing

This company develops hearing aids and tinnitus maskers.

Stat Medical Corporation
200 Debusk Lane
Powell, TN 37849
800-251-9864
Disability Served: physically disabled

This company makes foam wheelchair cushions.

Steelcraft Inc.
Burbank Street
Millbury, MA 01527
508-865-4445
Disability Served: physically disabled

Steelcraft manufactures walkers, commodes, support chairs, and bath aids.

Steridyne Corp.
3725 Investment Lane
Riviera Beach, FL 33404
407-844-3486, 800-327-6185
Disability Served: all

This company makes thermometer strips that attach to the forehead and a gel flotation cushion.

Stern Williams Co. Inc.
PO Box 8004
Shawnee Mission, KS 66208
913-362-5635
http://www.sternwilliams.com
Disability Served: physically disabled

This company makes bath aids, including shower cabinets and shower floors. The company also makes wheelchair-accessible water fountains.

Sticky Situations
244 Madison Avenue, Suite 9H
New York, NY 10016
212-983-1212
Disability Served: all

This company produces a parent/child interactive communication tool.

Stimwear Inc.
33161 Camino Capistrano, Suite J
San Juan Capistrano, CA 92675
714-248-2443
Disability Served: physically disabled

Stimwear makes neuromuscular electrical system stimulators for home use. They are designed to stimulate the muscles of paralyzed persons.

Stoma Button Co. Inc.
PO Box 984
Baker, OR 97814
541-894-2367
Disability Served: all

This company manufactures stoma buttons and personal identification tags.

Streamlight Inc.
1030 West Germantown Pike
Norristown, PA 19403
215-631-0600
Disability Served: vision

Streamlight manufactures professional flashlights to assist those with night blindness.

Street Thoma
8862 Willow Wood Way
Jessup, MD 20794
410-880-0056
Disability Served: vision

This company produces tactile models, diagrams, and verbal descriptions to help visually impaired people examine art and buildings.

Stretch Forming Corp.
PO Box 686
Murrieta, CA 92362
714-677-8651, 800-854-2461
Disability Served: all

This company develops a gravity traction system.

Strong Arm Fishing Products
2046A Pharmacy Avenue
Scarborough, ON M1T 1H8 Canada
416-756-1379
http://www.strongarmfishing.com
Disability Served: all

Fishing rod holders designed for persons with limited grip are manufactured by this company.

Stryker Corporation
420 Alcott Street
Kalamazoo, MI 49001
616-381-3811, 800-253-3210
Disability Served: all

Among the products this company manufactures are a foam heel protector, a circle bed, and a gel flotation seat cushion.

Suffridge and Treni Communications, Inc.
PO Box 1226
Ridgewood, NJ 07451
201-445-5052
Disability Served: hearing

This company makes a wireless microphone designed to be used in conjunction with a personal amplification system.

Summitville Tiles, Inc.
State Highway 644
Summitville, OH 43962
216-223-1511
Disability Served: vision

This company manufactures a tactile flooring surface designed to alert and warn persons with visual disabilities.

SunBelt Industries, Inc.
1254 Fish Hook Way
Ponte Verde Beach, FL 32082
904-285-4788
Disability Served: hearing

This company develops a closed-caption decoder for hearing impaired television viewers.

SunBox Company (The)
19217 Orbit Drive
Gaithersburg, MD 20879
301-869-5980, 800-548-3968
Disability Served: all

This company manufactures lights for the treatment of seasonal affective disorder.

Sunnyfield Supplies Inc.
4821 Elk Road, RR #5
Victoria, BC V8X 4M6 Canada
250-727-3254
Disability Served: physically disabled

This company makes a manual transfer apparatus that is a sling. The sling requires two attendants for proper transferring.

Sunrise Mobility
Kidkart Division
732 Cruiser Lane
Belgrade, MT 59714
406-388-1080
http://kidkart.avicom.net
Disability Served: physically disabled

Sunroc Corp.
Route 452
Glen Riddle, PA 19037
215-459-1100
Disability Served: physically disabled

Sunroc manufactures wheelchair-accessible drinking fountains.

Sunshine Brothers Inc.
4521 Emery Industrial Parkway
Cleveland, OH 44128
800-428-8000
Disability Served: all

This company manufactures adaptive clothing for men and women.

Supersine Company
6000 East Davison Avenue
Detroit, MI 48212
313-892-6200
Disability Served: all

This company manufactures access signs.

Superwinch
Connecticut Route 52
Putnam, CT 06260
203-928-7787
Disability Served: all

This company manufactures electric winches and hoists.

Support Engineering Associates
PO Box 7184
109 Fourth Street, Suite 44
Garden City, NJ 11530
516-741-7560
Disability Served: physically disabled

This company makes a wheelchair accessible computer work station.

Support Plus
99 West Street
PO Box 500
Medfield, MA 02052
508-359-2910
Disability Served: all

This company sells daily living aids, support hosiery, and comfort shoes.

SUREHANDS
982 Route 1
Pine Island, NY 10969-1205
914-258-6500, 800-724-5305
http://www.surehands.com
Disability Served: physically disabled

This company distributes patient lift and transfer systems for the motor disabled. A variety of permanent and portable lifts and accessories are available: ceiling-mounted track systems, wall lifts, mobile units, and pool lifts. Wall-mounted electric changing tables and mobile electric changing tables are also available.

Susquehanna Rehab Products
Road 2, Box 41
9 Overlook Drive
Wrightsville, PA 17368
717-252-4672, 800-233-2011
Disability Served: all

This company manufactures a stocking aid, a bathtub transfer bench chair, and a weighted ballpoint pen.

Sutter Corp.
9425 Chesapeake Drive
San Diego, CA 92123
619-569-8148
Disability Served: all

This company manufactures continuous passive motion devices. They are designed to assist in the recovery of joint injuries by maintaining range of motion and preventing swelling.

Swede-O-Inc.
6459 Ash Street
PO Box 610
North Branch, MN 55056
651-674-8301, 800-525-9339
http://www.swedeo.com
Disability Served: all

This company manufactures ankle supports, braces, and splints.

Sylvia Becker
6020 Nevada Avenue, #17
Woodland Hills, CA 91367
818-702-0562
Disability Served: all

Sylvia Becker provides beaded neckpieces for female laryngectomees.

Symmetric Designs Ltd.
2059 North End
Box 66
Ganges, BC V8K1C9 Canada
250-537-2177
Disability Served: all

This company manufactures orthotics and wheelchair supports.

T. L. Shield & Associates, Inc.
PO Box 6845
Thousand Oaks, CA 91359-6845
805-509-8228
Disability Served: physically disabled

This company manufactures an interior seat lift for wheelchair users.

Tag Toys
3330 El Segundo Boulevard
Hawthorne, CA 90250
800-488-4TAG
Disability Served: all

This company develops wooden puzzles designed to teach shapes, names, and numbers.

Tagg Industries
23210 Del Lago
Laguna Hills, CA 92653
714-770-9029, 800-548-3514
Disability Served: all

This company manufactures a skin coating designed to prevent itching inside casts.

Talcott Laboratories Inc.
455 Route 30
Imperial, PA 15126
412-695-1890, 800-332-8018
Disability Served: all

This company manufactures a portable whirlpool and a portable paraffin bath.

Talking and Visual Aids
8136 Appoline
Detroit, MI 48228
313-935-1266
Disability Served: vision

This company manufactures a low-vision reading system that magnifies the reading material onto a monitor.

Tallahassee Therapeutic Equipment
9601 Miccosukee Road, Lot 13
Tallahassee, FL 32308-9609
850-877-0488, 800-476-0487
Disability Served: physically disabled

This company manufactures a wheelchair base that allows wheelchair users to tilt forwards and backwards, a seating simulator, and a seating interface that allows seating adjustments.

Tamarack Habilitation Technologies, Inc.
1471 Energy Park Drive
St Paul, MN 55108-5204
612-644-9950
http://www.oandp.com/tamaracktamarack
Disability Served: all

This company provides orthotic and prosthetic services with a focus on the pediatric age group. They also do custom orthotic seating for children and adults with special needs for postural stability and/or pressure management.

Tamiko Corporation
15020 Delano Street
Van Nuys, CA 91411
818-782-7720, 800-222-4687
Disability Served: all

This company manufactures a therapeutic massage unit.

Tasco
7600 NW 26th Street
PO Box 520080
Miami, FL 33152
305-591-3670
Disability Served: vision

This company makes hand-held microscopes.

Taylor Made Healthcare

10 West 9th Avenue
PO Box 1190
Gloversville, NY 12078
518-725-0681, 800-258-0942
Disability Served: physically disabled

This company manufactures pediatric positioning chairs and strollers and an adjustable mobile standing aid for children.

Te Deum

Alice East Taraschke
23540 Poe Road
Grand Rapids, OH 43522
419-832-1762
Disability Served: physically disabled

This company manufactures carrying bags for walkers.

TechLite Products Corporation

4546 IDS Center
80 South Eighth Street
Minneapolis, MN 55402
612-371-4446, 800-879-9729
Disability Served: all

This company manufactures a motion detector switch that automatically turns on the lights when motion is detected in a room.

TechnaCrutch Inc.

3 Henry Drive
Barrington, RI 02806
401-245-2617
Disability Served: all

This company makes crutch extensions that act as shock absorbers.

Techni-Flair Corp.

Box 40
Cotter, AR 72626
800-643-5656
Disability Served: all

This company manufactures clothing for men and women.

Technical Resources Inc.

PO Box 1613
Waltham, MA 02254-1613
781-239-0440
Disability Served: all

This company manufactures an electronic pulse monitor and a transcutaneous electrical nerve stimulator (TENS) unit.

Technology for Independence

529 Main Street
Boston, MA 02129
617-242-7007, 800-331-TALK
Disability Served: vision

This company makes numerous items for individuals with visual impairments. Products include talking alarm clocks, watches, calculators, beeping balls, and more.

TecRec

30 River Drive
Titusville, NJ 08560
609-291-0490, 888-4-TECREC
Disability Served: all

This company manufactures fishing rod holders, fishing reels, and fishing accessories for persons with disabilities.

Ted Hoyer and Company

2222 Minnesota Street
Oshkosh, WI 54901
920-236-3460, 800-255-5022
Disability Served: physically disabled

This company manufactures a variety of lifts, including pool lifts, bath lifts, and travel lifts.

Teddy Tuckers, Inc.

551 Blackburn Road
Friedens, PA 15541
814-443-3106, 800-776-0407
Disability Served: all

This company manufactures back support cushions and infant support cushions.

Telcom International

28302 Industrial Boulevard, Suite H
Hayward, CA 94545
510-785-4000, 800-376-3323
Disability Served: hearing

This company repairs and sells TTY/TDD devices.

Teledyne Brown Engineering

PO Box 070007
Huntsville, AL 35807-7007
205-726-1000, 800-944-8002
Disability Served: all

This company manufactures an environmental control unit that is operated by remote control.

Telephone Extension Corporation

83 East Central Avenue
Pearl River, NY 10965
914-735-7877
Disability Served: hearing

This company manufactures various phone ringers and flashers to alert persons with hearing impairments of incoming calls.

Telephone Pioneers of America De Anza

950 West Washington, Room 210
Escondido, CA 92025
760-489-3305
Disability Served: vision

This company manufactures an auditory signal device for golf. The device is attached to the golf cup and beeps when a ball enters the hole.

Telephone Pioneers of America New England

Vermont New Hampshire Chapter
1228 Elm Street
Manchester, NH 03101
603-645-2666
Disability Served: hearing

This company manufactures a helmet fitted with a hearing aid.

Telex Communications Inc.

9600 Aldrich Avenue South
Minneapolis, MN 55420
612-884-4051, 800-328-3102
Disability Served: hearing

This company manufactures amplification systems and hearing aids.

Temasek Telephone Inc.

21 Airport Boulevard, Suite G
San Francisco, CA 94080
415-875-6666, 800-647-8887
Disability Served: physically disabled

This company manufactures voice-activated telephones.

Temco Healthcare Industries

PO Box 328
125 South Street
Passaic, NJ 07055
201-472-3173, 800-631-0170
Disability Served: all

This company offers a wide variety of daily living and health care aids, including adjustable canes, grab bars, commodes, shower and tub chairs and benches, walkers, and bed rails.

Tescor Technology Inc.

PO Box 606
Cedarburg, WI 53012
414-377-4208
Disability Served: all

This company manufactures a strobe light that can be connected to security systems.

Tetra Society of North America

Plaza of Nations, Box 27
770 Pacific Boulevard South
Vancouver, BC V6B 5E7 Canada
604-688-6464
http://orcn.ahs.uwo.ca/TETRA/
Disability Served: all

This nonprofit organization recruits skilled volunteer engineers and technicians to create assistive devices for people with disabilities. The products are not commercially available.

Texal Company

510 1st Avenue North
Minneapolis, MN 55403
612-332-5865
Disability Served: all

This company makes arm slings and splints.

Texas Greenhouse Co. Inc.

2524 White Settlement Road
Ft Worth, TX 76107
817-335-5447
http://www.texasgreenhouse.com
Disability Served: all

This company manufactures greenhouses.

Texas Instruments

Accessory Department
PO Box 53
Lubbock, TX 79408
800-842-2737
Disability Served: communication

This company manufactures a spelling tutorial device and an electronic communication unit.

Texas Instruments Inc.

PO Box 202230
Austin, TX 78720
800-527-3500
Disability Served: all

This company manufactures educational toys and devices.

Texim International

17777 Main Street, Suite H
Irvine, CA 92714
714-852-1360, 800-942-4249
Disability Served: all

Texim manufactures a magnetic latch for doors.

TFH (USA) Ltd.

4537 Gibsonia Road
Gibsonia, PA 15044
724-444-6400, 800-467-6222
http://www.tfhusa.com
Disability Served: all

This company manufactures adapted toys and products for education, rehabilitation, recreation, and fun.

TH Charters Inc.

9985 SW Heather Lane
Beaverton, OR 97005
503-643-9888, 800-252-1232
Disability Served: physically disabled

This company makes muscle and electrical nerve stimulators.

Thames Valley Children's Centre

779 Base Line Road East
London, ON N6C 5Y6 Canada
519-685-8680
http://www.tvcc.on.ca
Disability Served: all

The Centre makes a plastic floor sitter with a lapboard tray for children.

The Dorma Group

Dorma Drive, Drawer AC
Reamstown, PA 17567-0411
717-336-3881, 800-523-8483
http://www.dorma-usa.com
Disability Served: physically disabled

This company manufactures and markets a line of surface and concealed door closers, low energy operators, a coordinator system and closer-holder-release devices, pivots, stops/holders, exit devices, and security hardware.

The Endorphin Corporation

6901 90th Avenue North
Pinellas Park, FL 33782
727-545-9848
http://www.endorphin.net
Disability Served: physically disabled

This company makes exercise equipment accessible for wheelchair users, including treadmills, bicycle exercisers, and weight machines.

The New Vision Store

919 Walnut Street, 1st Floor
Philadelphia, PA 19107
215-629-2990
Disability Served: vision

This organization sells products for the visually impaired, including talking clocks, magnifiers, canes, calculators, and more.

The Speech Bin, Inc.

1965 25th Avenue
Vero Beach, FL 32960
561-770-0007
http://www.speechbin.com
Disability Served: all

This company publishes and distributes books and materials for professionals and individuals who are interested in rehabilitation, speech-language pathology, special education, and related fields. Among the major product lines are professional and children's books, computer software, diagnostic tests, educational games and materials, and specialty items. A catalog is available.

Theodore N. Vail State Chapter Telephone

529 South 7th Street, 4A
Springfield, IL 62721
217-789-8066
Disability Served: communication

This company manufactures sound-activated speech aids.

Thera P Cushion Inc.

210 South 8th Street
Lewiston, NY 14092
716-784-3727
Disability Served: all

This company provides support cushions, including anti-snoring pillows.

Thera P Equipment Company

PO Box 1
Snyder, NY 14226
716-833-5960
Disability Served: all

This company makes overhead suspension slings that provide support for arms.

Theradapt Products Inc.

17 West 163 Oak Lane
Bensenville, IL 60106
630-834-2461
Disability Served: physically disabled

This company manufactures a number of daily living aids. Products include prone and supine standers, chairs, easels and trays, benches, and walkers.

Therafin Corporation

PO Box 848
19747 Wolf Road
Mokena, IL 60448-0848
708-479-7300, 800-843-7234
Disability Served: all

This company offers more than 130 aids to daily living. Products range from dressing aids to kitchen utensils to armrests.

TheraMedic Products, Inc.

1110 Lexington Avenue
PO Box 1990
Mansfield, OH 44901
419-756-4660, 800-382-2919
Disability Served: all

This company makes a foam seat cushion for wheelchairs.

Therapeutic Alliances, Inc.

333 North Broad Street
Fairborn, OH 45324
937-879-0734
http://www.MusclePower.com
Disability Served: all

This company manufactures rehabilitation equipment for home and clinical use. Products are appropriate for those with head trauma, cerebral palsy, spinal cord injury, and others who need to restore muscle control.

Therapeutic Creations
544 Ygnacio Valley Road, #A-261
Walnut Creek, CA 94596
510-930-3460
Disability Served: all

This company manufactures a trunk support vest for children.

Therapeutic Health & Equipment Specialists
14000 NW 1st Avenue
North Miami, FL 33168
800-533-0178
Disability Served: all

This company manufactures therapeutic aids, including therapy mats, large foam shapes, side-lyers, wedges, rolls, and blocks.

Therapeutic Toys, Inc.
PO Box 418
Moodus, CT 06469-0418
203-873-9509, 800-638-0676
Disability Served: all

This company develops switches, including switches for telephones. The company also manufactures therapeutic activity boxes, communication boards, and battery-operated, voice-activated toys.

Therapy Air Support Systems Inc.
13912 Ponderosa, Unit H
Santa Ana, CA 92701
714-558-2490
Disability Served: all

This company develops air flotation mattresses that help prevent pressure sores.

Thermal Moldable Shoes Inc.
100 Deville Circle
Williamsville, NY 14221-4408
716-631-5611
Disability Served: all

This company manufactures orthopedic shoes.

Thermo-Electric Co.
455 Route 30
Imperial, PA 15126
412-695-1890, 800-633-8080
Disability Served: all

This company manufactures paraffin baths for paraffin therapy.

Thermoscan Inc.
10309 Pacific Center Court
San Diego, CA 92121
619-550-2100, 800-327-7226
Disability Served: all

This company develops digital, tympanic thermometers for home and institutional use.

Thetford Corp.
PO Box 1285
Ann Arbor, MI 48106
734-769-6000, 800-354-4135
Disability Served: all

This company manufactures hand-carried portable toilets.

Things from Bell Inc.
230 Mechanic Street
PO Box 206
Princeton, WI 54968
414-642-7337
Disability Served: all

This company manufactures exercise equipment and therapeutic aids, including balls, playground equipment, exercise mats, scooter boards, and balance boards.

Thirst Free
PO Box 9656
East Ridge, TN 37412
423-867-1759
Disability Served: physically disabled

Thirst Free makes a beverage holder that attaches to wheelchairs.

Thoele Manufacturing
RR 1, Box 116
Montrose, IL 62445
217-924-4553
Disability Served: physically disabled

This company manufactures a bicycle exerciser for wheelchair users.

Thomas Fetterman Inc.
1680 Hillside Road
Southampton, PA 18966
888-355-6941
http://www.fetterman-crutches.com
Disability Served: physically disabled

This company provides custom-made crutches, crutch tips, telescoping travel crutches, and accessories.

Thompson Medical Specialties
4301 Bryant Avenue South
Minneapolis, MN 55409
612-823-2058, 800-777-4949
Disability Served: physically disabled

This company manufactures wheelchair aids and accessories, including restraints, carrying bags, and support cushions and seats. The company also makes exercise weights and support slings.

Thought Technology Ltd.
RR #1 Route 9N, #380
West Chazy, NY 12992
514-489-8251, 800-361-3651
Disability Served: all

This company manufactures biofeedback systems.

ThreeM Company
3M General Office, Mail Stop 224-5M-38
St Paul, MN 55144
612-737-9587, 800-328-1063
Disability Served: vision

3M manufactures Braille labelers and accessories.

Tie Tech Inc.
PO Box 5226
Lynnwood, WA 98046
425-743-5863
http://tietechinc.com
Disability Served: physically disabled

This company manufactures wheelchair restraint systems for vehicles, emergency evacuation devices for removing physically disabled persons from emergency situations, and webbing cutters.

Timecal International Corp.
177 Main Street, Suite 363
Ft Lee, NJ 07024
201-836-0252
Disability Served: all

This company makes a pill organizer.

Tip Top Mobility, Inc.
PO Box 5009
Minot, ND 58702-5009
701-857-1182, 800-735-5958
http://www.minot.com/~tiptop/
Disability Served: physically disabled

This company manufactures the Tip Top Wheelchair Lift for use with automobiles.

TMI Healthcare Products
307 Bacon Road
Rougemont, NC 27572
919-477-1387, 800-550-4MOM
Disability Served: physically disabled

This company makes incontinence garments for children.

Today's Kids, Inc.
PO Box 207
2932 East State Highway 10
Booneville, AR 72927
501-675-2000, 800-258-8697
Disability Served: all

This company makes a rocking horse with a safety seat.

Tone Commander Systems

Box 97039
4320 150th Avenue NE
Redmond, WA 98052
425-883-3600
Disability Served: hearing

This company manufactures a telephone handset amplifier for persons with hearing disabilities.

Tonka

PO Box 200
Pawtucket, RI 02862
401-431-8697, 800-248-6652
Disability Served: all

Tonka manufactures touch-activated stuffed animals and toys.

Tootsietoy

600 North Pulaski Road
Chicago, IL 60624
773-638-1000, 800-944-TOYS
Disability Served: all

This company manufactures tactile toys designed to help children develop motor skills and eye-hand coordination.

Total Orthopedic/Total Care

18910 Bonanza Way
Gaithersburg, MD 20879
301-840-9027, 800-334-3802
Disability Served: all

This company manufactures orthopedic aids, including restraints, slings and supports, orthopedic shoes, and support cushions.

Total Support

Division of Parker Sales
1117 South B Street
San Mateo, CA 94401
650-574-1304, 800-344-4550
Disability Served: all

This company manufactures support pillows and finger splints.

Toto KiKi USA Inc.

1155 Southern Road
Morrow, GA 30030
770-282-8686
http://totousa.com
Disability Served: all

This company manufactures toilets, bidets, and electronic faucets and flush systems.

Toys For Special Children

385 Warburton Avenue
Hastings-on-Hudson, NY 10706
914-478-0960, 800-TEC-TOYS
http://www.enablingdevices.com
Disability Served: all

This company adapts toys for use by handicapped children. The company also provides augmentative devices, communication devices, and capability switches.

Trademark Medical

1053 Headquarters Park
Fenton, MO 63026-2033
636-349-3270, 800-325-9044
http://www.medicom.com/trademarktrademark
Disability Served: all

This company manufactures oral suction toothbrushes, waterproof cast covers, and fever strips for monitoring temperature as well as disposable wound-measuring guides.

Trail Ridge Products Inc.

112 Inverness Circle East, Suite E
Englewood, CO 80112
303-799-6900
Disability Served: all

This company makes an oxygen cylinder cart.

Transpo Industries, Inc.

20 Jones Street
New Rochelle, NY 10801-6024
914-636-1000, 800-321-7870
http://www.transpo-industries.com
Disability Served: vision

This company manufactures a tactile safety surface designed to help alert persons with visual disabilities.

Travel Ramp, Inc.

PO Box 2015
13818 NW 126th Terrace
Alachua, FL 32616
904-462-5267, 888-661-7267
Disability Served: physically disabled

This company manufactures lightweight fiberglass ramps for wheelchair and scooter users.

Travis International Inc.

100 Main Sumner
Coos Bay, OR 97420
541-269-6900, 800-437-9233
Disability Served: physically disabled

This company manufactures incontinence alarms to prevent bed wetting.

Treadle Power, Inc.

PO Box 180
Cedar Beach Road
Charlotte, VT 05445
802-425-2264, 800-648-7335
Disability Served: all

This company manufactures a three-wheeled cycle.

Trendware Phone Systems

4448 West El Segundo Boulevard, Suite 165
Hawthorne, CA 90250
310-644-3014, 800-644-3014
TTY/TDD: 310-644-3014
Disability Served: hearing

This company manufactures a telecommunications device that works as a standard telephone and can also record TTY calls for persons with hearing impairments.

Tri Hawk Corp.

849 South Broadway
Los Angeles, CA 90014
213-622-0143
Disability Served: all

Tri Hawk makes a thumb splint.

TRI KING Corporation

10 Drake Terrace
Prospect Heights, IL 60070
847-537-6032
Disability Served: all

TRI KING develops a hand-propelled tricycle.

Tri WG Inc.

PO Box 905
Valley City, ND 58072-0905
701-845-3984, 800-437-8011
Disability Served: all

This company manufactures parallel bars and powered treatment tables for use in therapy.

Tri-Sport Hand Trikes

8924 Columbus Road
Mt Vernon, OH 43050
614-392-9555
Disability Served: all

This company manufactures hand-propelled tricycles.

Triad Technologies, Inc.

219 Lamson Street
Syracuse, NY 13206
315-437-4089, 800-729-7514
Disability Served: physically disabled

This company manufactures the Transfer Tier, a fiberglass, stainless steel system that enables users to enter and exit a swimming pool.

Trident Technologies

3309 Winthrop, #85
Ft Worth, TX 76116
817-738-2485, 800-366-9950
Disability Served: hearing

Trident manufactures a portable TDD device that can be used with mobile phones and in phone booths.

TRS Inc.

2450 Central Avenue Unit D
Boulder, CO 80301-2844
303-444-4720, 800-279-1865
http://www.oandp.com/trstrs
Disability Served: physically disabled

This company manufactures prosthetic devices and recreational items for persons with disabilities who are missing a hand or hands. Products include prosthetic devices for skiing, camera mounts for prosthetic arms, amputee golf grips, bicycle brakes, and more.

Tru Fit

680 Lynnway
Lynn, MA 01905
617-592-6544, 800-225-6848
Disability Served: all

This company makes an ankle support.

Tru Trac Therapy Products Inc.

104 Industrial Boulevard
Sugar Land, TX 77478-3128
713-240-2442, 800-321-0918
Disability Served: all

This company manufactures therapeutic aids, including home traction systems, hot and cold packs, and therapy pillows.

Truxes Company

PO Box 265
Oswego, IL 60543
773-961-9495
Disability Served: vision

Truxes makes Braille signs for commercial use.

TT Systems Corp.

7 Oden Plaza
Yonkers, NY 10701
914-968-2100
Disability Served: all

This company makes a remote touch tone transmitter for use with rotary dial telephones, answering machines, and wireless intercoms.

Tub-Master Corp.

413 Virginia Drive
Orlando, FL 32803
407-898-2881
Disability Served: physically disabled

This company manufactures folding tub and shower doors, folding wheelchair-accessible shower doors, grab bars, folding shower seats, showerheads, and barrier-free bases.

Tubular Fabricators Industry Inc.

600 West Wythe Street
Petersburg, VA 23803
800-526-0178
Disability Served: physically disabled

This company manufactures bathroom fixtures, including commodes, bathtub and shower benches, stools, and toilet rails. The company also makes canes and walkers.

Tubular Specialties Manufacturing, Inc.

13011 South Spring Street
Los Angeles, CA 90061
310-515-4801, 800-225-5876
http://www.calltsm.com
Disability Served: all

This company manufactures grab bars, shower seats, commercial washroom accessories, corner guards, and railing systems in stainless steel, aluminum, brass, and bronze.

Tucker Designs Ltd.

PO Box 740031
New Orleans, LA 70114
504-464-7479
Disability Served: all

This company makes an infant positioning system to elevate infants while they sleep.

Tuffcare

420 West Crowter
Placentia, CA 92670
714-524-1133, 800-367-6160
Disability Served: physically disabled

This company manufactures wheelchairs, walkers, canes, and bath equipment, including shower benches, grab bars, and commodes.

Tysinger Sewing Machine Co.

Route 9, Box 567
Highway 64 West
Asheboro, NC 27203
910-629-2825
Disability Served: all

This company manufactures hand controls for sewing machines.

Udofot Enterprises, Inc.

PO Box 581733
Minneapolis, MN 55458
612-869-4333
http://www.litealert.com
Disability Served: physically disabled

This company manufactures and sells safety devices such as signs, lights, and sensory/wheelchair aids for use during dark hours or at night. One of the devices produced by this company is the Lite-A-Lert Safety Light.

Ulster Scientific Inc.

PO Box 819
New Paltz, NY 12561-0819
914-255-2200, 800-431-8233
Disability Served: all

This company manufactures syringe injection aids that can be operated with one hand and a blood test puncture device for home use.

Ultratec, Inc.

450 Science Drive
Madison, WI 53711
608-238-5400, 800-482-2424
TTY/TDD: 800-482-2424
Disability Served: hearing

This company manufactures text telephones for use by individuals who are deaf or hard of hearing.

UltraVoice

19 East Central Avenue
Paoli, PA 19301
800-721-4848
http://www.ultravoice.com
Disability Served: communication

Ultravoice manufactures a speech aid for laryngectomees. The aid consists of a unit that fits inside the mouth and a hand-held controller that transmits radio waves to the oral unit.

Ulverscoft Charnwood Linford

Large Print Books—Helen Boyle
279 Boston Street
Guilford, CT 06437
203-453-2080
Disability Served: vision

This company manufactures large-print books and books on audiocassettes.

UNI Manufacturing Co.

PO Box 607
Ontario, OR 97914
800-438-7757
Disability Served: communication

This company manufactures communication devices to assist nonspeaking persons.

Uni-Patch, Inc.

1313 West Grant Boulevard
Wabasha, MN 55981-0271
612-565-2601, 800-328-9454
Disability Served: all

This company manufactures a back support cushion.

Unique Bathing Systems, Inc.

7 Monroe Street
Troy, NY 12180
518-274-BATH
Disability Served: physically disabled

This company manufactures bathing equipment.

United Canvas & Sling Inc.

1 Olympic Drive
Orangeburg, NY 10962-2514
914-365-2333, 800-526-4856
Disability Served: all

This company manufactures a number of therapeutic aids, including items for children. Products include foam wedges, inflatable balls, balance training devices, play mats, and therapy rolls.

United Hearing Systems, Inc.
731 B Norwich Road
PO Box 122
Plainfield, CT 06374
860-564-4130
http://www.unitedhearing.com
Disability Served: hearing

This company manufactures hearing aids.

United States Manufacturing Company
PO Box 5030
180 North San Gabriel Boulevard
Pasadena, CA 91107
626-796-0477
Disability Served: all

This company manufactures prosthetics, orthotics, orthopedic bracing, and supports.

United Steel & Wire Company
PO Box 256
Battle Creek, MI 49016
616-962-5571
http://unitedsteelandwire.com
Disability Served: physically disabled

This company manufactures a shopping basket that attaches to wheelchairs.

Universal Rundle
303 North Street
PO Box 29
New Castle, PA 16103
412-658-6631
Disability Served: physically disabled

This company manufactures accessible bathroom fixtures, such as toilets and showers.

Universal Security Instruments, Inc.
10324 South Dolfield Road
Owings Mills, MD 21117-3586
410-363-3000
Disability Served: hearing

This company develops closed-caption readers and decoders for persons with hearing impairments who wish to watch television.

Universal Technology Systems, Inc.
PO Box 7908
Jacksonville, FL 32208-0908
904-778-8614
Disability Served: all

This company manufactures a galvanic stimulator designed to alleviate pain.

Urinette Inc.
7012 Pine Forest Road
Pensacola, FL 32526
850-944-9779
Disability Served: physically disabled

This company manufactures a wheelchair urinal.

Urocare Products Inc.
2735 Melbourne Avenue
Pomona, CA 91767
909-621-6013, 800-423-4441
Disability Served: all

This company manufactures health care aids, including skin care products, leg and drainage bags, and catheters.

US Mat and Rubber Company
PO Box 152
Brockton, MA 02403
800-343-5955
Disability Served: all

This company manufactures a nonslip floor covering.

Vail Products, Inc.
235 First Street
Toledo, OH 43605
419-698-3200, 800-235-8245
http://www.vailbed.com
Disability Served: all

This company manufactures enclosed beds, an alternative to physical and chemical restraints.

Valiant Educational Videos
18210 Sherman Way, Suite 106
Reseda, CA 91335-4554
818-996-9512
Disability Served: hearing

This company produces American Sign Language tutorial video tapes.

Variety Ability Systems Inc.
3701 Danforth Avenue
Scarborogh, ON M1N 2G2 Canada
416-698-1415
Disability Served: all

This company manufactures electric prosthetic limbs for children, walkers, communication boards, parapodiums, and mounting hardware for wheelchair accessories.

Vecta Contract
1800 South Great Southwest Parkway
Grand Prairie, TX 75051
972-641-2860
Disability Served: all

This company manufactures an ergonomically designed office chair that provides lower back support.

Vega Enterprises Inc.
RR #3, Box 193
Decatur, IL 62526
217-963-2232
Disability Served: physically disabled

This company makes a height-adjustable work table.

Velcro USA, Inc.
406 Brown Avenue
PO Box 5218
Manchester, NH 03108-5218
603-669-4892, 800-225-0180
Disability Served: all

This company makes Velcro straps, Velcro tape, and splints.

Ventek, Inc.
4137 White Oak Drive
PO Box 43527
Birmingham, AL 35243
800-233-4099
Disability Served: hearing

This company makes flashing smoke alarms for persons with hearing impairments.

Verimed International Inc.
11950 NW 39th Street, Suite D
Coral Springs, FL 33065-2564
305-344-2454, 800-999-9797
Disability Served: all

This company makes portable EMG biofeedback units.

Verite
PO Box 697
Harbor City, CA 90710-0697
213-832-1100
Disability Served: all

Verite manufactures transcutaneous electrical nerve stimulator (TENS) units.

Vesture Corporation
PO Box 791
202 Commerce Place
Randleman, NC 27317
919-498-7001, 800-462-4201
Disability Served: all

This company manufactures hot and cold packs, support pillows, and cushions.

VET-Co, Inc.
3700 Fifth Avenue South
Birmingham, AL 35222
205-595-3838, 800-827-8382
Disability Served: physically disabled

This company manufactures and markets the V.E.T. (Vacuum Erection Technology) for impotence management. It is available by prescription only.

Vicon Motion Systems
12309 East Florence Avenue
PO Box 3905
Santa Fe Springs, CA 90670
562-903-1219
Disability Served: all

This company manufactures a pinch gauge and a scoop dish to facilitate eating.

Victor Systems & Equipment
PO Box 171
Marietta, OH 45750
614-374-9300, 800-234-3654
Disability Served: all

This company makes desktop frame holders that hold index strips.

Viking Sewing Machine Co.
11760 Berea Road
Cleveland, OH 44111
216-252-3300
Disability Served: all

Viking manufactures sewing machines.

Villeroy and Boch
I80 at New Maple Avenue
PO Box 103
Pine Brook, NJ 07058
201-575-0550
Disability Served: all

This company manufactures a height-adjustable sink.

Vireo Inc.
PO Box 560
109 West Front Street
Annawan, IL 61234
309-935-6151
Disability Served: all

This company manufactures health care aids, including I.V. stands, oxygen cylinder carts, tables, and wheelchair I.V. stands.

Viscot Industries, Inc.
PO Box 351
East Hanover, NJ 07936-0351
201-887-9273, 800-221-0658
Disability Served: all

This company manufactures both male urinals and a female urinal designed to be used while in a prone position.

Vitajet Corporation
26941 Cabot Road, Suite 105
Laguna Hills, CA 92653
714-582-0713, 800-848-2538
Disability Served: diabetes

This company manufactures an insulin syringe infuser.

Vitalcall
PO Box 80475
Lincoln, NE 68501
402-475-4002, 800-824-2996
Disability Served: all

This company manufactures a wireless personal emergency alert system. Users wear a pendant that can be activated to call for assistance.

Vitalograph Medical Instrumentation
8347 Quivira Road
Lenexa, KS 66215
800-255-6626
Disability Served: all

This company manufactures pulmonary monitors and computerized spirometers.

Voice Control Systems VCS
14140 Midway Road, Suite 100
Dallas, TX 75244
214-386-0300
Disability Served: all

This company manufactures voice activated telephones.

Voicing!
3857 Birch, Suite 194
Newport Beach, CA 92660
714-833-2710
Disability Served: all

This company manufactures exhalation therapy toys for children with tracheostomies.

Vollrath Group Inc.
209 Vollrath Drive
Gallaway, TN 38036
901-867-2951, 800-233-1987
Disability Served: all

This company manufactures bedpans, urinals, shampoo basins, and bucket stands.

Von Duprin Inc.
2720 Tobey Drive
PO Box 6023
Indianapolis, IN 46206
317-897-9944
Disability Served: all

This company manufactures panic bars for doors.

Walk Easy, Inc.
2915 South Congress Avenue
Delray Beach, FL 33445
800-441-2904
http://www.walkeasy.com
Disability Served: all

This company manufactures crutches and crutch tips.

Walker Equipment Corp.
PO Box 829
Highway 151 South
Ringgold, GA 30736
706-935-2600, 800-426-3738
Disability Served: hearing

This company manufactures amplifiers for telephones.

Walter Nicke
36 McLoed Lane
PO Box 433
Topsfield, MA 01983
978-887-3388
http://gardentalk.com
Disability Served: all

This company offers ergonomically designed gardening tools and a water-saving hose nozzle.

Wardrobe Wagon, Inc.
555 Valley Road
West Orange, NJ 07052-5115
800-992-2737
http://www.wardrobewagon.com
Disability Served: physically disabled

This company designs, produces, and sells adaptive clothing and footwear for people with limited mobility. A free catalog is available.

Water Sport Industries
765 North Dodsworth Avenue
Covina, CA 91724-2408
818-967-1351
Disability Served: physically disabled

This company makes a water ski designed for persons with physical disabilities.

Waupaca Elevator Company
PO Box 246
Waupaca, WI 54981
715-258-5581, 800-238-8739
Disability Served: physically disabled

This company manufactures home elevators and dumb waiters.

Wayne County R.E.S.A.
ADAMLAB
33500 Van Born Road
Wayne, MI 48184-2497
734-334-1610
http://www.resa.net/adamlabadamlab
Disability Served: communication

This organization sells augmentative communication devices for individuals with no speech.

Wayne Engineering
1825 Willow Road
Northfield, IL 60093
847-441-6940
Disability Served: all

This company manufactures an electronic pen with an infrared sensor that produces auditory feedback and an exercise unit designed for eye-hand coordination training.

WearABLES

2200 North George Mason Drive
PO Box 7407
Arlington, VA 22207
703-841-7274
http://www.blvd.com/wearables
Disability Served: physically disabled

This company is dedicated to developing sewing patterns for adaptive clothing. Patterns can be purchased by mail order. Designs cater to the wheelchair bound and those with multiple sclerosis, cerebral palsy, polio, arthritis, spinal cord injuries, and more.

Weider Health and Fitness

Industrial & Safety Division
391 Airport Park
Lincoln, AL 35096
205-362-3411, 800-345-8590
Disability Served: all

This company manufactures a back support.

Weil Service Products Corp.

2434 West Fletcher Street
Chicago, IL 60618
773-528-6800
Disability Served: all

This company manufactures a tactile padlock.

Wenzelite Corporation

261 Broadway
Huntington Station, NY 11746
516-673-7022
Disability Served: physically disabled

This company manufactures wheeled walkers, walker hand brakes, I.V. poles that attach to walkers, and portable ventilator carriers that attach to wheelchairs.

Westek

9295 Farnham Street
San Diego, CA 92123-1201
619-268-3422, 800-331-3366
Disability Served: all

Westek manufactures automatic light sensor controls that turn lights on and off when motion is detected, lamp dimmers, and touch lamps.

Western States Manufacturing Corp.

1559 Sunland
Costa Mesa, CA 92626-1514
714-557-1933
Disability Served: all

This company manufactures kitchen faucet levers and hand showers.

Western Telematic Inc.

5 Sterling Street
Irvine, CA 92718
714-586-9950, 800-854-7226
Disability Served: all

This company manufactures a timing switch used for personal computers.

Westinghouse Security Electronics

5452 Betsy Ross Drive
Santa Clara, CA 95054-1102
408-727-5170, 800-624-8999
Disability Served: all

This company manufactures a door opener that can be used in the workplace by persons with physical disabilities.

Wheelchair Carrier Inc.

726 Farnsworth Road
PO Box 79
Waterville, OH 43566
419-878-8511, 800-541-3213
http://www.wheelchaircarrier.com
Disability Served: physically disabled

This company manufactures wheelchair carriers, including hitch-mounted carriers, and portable ramps. It also manufactures the ROAMER Riding Chair, a lightweight, foldable, electric mobility chair.

Wheelchairs of Kansas

204 West Second Street
Ellis, KS 67637
800-537-6454
Disability Served: physically disabled

This company manufactures wheelchairs, electric beds, bath aids, and powered transfer lifts for baratric (obses) individuals.

Wheelies Bentwear

647 West Luellen Drive
Roseburg, OR 97470
541-673-8726
Disability Served: physically disabled

This company develops children's clothes designed for wheelchair users.

Wheelin' Wear Products

PO Box 545
Coburg, ON K9A 4L3 Canada
905-373-4941
Disability Served: physically disabled

This company makes push gloves and arm protectors for children in wheelchairs.

Whelen Engineering Co.

Route 145, Winthrop Road
Chester, CT 06412
203-526-9504
Disability Served: hearing

This company manufactures a flashing smoke alarm for individuals with hearing impairments.

Whirlpool Corporation

Appliance Information Service
2000 M-63
Benton Harbor, MI 49022
616-926-5094, 800-253-1301
Disability Served: all

This company manufactures home appliances such as cooktops and ovens.

Whitaker Company

1 Odell Plaza
PO Box 1061
Yonkers, NY 10703
914-423-4200, 800-445-4387
Disability Served: physically disabled

This company manufactures interior stair lifts, recliner chairs with seat lifts, motorized beds, portable ramps, and mobile home lifts.

White Cap Enterprises Corp.

133 Beach Avenue
Hull, MA 02045
617-925-3705
Disability Served: physically disabled

This company makes a folding, wheeled walker.

White Home Products Inc.

2401 Lake Park Drive
Atlanta, GA 30080
404-431-0900
Disability Served: all

This company manufactures a motorized clothing rack and a rotating kitchen shelving system.

Whitestone Products

40 Turner Place
Piscataway, NJ 08854
201-752-2700
Disability Served: physically disabled

This company manufactures incontinence garments and pads, as well as bed underpads.

Whitmyer Biomechanix Inc.

848 Blountstown Highway, Suite H
Tallahassee, FL 32304
850-575-5510
Disability Served: physically disabled

This company manufactures head supports, wheelchair bases, and mounting hardware for wheelchairs.

Whitney Brothers Company

PO Box 644
Keene, NH 03431
800-225-5381
Disability Served: all

This company manufactures wooden educational toys and activities, such as balance beams, puzzles, shoes for teaching children how to tie shoes, and blocks.

Wickliffe Industries Inc.

PO Box 286
Wickliffe, OH 44092
216-256-1030
Disability Served: all

Wickliffe offers a breathing mask designed to provide air at a comfortable temperature in cold conditions.

Wild International Corp.
PO Box 8482
Asheville, NC 28814
704-254-5000
Disability Served: all

This company manufactures accessible windows for the home.

Williams Sound Corp.
10399 West 70th Street
Eden Prairie, MN 55344-3459
612-943-2252, 800-328-6190
http://www.williamssound.com
Disability Served: hearing

This company manufactures amplification systems, including FM, personal, and infrared, telephone amplifiers, auxiliary bells, and speech amplifiers.

Willow Pond Tools Inc.
Adaptive Division
435 Deerpath Lane
PO Box 544
Pembroke, NH 03275
603-485-2321
Disability Served: all

This company makes forearm supports for persons with repetitive motion disorders and height-adjustable work tables.

Wimmer Ferguson Child Products Inc.
PO Box 100427
Denver, CO 80250
303-733-0848
Disability Served: all

This company makes products for infants and children, including activities and mobiles for developing gross motor skills and visual development.

Winco Inc.
5516 SW First Lane
Ocala, FL 34474-9307
352-854-2929, 800-237-3377
http://www.winco-medquip.com
Disability Served: all

This company manufactures bath and home equipment, including height-adjustable commode chairs, recliner chairs, shower chairs, footstools, grab bars, and walkers.

Winganna Care Products
6520 US Highway 10 West
Missoula, MT 59802-9364
406-883-2337
Disability Served: all

This company manufactures decubitus pads, sheepskin elbow and heel protectors, and other medical sheepskins.

Wise Enterprises
3500 Bridgeford Drive
Sacramento, CA 95834
916-927-7203, 888-947-3368
http://www.wisent.com/
Disability Served: all

This company features a catalog of adaptive daily living, communication, and mobility products for the physically challenged.

Won-Door Corporation
3609 Fox Glove Drive
Mid-Atlantic Branch Office
Huntingtown, MD 20639
410-535-8620
Disability Served: all

This company manufactures fire doors.

Woodbury Products, Inc.
3580 Oceanside Road
Island Park, NY 11572
800-777-1111
http://www.woodburycares.com
Disability Served: all

This discount mail order company offers savings of up to 50 percent on products for anyone suffering from incontinence. Products include adult disposable diapers, briefs, pads, and more. The company offers a free sample program.

Woodcraft Creations

Route 5, Box 442A
Salem, MO 65560
314-729-2258
Disability Served: all

This company manufactures rocking horses with safety seats.

Words +, Inc.

1220 W. Avenue J
Lancaster, CA 93534
800-869-8521
http://www.words-plus.com
Disability Served: all

Words +, Inc. provides augmentative and alternative communications systems as well as computer access programs, input switches, and wheelchair mounting.

Work Connections

525 Wall Street
Tiffin, OH 44883
419-448-4655, 800-589-2572
Disability Served: all

This company manufactures an ergonomically designed office chair.

Work Stations Inc.

11 Silver Sreet
South Hadley, MA 01075
413-535-3340, 800-759-6948
Disability Served: all

This company manufactures height-adjustable desks, office chairs, and other ergonomic office equipment, as well as powered elevating toilet seats and folding walkers with powered lifting arms.

Workstation Environments

1075 13th Street South
Birmingham, AL 35205
205-934-3136
Disability Served: physically disabled

This company manufactures an ergonomically designed computer work station.

WR Medical Electronics Co.

123 North Second Street
Stillwater, MN 55082
612-430-1200
Disability Served: all

Whirlpools and paraffin baths are manufactured by this company.

Wright Linear Pump

185A Robinson Road
Imperial, PA 15126
412-695-0800, 800-631-9535
Disability Served: all

This company makes an electrically-operated pressure system designed to reduce lymphedema.

WWRC Council of Organizations

Woodrow Wilson Rehabilitation Center
Fishersville, VA 22939
540-332-7149
Disability Served: all

This company manufactures mouthsticks and mouthstick holders.

X-10 (USA) Inc.

91 Ruckman Road
Closter, NJ 07624-0420
201-784-9700, 800-526-0027
Disability Served: all

This company manufactures a variety of environmental control units and switches designed to control appliances and lights. X-10 also makes flashing telephone signalers, timing switches, security systems and alarms, and thermostat controllers.

Zackback International

PO Box 9100
Rochester, MN 55903
507-281-7928
Disability Served: all

This company makes a back support system designed to fit office chairs.

Zero International Inc.

415 Concord Avenue
Bronx, NY 10455-4801
718-585-3230
Disability Served: physically disabled

This company manufactures accessible thresholds and portable ramps to facilitate wheelchair access.

ZiCom Technologies Inc.

576 Via Colinas
Thousand Oaks, CA 91362-5030
805-727-7110
Disability Served: hearing

This company manufactures an internal modem card that allows a computer to function as a telecommunication device for the deaf. The company also makes a portable TDD device.

Zim Manufacturing Co.

6100 West Grand Avenue
Chicago, IL 60639
773-622-2500
Disability Served: all

Zim makes kitchen tools, including basters and jar openers.

Zimmer Patient Care Systems

200 West Ohio Avenue
Dover, OH 44622
800-348-2759
Disability Served: all

This company manufactures cold packs and neoprene support systems for the knee, ankle, wrist, and elbow.

Zinco Industries, Inc.

180 North San Gabriel Boulevard
PO Box 5030
Pasadena, CA 91107-3488
626-405-0660, 800-228-5448
Disability Served: all

This company manufactures specialty orthotics, braces, and supports.

Zygo Industries, Inc.

PO Box 1008
Portland, OR 97207-1008
503-684-6006, 800-234-6006
http://www.zygo-usa.com
Disability Served: communication

This company manufactures and distributes communication systems for nonspeaking persons as well as environmental controls for electrical appliance access, including elevator control.

Mobility & Transportation

These companies develop, design, or sell wheelchairs, carts, vehicles, driving aids, and other items designed to increase the mobility of persons with disabilities.

Accumec Corp.

32 Race Street
San Jose, CA 95126
408-294-3100
Disability Served: physically disabled

This company manufactures wheelchairs, including wheelchairs with elevating seats and powered reclining wheelchairs. Accumec also makes powered chairs, wheelchair lapboards, and wheelchair accessories.

Adaptive Engineering Lab Inc.

4493 Russell Road, #113
PO Box 66
Mukilteo, WA 98275-0066
206-353-1335, 800-327-6080
Disability Served: physically disabled

This company manufactures abductor pads, mounting hardware for wheelchairs, restraints, and support systems.

Advanced Mobility Inc.
12555 Sherman Way
North Hollywood, CA 91605
818-982-1004
Disability Served: physically disabled

This company manufactures a portable, aluminum wheelchair ramp, a powered van seat that moves the driver's seat to accommodate wheelchairs, and passenger wheelchair restraint systems.

Advanced Technology Corporation
1601 Charlotte Street
Kansas City, MO 64108
816-421-6688, 800-785-9108
Disability Served: physically disabled

This company manufactures a motorized standing device called the Moto-Stand. This unit enables a paraplegic to stand and move about at work or at home. It also manufactures the Power-Stand, which is equipped with an electric lift assist and is used for standing therapy.

Advantage Bag Company
22633 Ellinwood Drive
Torrance, CA 90505
310-540-8197, 800-556-6307
Disability Served: physically disabled

This company manufactures backpacks and other carrying devices for use on wheelchairs, walkers, and crutches.

Ahnafield Corp.
3219 West Washington
Indianapolis, IN 46222
317-636-8061
Disability Served: physically disabled

This company manufactures driving aids and accessories for persons with disabilities. Products include hand controls, restraint systems, raised doors and tops, foot steering aids, and vehicle conversions and modifications.

All Purpose Manufacturing Corp.
3451 Merlin Drive
Clearwater, FL 34621
813-725-3144
Disability Served: physically disabled

This company manufactures hitch-mounted platform lifts and bumper-mounted lifts for scooters.

Alloy Graphics
8145 North Weirick Road
Corona, CA 91719
909-737-2545
Disability Served: physically disabled

This company manufactures push rims for racing wheelchairs.

Alpha Kinetics, Inc.
220 Water Street West
Cannon Falls, MN 55009
507-263-4774
Disability Served: physically disabled

This company manufactures a wheelchair crank that allows the user to crank the wheels rather than push them. The crank is ideal for racing wheelchairs.

Alshin Tire Corporation
8767 Onyx Street
Rancho Cucamonga, CA 91730
909-989-0604
Disability Served: physically disabled

This company manufactures urethane tires and caster assemblies for wheelchairs.

American Walker, Inc.
900 Market Street
Oregon, WI 53575
608-835-9255, 800-828-6808
Disability Served: physically disabled

This company manufactures and markets a line of patented, wheeled walkers. All have locking handbrakes, and two units have seats for resting.

Amigo Mobility International, Inc.
6693 Dixie Highway
Bridgeport, MI 48722-0402
517-777-0910, 800-821-2710
Disability Served: physically disabled

This company manufactures scooters, scooter accessories, a transport wheelchair, and a trunk-mounted wheelchair loader.

An-T-Roll, Inc.
PO Box 10054
Lynchburg, VA 24506
804-933-4400, 800-440-9588
Disability Served: physically disabled

This company makes an anti-tipping device for wheelchairs.

Angeles Group
PO Box 508
Pacific, MO 63069-0508
314-257-0533
Disability Served: all

This company manufactures wheeled walkers for toddlers.

Angle Lake Cyclery
20840 Pacific Highway South
Seattle, WA 98188
206-878-7457
Disability Served: physically disabled

This company develops semirecumbent tandem bicycles and recumbent bicycles.

Anthony Brothers Manufacturing
1945 South Rancho Santa Fe Road
San Marcos, CA 92069-5195
619-744-4763
Disability Served: physically disabled

This company manufactures hand-propelled tricycles for children and adults.

Arizona Freedom Wheels
PO Box 42982
Phoenix, AZ 85080
602-582-2399
Disability Served: physically disabled

This company manufactures a wheelchair accessory that converts a manual wheelchair into a lever-driven wheelchair.

Baby Jogger Company
PO Box 2189
2609 River Road
Yakima, WA 98907
509-457-0925, 800-241-1848
http://www.babyjogger.com
Disability Served: all

This company develops racing and heavy-duty strollers.

Bayview Manufacturing
Division of Dura-Tec Engineering, Inc.
2795 East Grand Boulevard
Detroit, MI 48211
313-891-7722, 800-966-9002
Disability Served: physically disabled

This company manufactures a wheelchair lift for vehicles. The lift loads the wheelchair behind the front seat.

Beach Wheels Inc.
1555 Shadowlawn
Naples, FL 33942
941-775-1078
Disability Served: physically disabled

This company offers a beach wheelchair.

Biomedical Horizons, Inc.
PO Box 889
Jackson, MI 49204
517-789-3216, 800-788-0889
Disability Served: physically disabled

This company manufactures a tilt and recline conversion system for manual wheelchairs.

BlackBerry Technologies Inc.
3813 Coventryville Road
Pottstown, PA 19465-8905
610-469-2151, 800-413-4824
Disability Served: physically disabled

This company manufactures lifestyle products for the disabled, including wheelchair brakes and locks.

Blatnik Precision Controls

1525 Cota Avenue
Long Beach, CA 90813
562-590-0445
Disability Served: physically disabled

Blatnik manufactures hand controls for vehicles.

Braun Corporation

1014 South Monticello
PO Box 310
Winamac, IN 46996
219-946-6153, 800-843-5438
Disability Served: physically disabled

Braun offers vehicle accessories, including lifts, ramps, powered seat bases for wheelchair drivers, automatic door controls, and vans.

Burr Engineering Company

730 East Michigan Avenue
PO Box 460
Battle Creek, MI 49016-0460
800-537-9940
Disability Served: physically disabled

This company manufactures vehicle accessories, including bumper-mounted scooter carriers, wheelchair alternative lifts for vans, and hitch-mounted scooter carriers.

California Cruisers, Inc.

8334 Amigo Avenue, Apartment 12
Northridge, CA 91324-4704
Disability Served: physically disabled

This company manufactures a manual, sport wheelchair.

Calley & Currier Co.

Old Bristol Road
Bristol, NH 03222
603-744-5151, 800-762-5500
Disability Served: all

This company provides crutches and crutch accessories such as handgrip pads, tips, and underarm cushions.

Cameron Enns Company

PO Box 5019
Fresno, CA 93755-5019
209-222-2922
Disability Served: physically disabled

This company manufactures foot controls to accommodate drivers with upper extremity disabilities.

Care Concepts

3145 West Lewis Avenue
Phoenix, AZ 85009
602-274-1432, 800-322-1432
Disability Served: physically disabled

This company provides wheelchair-accessible vans and vehicles.

Casa De Gutierrez

52 Englewood Hill
Pittsford, NY 14534-2517
716-334-8986
http://www.rit.edu/~dp94057/FVM.html
Disability Served: hearing

This company sells rearview mirrors for deaf drivers, wheelchair operators, and bed-confined persons.

Castleton Inc.

11300 Coloma, #A6
Rancho Cordova, CA 95670
916-638-8291
Disability Served: all

This company manufactures a driving aid that mounts on vehicles and detects objects near the rear of the vehicle by using ultrasound.

Chuck Chevillon & Associates Inc.

413 North Mannheim Road, Suite 2
Bellwood, IL 60104
708-544-0080
Disability Served: physically disabled

This company produces a wheelchair footrest.

Colours 'N Motion
1591 South Sinclair Street, Suite A
Anaheim, CA 92806
714-978-1440, 800-892-8998
Disability Served: physically disabled

This company manufactures a lightweight sport wheelchair.

Colson Caster Corporation
3700 Airport Road
Jonesboro, AR 72401
800-643-5515
http://www.colsoncaster.com
Disability Served: physically disabled

This company manufactures casters and wheels for industrial and institutional applications.

Complete Mobility
1901 Oakcrest
Roseville, MN 55113
612-635-0655
Disability Served: physically disabled

This company manufactures vehicle accessories, including electric-powered seats, automatic van door controls, powered parking brakes, and van lifts.

Concept Solutions Inc.
1 Wander Way
Lake in the Hills, IL 60102
847-658-8846
Disability Served: physically disabled

This company manufactures the Ivee Lift, an I.V. stand that attaches to the back of a standard wheelchair.

Concorde Battery Corporation
2009 San Bernardino Road
West Covina, CA 91790
626-962-4006
Disability Served: physically disabled

This company is a manufacturer of wheelchair batteries.

Conkle & Conkle Manufacturing
212 Walnut Street
Harrod, OH 45850
419-648-3328
Disability Served: physically disabled

This company produces a night light for use with walkers, crutches, or wheelchairs.

Convaquip Industries, Inc.
1102 Oak Street
Abilene, TX 79602
915-677-4177, 800-637-8436
http://www.convaquip.com
Disability Served: physically disabled

This company manufactures aids for obese patients. Items offered include wheelchairs, commodes, bath seats, crutches, canes, and more. Product weight specifications range from 250 pounds to 1,500 pounds.

Creative Controls Inc.
32450 Dequindre
Warren, MI 48092
313-979-3500
Disability Served: physically disabled

This company develops vehicle and driving accessories, such as a hardware kit with tools for installing a wheelchair restraint system in vehicles and hand controls.

Curtis Instruments Inc.
200 Kisco Avenue
Mt Kisco, NY 10549
914-666-2971
Disability Served: physically disabled

This company manufactures a speed limiter for wheelchairs and a battery fuel gauge.

Cyclo Manufacturing Company
1438 South Cherokee Street
Denver, CO 80223
800-525-0701
Disability Served: physically disabled

This company manufactures a pneumatic tire for wheelchairs.

D & D Advanced Technologies
PO Box 1077
Wayne, MI 48184
313-320-1173
Disability Served: physically disabled

This company develops a boost charger for electric wheelchair batteries.

Damaco Inc.—Freedom on Wheels
5105 Maureen Lane
Moorpark, CA 93021
805-532-1832, 800-432-2434
Disability Served: physically disabled

This company manufactures various wheelchairs.

Deming Designs
141 West Pinestead Road
Pensacola, FL 32503
850-478-5765
http://www.AIAweb.com
Disability Served: physically disabled

This company manufactures beach wheelchairs.

Donley Battery Company
7521 East Slauson Avenue
Los Angeles, CA 90040
213-728-2262
Disability Served: physically disabled

This company distributes wheelchair and motive power batteries.

Door-Aid Corporation
7700 Sprinkle Road
Portage, MI 49002
800-493-8377
http://www.door-aid.com
Disability Served: all

This company manufactures and markets the Retro-fit Automatic Door Opener.

Doron Precision System Inc.
PO Box 400
Binghamton, NY 13902
607-772-1610
Disability Served: physically disabled

This company manufactures a driving simulator to be used in training persons with disabilities to drive.

Drive Master Company, Inc.
9 Spielman Road
Fairfield, NJ 07004
973-808-9709
http://www.drivemaster.net
Disability Served: physically disabled

This company manufactures a number of driving and vehicle accessories, including hand and foot controls, wheelchair and scooter lifts, electronic driving aids, sensitized steering and braking, home modification.

Dynamo Aid Manufacturing Ltd.
577 Hanley Crescent
Windsor, ON N9G 1M5 Canada
519-252-2800
Disability Served: physically disabled

This company manufactures a four-wheel cycle for children.

Eagle Sportschairs
2351 Parkwood Road
Snellville, GA 30039
770-972-0763
http://www.harb.net/EagleSportschairs/
Disability Served: physically disabled

This company sells lightweight sports wheelchairs and products.

Easy One Corporation
Box 26244
Phoenix, AZ 85020
602-996-6123
Disability Served: physically disabled

This company manufactures a manual wheelchair loader designed to allow persons with limited strength to load and unload wheelchairs from vehicle trunks.

El Dorado National
13900 Sycamore Way
Chino, CA 91710
714-591-9557
Disability Served: physically disabled

This company manufactures the Aerotech, a public transport van for commercial bus use.

Elastocraft
7389 Kimbel Street, Unit 6-7
Mississauga, ON L4T 3M6 Canada
416-678-1466
Disability Served: physically disabled

This company manufactures accessories for wheelchairs, including calf rests and arm rest pads.

Electric Mobility Corp.
#1 Mobility Plaza
Sewell, NJ 08080
609-468-0270, 800-662-4548
Disability Served: physically disabled

This company produces wheelchair alternatives, including the Sparky Joystick Powerchair and the Electro Ped Trike.

Eliminator Airless Division
Anaheim Custom Extruders, Inc.
4640 East La Palma Avenue
Anaheim, CA 92807-1910
714-693-7577, 800-229-2760
Disability Served: physically disabled

The Eliminator is an airless cushion innertube for wheelchairs and bicycles.

Elite Wheelchair Products
2884 Melissa Court
Snellville, GA 30278
770-972-3757, 800-824-7903
Disability Served: physically disabled

This company manufactures wheelchairs, including sport and racing wheelchairs.

Environmental Coating Systems, Inc.
3321 South Susan Street
Santa Ana, CA 92704
714-641-1340
http://www.alldeck.com
Disability Served: physically disabled

This company manufactures nonslip floor-covering systems for indoor or outdoor use.

Equalizer Sport Tractor Company
Route 1, Box 1324
Elk Mound, WI 54739
715-897-5636
Disability Served: physically disabled

This company manufactures a four-wheel drive sport tractor for persons with mobility impairments.

Eric's House Inc.
12503 44th Drive SE
Everett, WA 98203-9000
Disability Served: physically disabled

This company manufactures a powered wheelchair for children.

EVAC+CHAIR Corporation
17 East 67th Street
New York, NY 10021
212-734-6222
http://www.evac-chair.com
Disability Served: physically disabled

This company manufactures an emergency wheelchair for stairway evacuation.

Ez Lift & Carrier Company
10609 Boedeker
Dallas, TX 75230
214-363-4820, 800-527-5239
Disability Served: physically disabled

This company manufactures the Kar Kady, a wheelchair carrier that attaches to a standard trailer hitch.

EZ Lock Inc.
2001 Wooddale Boulevard
Baton Rouge, LA 70806
225-214-4620
http://www.ezlock.net
Disability Served: physically disabled

This company manufactures an electric docking wheelchair restraint system that secures wheelchairs to vehicle floors.

Ferguson Auto Service
1112 North Sheppard Street
Richmond, VA 23230
804-358-0006
Disability Served: physically disabled

This company handcrafts and installs hand controls in automobiles.

Forth Research, Inc.
1435 North Hayden Road
Scottsdale, AZ 85257
602-423-2998
Disability Served: physically disabled

This company develops adult wheelchairs designed for controlled environments, such as laboratories and clean rooms.

Forward Motion, Inc.
Route 15, Box 125
Mechanicsville, VA 23111
804-746-4088
Disability Served: physically disabled

This company manufactures a beach wheelchair.

Forward Motions, Inc.
214 Valley Street
Dayton, OH 45404-1839
937-222-5001
Disability Served: physically disabled

This company modifies vehicles for people with physical disabilities.

G & R Specialties
Route 2, Box 140
Elgin, TX 78621
512-285-5379
Disability Served: physically disabled

This company manufactures chains for wheelchair tires that provide traction in snow, ice, mud, or sand.

Gadabout Wheelchairs
1165 Portland Avenue
Rochester, NY 14621
716-544-9060
Disability Served: physically disabled

This company manufactures portable, manual wheelchairs.

Gandy Company
528 Gandrud Road
Owatonna, MN 55060-0528
507-451-5430
http://www.gandy.net
Disability Served: physically disabled

This company manufactures a tandem bicycle adapter kit designed to convert two two-wheel bicycles into a stable four-wheel unit.

Gary E. Colle Inc.
5457 Ruffin Road, Suite B
San Diego, CA 92123
619-279-9710
Disability Served: physically disabled

This company manufactures a car-top wheelchair carrier that is powered by a car battery or the car cigarette lighter.

Genus Medical Inc.
203 Eggert Road
Buffalo, NY 14215
716-660-4005, 800-472-2549
Disability Served: physically disabled

This company distributes powered reclining and tilt systems for wheelchairs.

Global Research Inc.

201 East Washington Center Road
Fort Wayne, IN 46825
800-554-8044, 219-373-0075
http://globalpowersystems.com
Disability Served: physically disabled

This company manufactures powered wheelchairs for adults and children.

Goshen Coach

Division of Warrick Industries, Inc.
1809 West Hively Avenue
Elkhart, IN 46517
219-293-3500
Disability Served: physically disabled

This company manufactures public transport vans.

Gresham Driving Aids

30800 Wixom Road
PO Box 405
Wixom, MI 48393
810-624-1533, 800-521-8930
Disability Served: physically disabled

This company manufactures driving aids, including steering devices, extension levers for parking brakes and gear selectors, hand controls, and restraint systems.

Grove Innovations, Inc.

120 West Church Street
Centre Hall, PA 16828
814-364-2677
Disability Served: physically disabled

This company manufactures sport wheelchairs, mono-skis, and hand-propelled bicycles.

Hand Drive Company

211 Orchard Street
Golden, CO 80401
800-224-8156
http://www.handdrive.com
Disability Served: physically disabled

This company manufactures hand controls, a hand clutch, automotive accessories, and joy stick controls.

Handi Cap Aids of Oklahoma Inc.

223 West Britton Road
Oklahoma City, OK 73114
405-842-0511
Disability Served: physically disabled

This company manufactures a bumper-mounted wheelchair carrier.

Handi-Trak, Inc.

5150 North 32nd Street
Milwaukee, WI 53209
414-466-8725, 800-726-7718
Disability Served: physically disabled

This company makes snow chains for the tires of wheelchairs and scooters.

Haul Master Inc.

1501 1st Avenue
Mendota, IL 61342
815-539-7422, 800-848-42850
Disability Served: physically disabled

This company manufactures a gas-powered, all-terrain mini truck.

Haverich Ortho Sport, Inc.

165 Martell Court
Keene, NH 03431
603-358-0438, 800-529-9444
http://www.haverich.com
Disability Served: physically disabled

This company manufactures tricycles and bicycles for physically challenged individuals, for both single and tandem riders. Cycles are available to fit children from one and a half years to adults. Senior Cycles and Tri-Mountain models are available, along with numerous accessories.

Hoveround Corporation

8135 25th Court East
Sarasota, FL 34243-2800
941-359-3075, 800-96-HOVER
Disability Served: physically disabled

This company manufactures a powered wheelchair that has an elevating seat.

Imex Healthcare Inc.
1671 Dell Avenue, Suite 202
Campbell, CA 95008-6903
408-358-6320
Disability Served: physically disabled

This company manufactures a manual stand-up wheelchair.

IMS & Associates
4100 West Piedras Street
Farmington, NM 87401-3653
505-326-4538, 800-622-0623
Disability Served: physically disabled

This company manufactures a minivan with a ramp system to accommodate wheelchairs.

Innovative Products Inc.
830 South 48th Street
Grand Forks, ND 58201
701-772-5185
http://www.iphope.com
Disability Served: physically disabled

This company manufactures mobility equipment for children with disabilities.

Innovative Specialties Inc.
Route 1
PO Box 75
Harriman, TN 37748
615-882-5949
Disability Served: physically disabled

This company manufactures a hitch-mounted wheelchair carrier.

International Mobility Products Inc.
3915 San Pedro
San Antonio, TX 78212
210-732-1211, 800-533-5990
Disability Served: physically disabled

This company manufactures a car door opener to accommodate persons with limited hand strength.

Iron Horse Productions, Inc.
2624 Conner Street
Port Huron, MI 48060
810-987-6700, 800-426-0354
Disability Served: physically disabled

This company manufactures the Iron Horse, a folding frame wheelchair with a four-wheel suspension system.

Jaken Medical—New Horizons
2310 East Orangethorpe Avenue
Anaheim, CA 92806
714-447-4625, 800-678-4499
Disability Served: physically disabled

This company manufactures adult wheelchairs.

Kareco International Inc.
299 Route 22 East
Green Brook, NJ 08812
732-752-9292, 800-8KARECO
Disability Served: physically disabled

This company manufactures adult wheelchairs.

Kempf
1080 East Duane Avenue, Suite E
Sunnyvale, CA 94086
408-773-0219
Disability Served: physically disabled

This company manufactures an adapted Mercedes Benz that is foot and voice controlled. The company also offers a voice input-powered wheelchair.

Kettler International, Inc.
1355 London Bridge Road
Virginia Beach, VA 23456
757-427-2400
http://www.heinz-kettler.de
Disability Served: all

This company manufactures a pedal-powered car for children.

Kid-Kart Inc.
126 Rosebud, Suite #1
Belgrade, MT 59714
406-388-1080, 800-388-5278
Disability Served: all

This company manufactures a variety of child and infant strollers.

Kik Tire Inc.
590 Airport Road
Oceanside, CA 92054
760-967-2777
http://kiktire.com
Disability Served: physically disabled

This company manufactures tires for wheelchairs, scooters, and powerchairs.

Kinedyne Corporation
3701 Greenway Circle
Lawrence, KS 66046-5442
913-841-4000
Disability Served: physically disabled

This company designs and manufactures mobility aid (wheelchair) securement and occupant restraint systems.

Kroepke Kontrols Inc.
104 Hawkins Street
Bronx, NY 10464
718-885-1100
Disability Served: physically disabled

This company manufactures hand controls for automobiles.

Lark of America
West 220 North 507 Springdale Road
PO Box 1647
Waukesha, WI 53187
800-446-4522
http://www.larkofamerica.com
Disability Served: physically disabled

This company manufactures a powered scooter.

Lazy Days RV Center
11028 North Florida Avenue
Tampa, FL 33612
813-933-7613, 800-626-7800
Disability Served: physically disabled

This company manufactures a motor home that is wheelchair accessible.

LDC Corporation of America Inc.
780 Unit B2, Primos Avenue
Folcroft, PA 19032
610-586-0986, 800-782-6324
Disability Served: physically disabled

This company manufactures a wheelchair with a stand-up mechanism.

Le Mans Industries Corporation
79 Express Street
Plainview, NY 11803
516-942-9800, 800-289-5667
Disability Served: physically disabled

This company manufactures a wheelchair cover made of clear plastic.

Lester Electrical, Inc.
625 West A Street
Lincoln, NE 68522
402-477-8988
Disability Served: physically disabled

This company manufactures battery chargers for wheelchairs.

Levo USA
21050 Superior Street
Chatsworth, CA 91311
818-882-6944, 800-882-6944
Disability Served: physically disabled

This company manufactures manual wheelchairs that have power lifting features so the user can stand up.

Love Lift of Michigan
6270 Newholland Street
Hudsonville, MI 49426
616-875-6054, 800-218-8353
Disability Served: physically disabled

This company manufactures a transport wheelchair.

Manufacturing & Production Services Corp.
7948 Ronson Road
San Diego, CA 92111
619-292-1423, 800-243-4051
Disability Served: physically disabled

This company develops a left foot gas pedal to enable persons with limited or no use of the right leg to drive with the left leg. The company also manufactures a hand control for driving without the use of legs.

Martin Technology Inc.

29 North Main Street
Gloversville, NY 12078-3093
518-725-1837, 800-800-1410
Disability Served: physically disabled

This company manufactures a walker designed to climb stairs and traverse rough terrain.

Mason Corp.

7104 Crossroads Boulevard, Suite 108
Brentwood, TN 37027
615-373-8787, 800-821-4141
Disability Served: physically disabled

This company manufactures the Roller Racer, a riding toy propelled by pushing and pulling the handlebars.

Master Mobility Manufacturing

PO Box 127
Columbus, TX 78934
409-732-6638
Disability Served: physically disabled

This company modifies jeeps to make them wheelchair accessible.

Medical Lab Automation Inc.

8110 Ulmerton Road
Largo, FL 34641-3970
800-237-1162
Disability Served: physically disabled

This company manufactures a manual wheelchair and a combination wheelchair stretcher.

Medical Resource Companies of America

4265 Kellway Circle
Addison, TX 75244
214-407-8400, 800-583-6565
Disability Served: physically disabled

This company manufactures a three-wheeled, powered scooter.

Mednet Ketronic Inc.

555 Industrial Park Drive
Battle Creek, MI 49015
616-962-3800
Disability Served: physically disabled

This company manufactures the Kneelkar, a Dodge Caravan or Plymouth Voyager van with a rear ramp for wheelchair access.

MidWest Mobility, Inc.

401 South Schubert
11579 Kaw Drive (K-32 Highway)
Bonner Springs, KS 66012
888-640-1950
Disability Served: physically disabled

This company adapts vehicles for the disabled, adding or altering such features as wheelchair lifts, hand controls, power seats, raised roofs and doors, lowered floor minivans, door openers, and manual and electric wheelchair tie-downs.

MK Battery

13752 Harbor Boulevard
Garden Grove, CA 92643
714-554-9903, 800-372-9253
Disability Served: physically disabled

This company manufactures batteries for powered wheelchairs.

Mobilchair Corporation

8250 Vickers Street, Suite D
San Diego, CA 92111
619-292-4865
Disability Served: physically disabled

This company manufactures a geriatric chair designed for indoor use. The chair is on a powered wheel base.

Mobile Tech Inc.

PO Box 2326
Hutchinson, KS 67504-2326
316-663-4441, 800-835-5007
Disability Served: physically disabled

This company makes vehicle and transportation aids for persons with disabilities, including folding seats, ramps, platform lifts, and restraints.

Mobility Concepts
10 Maclaine Drive
North Providence, RI 02904-5210
Disability Served: physically disabled

This company manufactures manual wheelchairs.

Mobility Works
810 Moe Drive
Akron, OH 44310
330-633-1118, 800-638-8267
http://www.mobilityworks.com
Disability Served: physically disabled

This company builds and adapts vehicles for the handicapped.

Modern Mobility
8510 Rayburn Road
Bethesda, MD 20817
301-897-5541, 800-848-9255
Disability Served: physically disabled

This company offers folding, wheeled walkers and wheeled walkers with platform arm supports.

Morgan Technology, Inc.
2230 Wisconsin Avenue
Downers Grove, IL 60515
630-963-3210, 800-906-LITE
Disability Served: physically disabled

This company manufactures lightweight, manual wheelchairs for adults.

Motovator
1732 Border Avenue
Torrance, CA 90501-3601
310-320-5941
Disability Served: physically disabled

This company manufactures a three-wheeled, electric-powered scooter.

MSE Corporation
2546-A Mercantile Drive
Rancho Cordova, CA 95742
916-635-8284
Disability Served: physically disabled

This company makes a suspension caster fork for wheelchairs.

Mulholland Positioning Systems Inc.
PO Box 391
215 North 12th Street
Santa Paula, CA 93060
800-543-4769
http://mulhollandinc.com
Disability Served: physically disabled

This company designs, manufactures, markets, and sells pediatric seating and standing positioning devices for individuals with central nervous system deficits.

Natural Access
PO Box 2222
Princeton, NJ 08543
800-411-7789
http://www.natural-access.com/home
Disability Served: physically disabled

This company manufactures all-terrain wheelchairs for use on beaches and trails.

New England Handcycles Inc.
48 Bogle Street
Weston, MA 02193
508-237-7720
Disability Served: physically disabled

This company manufactures a hand-propelled cycle.

Newton Wheelchairs USA
21209 Lago Circle 12E
Boca Raton, FL 33433
561-483-7184
Disability Served: physically disabled

This company manufactures a folding transport wheelchair for adults that fits the aisles of commercial airplanes.

NobleMotion, Inc.
PO Box 5366
Pittsburgh, PA 15206
800-234-WALK
http://www.noblemotion.com
Disability Served: physically disabled

NobleMotion manufactures Swedish-style, four-wheeled roller walkers and other products for the walking impaired.

Normax Company

1040-35th Street
Columbus, GA 31904
706-596-1995, 800-392-1995
Disability Served: physically disabled

This company produces hand controls that allow persons with disabilities to drive automobiles with their hands.

Northern Wolf Enterprises

391 Page Street
Lunenburg, MA 01462
508-582-9057, 800-922-9057
Disability Served: hearing

This company provides assistive technology for automobiles, specifically alerting devices for vehicles driven by hearing impaired individuals. The cost of these devices may be reimbursed to qualified drivers.

On The Move Inc.

334 Franklin Street
Mansfield, MA 02048
508-339-4027
Disability Served: all

This company manufactures a walker for children.

One Step Beyond

80 Barbados Boulevard, Unit 30
Scarborough, ON M1J 1K9 Canada
416-267-6319
Disability Served: physically disabled

This company makes a heavy duty wheelchair suitable for rough terrain.

Ontario Drive & Gear Limited

PO Box 280
220 Bergey Court
Bleams Road
New Hamburg, ON N0B 2G0 Canada
519-662-2840, 800-561-9508
http://www.argoatv.com
Disability Served: physically disabled

This company manufactures and distributes amphibious all-terrain vehicles that can be operated with hand controls.

Optiway Technology Inc.

500 Norfinch Drive
Downsview, ON M3N 1Y4 Canada
416-739-8333, 800-514-7061
http://www.optiway.com
Disability Served: physically disabled

This company manufactures battery-powered scooters and wheelchairs.

Originator Corporation

832 Northwest 1st Street
Ft Lauderdale, FL 33311
954-463-7231, 888-859-5031
Disability Served: physically disabled

This company manufactures a rotary van lift called the Swing Out Lift.

Ortho Safe Systems, Inc.

6 B South Gold Drive
Robbinsville, NJ 08691
609-587-3859
Disability Served: physically disabled

This company manufactures a wheelchair-restraint system for vehicles.

Orthofab Inc.

2160 De Celies
Quebec, QC G2C 1X8 Canada
418-847-5225
Disability Served: physically disabled

This company manufactures powered wheelchairs.

Osprey Engineering

PO Box 511
15 Glengarry
Winchester, MA 01890
617-721-6737, 800-615-3305
Disability Served: physically disabled

Osprey makes an umbrella for wheelchairs.

Palmer Industries
PO Box 5707, Union Station
Endicott, NY 13763
607-754-1954, 800-847-1304
Disability Served: physically disabled

This company manufactures powered tricycles, manual tricycles, and all-terrain carts.

Paraglide Medical, Inc.
12001 31st Court North
St Petersburg, FL 33716
813-573-1010
Disability Served: physically disabled

This company manufactures a sports wheelchair for adults.

Permobil of America Inc.
6 B Gill Street
Woburn, MA 01801-1721
617-932-9009, 800-736-0925
Disability Served: physically disabled

This company manufactures powered wheelchairs as well as wheelchair restraint systems for automobiles.

Phil Wood and Co.
580 North 6th Street
San Jose, CA 95112
408-298-1540
Disability Served: physically disabled

This company manufactures wheels and hubs for wheelchairs.

Pop-Top Company
1895 Blase Nemeth Road, #6
Painesville, OH 44077
216-354-5231
Disability Served: physically disabled

This company manufactures a raised van top, which provides extra headroom in vans.

Power Technologies Inc.
Box 3244
201 Devil's Bedstead
Kethchum, ID 83340
208-726-3800, 800-228-8626
Disability Served: physically disabled

This company manufactures wheelchair batteries.

Precision Controls Inc.
PO Box 45
Haskell, NJ 07465
201-835-5000
Disability Served: physically disabled

This company manufactures hand controls for driving.

Precision Technology, Inc.
513 South Pine Street
Chelsea, OK 74016-1817
918-789-5505, 800-221-3433
Disability Served: physically disabled

This company manufactures a trunk-mounted scooter lift.

Prime Engineering
4838 West Jacquelyn, Suite 105
Fresno, CA 93722
209-276-0991, 800-827-8263
Disability Served: physically disabled

This company manufactures standing aids for children and adults.

Production Research Corp.
10217 Southard Drive
Beltsville, MD 20705
301-937-9633
Disability Served: physically disabled

This company makes wheels and specialty items for wheelchairs, such as handrims, camber plates, spoke protectors, and hubs.

Professional Service Unlimited
4418 NW 32nd Avenue
Gainesville, FL 32606
352-373-9810
Disability Served: physically disabled

This company makes a wheelchair narrowing device for standard wheelchairs so they can fit through narrow passages and entryways.

Pulsar/Antalco

PO Box 2706
Culver City, CA 90230
310-609-1584
Disability Served: physically disabled

This company manufactures a remote control unit used for operating van lifts.

Q'Straint

5553 Ravenswood Road, Suite 104
Ft Lauderdale, FL 33312
954-986-6665
http://qstraint.com
Disability Served: physically disabled

This company develops wheelchair restraint systems for vehicles.

Quantum Leap

974 Pinson Boulevard
Rockledge, FL 32955
407-631-5771
Disability Served: physically disabled

This company manufactures a hand-propelled, all-terrain tricycle for wheelchair users.

Quickie Designs, Inc./Shadow Products

A Division of Sunrise Medical
2842 Business Park Avenue
Fresno, CA 93727-1328
209-292-2171, 800-342-1579
Disability Served: physically disabled

This company manufactures wheelchairs, water skis, and mono-skis.

Ranger All Season Corp.

PO Box 132
2002 Kingbird Avenue
George, IA 51237
712-475-2811, 800-225-3811
http://www.rangerallseason.com
Disability Served: physically disabled

This company manufactures three-wheeled wheelchair alternatives.

RC Sales & Manufacturing Inc.

14726 Wake Street NE
Ham Lake, MN 55304
612-786-6504
Disability Served: physically disabled

This company manufactures wheelchair lifts and ramps for autos, driving aids, and wheelchair tie-down lifts for home use.

ReBike, Inc.

103 NW 43rd Street
Boca Raton, FL 33431
561-750-1304
Disability Served: all

This company manufactures a modified bicycle.

Recreatives Industries Inc.

60 Depot Street
Buffalo, NY 14206
800-255-2511
Disability Served: physically disabled

This company manufactures an all-terrain vehicle with hand controls.

Redman Wheelchairs

945 East Ohio Street #4
Tucson, AZ 85714-1694
520-294-2621, 800-727-6684
Disability Served: physically disabled

This company manufactures a number of wheelchairs.

Rehab 'n Motion Technologies, Inc.

67 Emerald Street
Keene, NH 03431
603-358-0439
Disability Served: physically disabled

This company manufactures a manual, adult wheelchair.

Rehabilitation Equipment & Supply

4804 North Sheridan Road
Peoria, IL 61614-5928
309-676-6054
Disability Served: physically disabled

This company makes a wheelchair-accessible motor home.

Renfroematics
PO Box 596
Kodak, TN 37764
800-53LIFTS
Disability Served: physically disabled

This company manufactures a hitch-mounted scooter carrier and wheelchair carriers for automobiles.

Roleez
5711A Sellger Drive
Norfolk, VA 23502
804-461-1122, 800-369-1390
Disability Served: physically disabled

This company manufactures all-terrain carts that are suitable for trails, beaches, and other terrains where conventional wheelchairs would not be suitable.

Rx Rocker Corporation
3541 Old Conejo Road, Suite 101
Newbury Park, CA 91320
805-499-0696, 800-ROCKER1
Disability Served: physically disabled

This company manufactures rocking wheelchairs.

Samhall Rehab
300 Long Beach Boulevard
Stratford, CT 06497-7153
203-380-0000, 800-882-0098
Disability Served: all

This company manufactures adjustable, wheeled walkers for children.

Schauer Manufacturing Corporation
4500 Alpine Avenue
Cincinnati, OH 45242
800-899-VOLT
Disability Served: physically disabled

This corporation manufactures a battery charger for wheelchair batteries.

Scooter Discounters
1601 Big Springs Place
Virginia Beach, VA 23456
800-229-1317
Disability Served: physically disabled

This company offers discount pricing on new electric scooters, ramps, scooter lifts, and gentle lift recliners.

SeatCase, Inc.
Division of Jarke-Thorsen Products
6407 Fair Valley Trail
Austin, TX 78749-1611
512-301-3703, 800-221-SEAT
Disability Served: physically disabled

This company manufactures a wheelchair and transfer chair that can be used during travel.

Seidel Electronics
466 West Market Street
Akron, OH 44303
330-376-3817
Disability Served: physically disabled

This company manufactures a powered wheelchair alternative.

Shade & Rain Umbrella Co.
11000 Highway 105W, Suite 105
Montgomery, TX 77356
409-588-3415
Disability Served: physically disabled

This company manufactures an umbrella designed to be attached to wheelchairs.

Skyway
4451 Caterpillar Road
Redding, CA 96003
916-243-5151, 800-332-3357
Disability Served: physically disabled

This company manufactures wheelchair wheels and casters.

Stand N Go Inc.
Route 5, Box 22A
Fergus Falls, MN 56537
218-739-5252
Disability Served: physically disabled

This company manufactures a mobile standing device that is powered by hand.

Starcraft Mobility—Consumer Division of National Mobility Corporation
2940 Dexter Drive
Elkhart, IN 46514
800-528-3769
http://www.starcraftcorp.com
Disability Served: physically disabled

This company manufactures lowered-floor, front wheel drive Chrysler, GM, and Ford minivans, as well as fully customized vans with power lifts.

Steven Motor Chair Company
120 North Gunter
Siloam Springs, AR 72761
501-524-8448
Disability Served: physically disabled

This company manufactures an electric powered wheelchair designed like a golf cart.

Style N Motion
17610 Ridge Top Drive
Houston, TX 77090
281-697-6688
Disability Served: physically disabled

This company provides upholstery and accessories for sports wheelchairs.

Summit Seating Systems
6310 Gross Point Road
Niles, IL 60648
847-647-2087
Disability Served: all

This company manufactures the Standing Bike, a standing aid that is available with or without wheels.

Sun Metal Products Inc.
PO Box 1508
Warsaw, IN 46581-1508
219-267-3281
Disability Served: physically disabled

This company manufactures wheels, tires, rims, bearings, and hubs for wheelchair wheels.

Supercruiser Inc.
23870 Pine Street, #1
Newhall, CA 91321-3111
805-255-6635
Disability Served: physically disabled

This company manufactures foot-powered scooters and carts for children and adults.

Tag Along Trailers, Inc.
Route 5, Box 184-2
Chippewa Falls, WI 54729
715-723-3060, 800-203-3060
Disability Served: physically disabled

This company manufactures a hitch-mounted scooter carrier.

Technical Engineering and Management (TEAM)
PO Box 15427
Augusta, GA 30919-1427
706-733-2727
Disability Served: physically disabled

This company manufactures a portable hand control for driving.

Technovation Inc.
6373 West Glenbrook Road
Brown Deer, WI 53223
414-354-8895
Disability Served: physically disabled

This company manufactures a manual, folding wheelchair.

Theradyne Corporation
21730 Hanover Avenue
Lakeville, MN 55044
612-469-4404, 800-328-4014
Disability Served: physically disabled

This company manufactures a wide variety of wheelchairs.

Tibby's
RR#4
7469 Rosevear Road
Duncan, BC V9L 3W8
604-748-2264
Disability Served: physically disabled

This company manufactures an all-terrain cart.

Time Savers Products Inc.
9210 Tokay Lane
PO Box 7147
Sacramento, CA 95826
916-383-2452
Disability Served: physically disabled

This company manufactures an electric lift for mobile homes and a hydraulic platform lift for vans.

Tiretyte International
66 East Santa Clara Street
San Jose, CA 95113
408-993-1010, 800-847-3898
http://www.tiretyte.com
Disability Served: physically disabled

This company manufactures flat tire sealant for wheelchair tires.

Top End by Action
4501-63rd Circle North
Pinellas Park, FL 34665
813-522-8677, 800-532-8677
Disability Served: physically disabled

This company manufactures sport wheelchairs, tricycles, and water skis for the physically disabled.

Trailex Aluminum Products
60 Industrial Park Drive
Canfield, OH 44406-0553
800-282-5042
http://www.trailex.com
Disability Served: physically disabled

This company manufactures hitch-mounted scooter carriers.

Trailmate
2359 Trailmate Drive
Sarasota, FL 34243
941-755-5511, 800-777-1034
Disability Served: physically disabled

This company manufactures tricycles and tandem bicycles for children and adults.

Triad Rehabilitation Products
PO Box 1364
Cumberland, MD 21502
301-759-3525
Disability Served: physically disabled

This company manufactures three-wheeled cycles.

Twenty-First Century Scientific Inc.
4915 Industrial Way
Coeur d'Alene, ID 83815
208-667-8800, 800-448-3680
http://www.wheelchairs.com
Disability Served: physically disabled

This company manufactures powered wheelchairs and replacement power drives for powered wheelchairs.

UNI-USA
8025 SW 185th
Aloha, OR 97007
503-649-7922
Disability Served: all

This company makes a three-wheeled stroller.

Union Battery Corporation
210 Dowdle Street, Unit #3
Algonquin, IL 60102
847-854-1295
Disability Served: physically disabled

This company makes rechargeable batteries for wheelchairs.

Up and Over Engineering
1509 Liberty Street
El Cerrito, CA 94530
510-233-1328
Disability Served: physically disabled

This company manufactures an off-road, sport wheelchair.

Uplift Mobility, Inc.
1625 Starkey Road
Largo, FL 33771
813-535-4645, 800-237-8268
Disability Served: all

This company sells, services, and rents medical equipment, including scooters, wheelchairs, liftchairs, walkers, and lifts.

USECO
4949 Everett Avenue
Los Angeles, CA 90058
Disability Served: all

This company manufactures an oil gauge that allows the driver to check the oil level of a vehicle from behind the wheel rather than under the hood.

Vantage Sales Inc.
5214 South 30th Street
Phoenix, AZ 85040
602-243-2700
Disability Served: physically disabled

This company offers modified vans for wheelchair accessibility.

Varna Cycles
Site 54-13, RR2
Gabriola Island, BC V0R 1X0 Canada
250-247-8379
Disability Served: physically disabled

This company makes hand-propelled bicycles, tricycles, and other cycles for the disabled.

Vartanian Industries, Inc.
PO Box 636
Switzgable Drive
Brodheadsville, PA 18322
717-992-5700, 888-242-4782
Disability Served: physically disabled

This company provides custom van conversions for physically challenged individuals.

Vector Mobility
5030 East Jensen
Fresno, CA 93725-1807
209-441-0358, 800-441-0358
Disability Served: physically disabled

This company manufactures manual and powered wheelchairs.

Vehicle Dynamics
291 Towers Road
Woodbridge, ON L4L 6A2 Canada
416-850-4440
Disability Served: physically disabled

This company develops a Chevrolet Blazer vehicle modified to accommodate wheelchair drivers.

Ventura Enterprises, Inc.
35 Lawton Avenue
Danville, IN 46122
317-745-2989
Disability Served: physically disabled

This company manufactures mobility aids.

Viking Formed Products
PO Box 319
Middlebury, IN 46540
219-825-8401
Disability Served: physically disabled

This company makes raised tops for vans.

Volkswagen United States Inc.
PO Box 2012
Bloomfield Hills, MI 48303-2012
800-444-8987
Disability Served: physically disabled

Volkswagen manufactures a wheelchair accessible minivan.

Voyager Inc.
68102 US Highway 31
Lakeville, IN 46536-9738
Disability Served: physically disabled

This company manufactures powered carts for outdoor use.

WalkerWorks
2101-1230 Nelson Street
Vancouver, BC V6E 1J6 Canada
604-944-8990, 800-667-4111
Disability Served: physically disabled

This company manufactures adjustable walkers.

WCMS Inc.
9920 Painter Avenue
PO Box 4023
Santa Fe Springs, CA 90670
562-944-8555
Disability Served: physically disabled

This company manufactures electric motors for powered wheelchairs.

Wells-Engberg Company, Inc.
PO Box 6388
Rockford, IL 61125-1388
815-874-5882, 800-642-3628
Disability Served: physically disabled

This company manufactures driving accessories, including hand controls, parking brake extensions, and pedal extensions.

Wheel Ring Inc./Enduro Wheelchairs
199 Forest Street
Manchester, CT 06040
203-647-8596
Disability Served: physically disabled

This company manufactures a variety of wheelchairs.

Wink Corporation
720 123st Street, SW, Suite 202
Everett, WA 98204
206-742-4145, 800-624-2101
Disability Served: all

Wink manufactures an extended rear view mirror for vehicles.

Winnie Walker Company
505 North Del Prado Boulevard
Cape Coral, FL 33909-2244
813-772-5155, 800-544-5155
Disability Served: physically disabled

This company manufactures adjustable wheeled walkers.

Worldwide Engineering Inc.
3240 North Delaware Street
Chandler, AZ 85225
602-545-0033, 800-848-3433
Disability Served: physically disabled

This company makes bumper- and trunk-mounted wheelchair and scooter carriers.

Wright Way Inc.
175 East I-30
Garland, TX 75043
214-240-8839
Disability Served: physically disabled

Wright Way manufactures driving aids for the physically disabled, including steering devices, restraint systems, vehicle modification kits, and hand controls.

Wy'East Medical Corporation
PO Box 1625
8850 SE Herbert Court
Clackamas, OR 97015
503-657-3101
Disability Served: physically disabled

This company manufactures a chair stretcher and transport wheelchair.

XL Manufacturing Co., Inc.
1020 Marauder Street, Suite 102
Chico, CA 95926
916-891-3535, 800-356-3554
Disability Served: physically disabled

This company manufactures a variety of wheelchairs for children and adults.

The Able and the Disabled

Communicating with People Who Have Disabilities

Martha Knowles of Orlando, Florida, will never forget the time she went to renew her driver's license at the Department of Motor Vehicles. When her number came up, she handed the clerk her paperwork and told him that she was deaf. He became flustered and asked, "And you currently have a driver's license?" Martha laughs about it now, but at the time, she was indignant. "He was clearly surprised that a person who was deaf could drive a car," she says. "Communication goes beyond just what people say; [it's] their attitudes and body language as well."

If you ask ten people who have disabilities to describe moments when communicating with other people has been strained or unpleasant, you'll hear certain themes repeat themselves in their stories. There's the recurring theme of being treated like a child. A middle-aged woman who has a speech impairment as the result of a stroke says she wishes that people wouldn't talk to her in a high-pitched, sing-song voice. Another woman who uses a wheelchair says she has been patted on the head countless times. Then there's being ignored in public. One man with muscular sclerosis who uses a wheelchair is not even taken aback anymore when waiters and waitresses hand a menu to his wife instead of directly to him.

If you haven't spent much time around people with disabilities, you might read these anecdotes and feel nervous about doing or saying the wrong thing yourself. But if you learn some very simple guidelines, communicating with people who have disabilities doesn't have to be awkward. Jude Monson, who works at the Summit Independent Living Center in Missoula, Montana, says, "The most common mistake people make is forgetting that it's a person they're dealing with, someone with feelings, thoughts, and their own personality." She offers an easy rule of thumb, which is to just relax and think how you would want to be treated. Instead of tiptoeing on eggshells and dwelling on the way that the person is different from you, focus on the many things you have in common.

Communication Basics

The best guide to communication is always the person you are communicating with. But there are some basic guidelines—specific to the type of disability—that you can follow as you're getting to know someone.

Visual Impairments. Be sure to identify yourself and anyone with you when you are meeting a person who is visually impaired. In talking to or working with people who have visual impairments, be as descriptive and specific as possible. For instance, say, "The chair is on your left, about two feet away." If you are guiding a person, don't grab or push. Instead, offer your arm and walk at their pace. In addition, remember that you should ask permission to interact with a person's guide dog.

Mobility Impairments. For people who are in wheelchairs, position yourself at eye level when you're speaking. Don't patronize someone by patting him or her on the head or shoulder. Treat the wheelchair as you would someone's personal body space, and don't lean on it. Feel free to offer assistance. After all, think about how grateful you are when someone holds open a door when you're carrying packages. Simply ask the person if he or she needs help and then act accordingly. If the answer is no, don't insist on it. Never move anyone's crutches, walker, cane, or other mobility aid without asking the person.

Speech Impairments. When you are talking to someone with a speech disability, don't pretend to understand what they've said if you haven't. The goal is communication. Repeat what you've understood, using a regular tone of voice, and let the person respond. Listen carefully. Be patient and wait for the person to finish. Don't step in to speak for him or her. If it's easier, the person can write it down. If you need to get information quickly, try to ask brief questions that can be answered by a nod of the head or a simple response. However, don't insult the person's intelligence by oversimplifying.

Hearing Impairments. To get the attention of a person who is deaf, tap him or her lightly on the shoulder. If the person can read lips, face the person so that he or she can see your mouth. Speak clearly and with natural expressiveness, but keep in mind that not all people who are deaf can read lips. If you are speaking through an interpreter, remember to pause occasionally to allow him or her to translate completely and accurately—particularly if there are technical terms or names that need to be fingerspelled. Even though the person you are speaking to will be looking at the interpreter, speak directly to the person who is deaf.

Cognitive Impairments. An adult with a cognitive disability should be treated as an adult. Use language that is concrete rather than abstract. People with brain injuries may have short-term memory deficits and will need information to be repeated. People with auditory perceptual problems might need to take notes to remember directions. They may benefit from having a task demonstrated. Other people have a problem with sensory overload and will find it disorienting to absorb too much information at once. As with speech impairments, don't pretend to understand someone with a cognitive impairment if you don't. Give the person time to respond and be supportive. Finally, don't interpret the person's distractedness as rudeness.

Language Matters

Are you worried about using the politically correct terminology and perhaps opting instead to say nothing at all? The more you work or talk with people who are disabled, the more of a handle you'll get on this. Generally speaking, however, remember this trick: put people first. That is, say "person with a disability" rather than "disabled person." Having a disability is just one aspect of a person's life. You want to use words that emphasize the wholeness of the person. After all, a woman with prosthetic arms might also be a mother, a skier, a singer, and a stockbroker. Think about how you would feel if people constantly referred to you as "the knock-kneed person," "the tea-drinking person," or "the shaky-hands person."

June Isaacson Kailes, a disability policy consultant in Los Angeles, California, was one of the earliest advocates for the thoughtful use of language about disabilities. She argues that while some people feel it's a trivial matter, "language plays a role in perpetuating negative stereotypes and in shaping ideas and attitudes." It really isn't any more complicated than learning the lingo of, say, a new sport, hobby, or job. Once you get used to phrasing things "people first," it will become second nature.

In considering the subtle power that words carry, it's worthwhile to take a look at a few other phrases that are inappropriate. The phrases "confined to a wheelchair" or "wheelchair bound" carry negative connotations. A person uses a wheelchair to increase his or her mobility and is anything but confined to it. Likewise, you've probably read articles in the newspaper that talked about how someone "overcame his or her disability." In fact, people live with disabilities. What they overcome are social, economic, psychological, architectural, transportation, educational, and employment barriers. Other terms that are considered outdated and even offensive are "handicapped," "sightless," "lame," "deformed," and "deaf mute."

Remember that the language that is considered appropriate now will not be so forever. It will change and evolve. But if you treat people who have disabilities as equal human beings, you will learn more along the way and forge the kind of relationships that have give and take. "I try to teach in my style of language," comments Jude Monson. "People who have the willingness to learn tend to pick up on it and begin mirroring how I've phrased things."

Some people with disabilities say that when you are in doubt about how to relate to a person, imagine how a child would handle the situation. A man who is deaf comments, "If I'm at the park, kids aren't afraid to walk over to me. They're curious, and they'll come right out and ask, 'Can you read my lips?'" Jude Monson reiterates that sentiment. As part of her job as educational coordinator for an independent living center, she goes into the local schools to do presentations. "Kids are great because they'll ask questions. Their parents are often the ones who are embarrassed or trying to be tactful," she says. "It's good to think that we can educate future generations to feel at ease with people who have disabilities."

Sources

Ten Commandments of Etiquette for Communicating with People with Disabilities
National Center for Access Unlimited
155 North Wacker Drive, Suite 315
Chicago, IL 60606

DO-IT
University of Washington
PO Box 354842
Seattle, WA 98195-4842
206-685-DOIT
doit@u.washington.edu
http://www.washington.edu/doit

Community Access Facts
Adaptive Environments Center
374 Congress Street, Suite 301
Boston, MA 02210
617-695-1225
http://www.adaptenv.org

This publication discusses the basic design needs of persons with disabilities in their homes.

Guidelines to Reporting and Writing and People with Disabilities
The President's Committee on Employment of People with Disabilities
1331 F Street NW, Suite 300
Washington, DC 20004
202-376-6200
TDD: 202-376-6205
info@pcepd.gov
http://www.pcepd.gov

Resources for Caregivers and Relatives

Activity-Based Approach to Early Intervention (An)
Paul H. Brookes Publishing Company
PO Box 10624
Baltimore, MD 21285
410-337-9580, 800-638-3775
http://www.pbrookes.com
Disability Served: all

This book helps parents and educators with activity-based intervention techniques for infants and young children.

Adaptable Housing
Rehabilitation Institute of Chicago
345 East Superior Street
Chicago, IL 60611
Disability Served: physically disabled

Attitudes Toward Persons with Disabilities
Springer Publishing Company
536 Broadway
New York, NY 10012
212-431-4370
Disability Served: all

This book discusses various attitudes that people hold regarding persons with disabilities.

Baby Power: A Guide for Families for Using Assistive Technology with their Infants
Center for Literacy and Disability Studies
University of North Carolina at Chapel Hill
Chapel Hill, NC 27599-8135
919-966-7486
Disability Served: all

This book provides basic information on assistive technology to aid parents of infants with disabilities.

Can't Your Child Hear? A Guide for Those Who Care About Deaf Children
Pro-Ed, Inc.
8700 Shoal Creek Boulevard
Austin, TX 78757-6897
512-451-3246, 800-897-3202
http://www.proedinc.com
Disability Served: hearing

This book is designed for parents of deaf children and provides answers to frequently asked questions concerning deafness.

Capsule
Children of Aging Parents
1609 Woodburne Road, Suite 302A
Levittown, PA 19057
215-945-6900
Disability Served: elderly

This bimonthly publication provides information and news for children of aging parents who are the caregivers.

Caretakers: The Forgotten People
1531 North Saddle Creek Road
Omaha, NE 68104
402-533-1200
Disability Served: all

This book discusses the role of the caretaker and its importance.

Caring Concepts
Centering Corporation
1531 North Saddle Creek Road
Omaha, NE 68104
402-533-1200
Disability Served: all

This quarterly publication recognizes the emotional aspects of living with family members with disabilities.

Center for Disability Information and Referral
Indiana Institute on Disability and Community
The University Affiliated Program of Indiana
2853 E. Tenth Street
Bloomington, IN 47408-2601
800-437-7924, 812/855-9396
http://www.isdd.indiana.edu/~cedir/familybib.html

This center has a bibliography of materials available to families of people with disabilities who are Indiana residents.

The Family Village
Waisman Center
University of Wisconsin-Madison
1500 Highland Avenue
Madison, WI 53705-2280
http://www.familyvillage.wisc.edu/index.html
Disability Served: all

This Internet community integrates information, resources, and communication opportunities for persons with cognitive and other disabilities, for their families, and for those that provide them services and support.

Golden Care Nurse's Registry
http://www.goldencares.com/
Disability Served: all

Golden Care Nurse's Registry, Inc. provides quality, experienced nursing services to hospitals and private residences in Southern California.

How to Write an IEP
Alliance for Parental Involvement in Education
PO Box 59
East Chatham, NY 12060
518-392-6900
Disability Served: all

This manual is designed to assist parents of children with disabilities.

Karri's Family Caregiver Support Page
http://www.geocities.com/HotSprings/Spa/2503/index.html
Disability Served: all

This Web site contains information on different aspects of care giving, from disabled children through elder care. The main interest on this site is husband/wife caregiving.

Making a Difference
L'institut Roeher Institute
4700 Keele Street
North York, ON M3J 1P3 Canada
416-661-9611
http://indie.ca/roeher/
Disability Served: all

This series of books discusses how to enhance the lives of the disabled.

Making Changes: Family Voices on Living with Disabilities
Brookline Books
PO Box 1046
Cambridge, MA 02238
617-868-0360, 800-666-BOOK
Disability Served: all

This book provides accounts of families caring for disabled members.

News Line
Federation for Children with Special Needs
135 Tremont Street, Suite 420
Boston, MA 02120
617-236-7210
http://www.fcsn.org
Disability Served: all

This monthly publication provides news and articles for parents of children with special needs.

Our Kids Magazine
Alexander Graham Bell Association of the Deaf
3417 Volta Place, NW
Washington, DC 20007
202-337-5220
Disability Served: hearing

This publication is designed for families of children with hearing impairments.

SCI Nursing
American Association of
Spinal Cord Injury Nurses
75-20 Astoria Boulevard
Jackson Heights, NY 11370
718-803-3782
Disability Served: physically disabled

This publication is designed for nurses of patients with spinal cord injuries.

So Your Child Has a Learning Problem?
CPPC, 4 Conant Square
Brandon, VT 05733
802-247-6871, 800-433-8234
Disability Served: all

This guide is written for parents of children who have learning problems.

Society's Assets
5200 Washington Avenue, Suite 225
Racine, WI 53406-4238
414-637-9128
Disability Served: all

Society's Assets, Inc. provides home care services for clients of all ages with an illness, injury, or disability.

Symptoms and Treatment of a Child's Learning and Academic Disorders
Psychological & Educational Publications, Inc.,
1477 Rollins Road
Burlingame, CA 94010
800-523-5775
Disability Served: learning disabled

This handbook is designed for parents of children with learning disabilities or other disorders.

Symptoms and Treatment of Child's Learning
Heath Publishing Company
PO Box 3805
San Francisco, CA 94119
415-750-6165
Disability Served: all

This book targets parents and provides descriptions and definitions of learning disabilities and disorders.

Web of Care
http://www.webofcare.com/
Disability Served: all

Web of Care is a home caregivers site providing support and information for people who are affected by various ailments, including Alzheimer's, cystic fibrosis, Down's Syndrome, muscular dystrophy, multiple sclerosis, Parkinson's, and cancer. The site is also intended for their caregivers, and their families.

Working Together: Workplace Culture, Employment and Disabilities
Brookline Books
PO Box 1046
Cambridge, MA 02238
617-868-0360, 800-666-BOOK
Disability Served: all

This book emphasizes the importance of collaboration between workplace members, service providers, and family in aiding disabled people to succeed in the workplace.

Funding Sources

Locating the Resources to Go to College

"I've always known I would go to college," says Joe Coombs, Jr., a freshman with cerebral palsy at Delaware Technical College. "To make decent money these days you really have to." Eric Patterson, a freshman at Mt. Hood Community College, echoes that sentiment. He began toying with the idea of going to college while he was a high school student at the Oregon School for the Blind. He explains, "I started researching careers and talking to a lot of people who worked in technology. Almost everyone had a college degree."

Joe and Eric are among an increasing number of people with disabilities who are heading off to college—and thriving there. The percentage of first-year college students who report having a disability has more than tripled since the late 1970s. A rise in the awareness and diagnosis of learning disabilities accounts for some of this tremendous enrollment jump. More significantly, however, students with disabilities who would have been steered away from college in the past now recognize that it's a great way to prepare for an interesting career and to take fuller control of their lives.

Nevertheless, heading off to college ranks right up there as one of life's major transitions. For the disabled student, it's particularly important to start laying the foundation for a good college experience early. This essay will provide some tips to help you get into the school of your choice, locate a variety of financial aid options, and make a smooth transition once you're on campus.

Starting Now

You can't start preparations too soon. Even if you're only in the ninth or tenth grade, it's time to begin considering your options. Get started by talking with school counselors or independent-living-center counselors about careers that pique your interest. Sign up for college-prep courses or consider taking a few college-level classes at a community college. Tackling tough courses now will make it easier once you're in college. And purchase the best computer you can afford, since they've become a necessity on most campuses.

Doing well on precollege exams such as the SAT and ACT is also going to give you a head start on getting into the college of your choice. If you need any sort of test-taking accommodations, don't be shy about asking for them. If you're disappointed with your score and feel you could improve on it, consider retaking the exam.

Choosing a School

You've decided what kind of career or degree program interests you. Now it's time to make a list of schools that offer those programs. Your high school counselor will have some suggestions, but you should also do your own research on colleges and universities by using reference books, using the Internet, and talking to people who have been to college about their experiences.

After you've made a preliminary list of schools that offer your chosen course of study, start narrowing the list based on other criteria. One of the things you'll need to decide is how important a school's disability services are to you. This question evokes strong reactions. "I feel that someone with a disability should not choose a school because of its disability services," says Jim Marks, Director of Disability Services for Students at the University of Montana. "They should choose one because it's in a cool city, or because the academic program is what they want, or because their friends are all going there." Carolyn Tyjewski, who is blind, wholeheartedly agrees. She has earned degrees in Black studies and English and is working toward a Ph.D. in Rhetoric at Ohio State University. She advises, "The law is quite clear that all schools have to make themselves accessible. Make your decision based on what you want to get out of the [college] experience."

Yet a number of students believe that the strength of a college's disability services can have a huge impact on their academic success or failure. Chuck Hurlburt was born with spina bifida and has learning disabilities. He earned an associate's degree from Mitchell College in New London, Connecticut, and a bachelor's degree from New Hampshire College. "I was not a terrific student and knew I needed to attend a college with small classes and lots of support," he says. "I worked with my guidance counselor to select a college that had excellent disability services."

Whatever the criteria on which you ultimately base your decision, you'll definitely want to inquire about disability services at all of the colleges on your list. Here are a few questions to ask:

- How much money does the school spend on its disability services? Is financial support available for continuing services?
- What's the enrollment of disabled students on campus? What is the graduation rate for students with disabilities?
- Is the staff knowledgeable about my disability?

Finding the Funds

If you're worried about how to foot the bill for college, you're not alone. Every three years, the Heath Resource Center publishes a statistical profile on first year college students with disabilities. Among its findings, the 1995 study showed that students with disabilities are more likely than their peers without disabilities to be significantly concerned about paying for their education's. The good news is that with some perseverance, you can find financial aid that will cover—or at least offset—the expense of college.

One of the sources that many college students with disabilities depend on is vocational rehabilitation (VR). The purpose of VR is to help individuals with disabilities maximize their employment, economic self-sufficiency, and integration into society. It's very important to contact your local VR office as early as possible. If you're a junior in high school, you should apply now to find out if you're eligible. Once VR determines your eligibility, you'll begin meeting with a counselor who will help you map out a long-term career plan. In most states, VR will pay for tuition, books, reader and interpreter services, and technological aids or devices. Kathy Cook, a disabled services counselor at the University of Washington, cautions that getting assistance from VR requires patience and persistence: "To go this route, you need to go through a lot of red tape, but it can definitely pay off. Last year, two of my students with learning disabilities had VR pay for their laptop computers."

It's unlikely, however, that all of your expenses will be covered by VR. You'll need to look into funding from other sources, too, such as grants, scholarships, loans, and work-study. The benefit of grants and scholarships is that they do not have to be repaid. Some scholarships are given to specific disability populations (contact the Heath Resource Center for a partial list). However, these scholarships are usually limited and in small amounts ranging from $500 to $1,000. Some colleges and universities also offer scholarships for students with disabilities, so it's important to make contact with disability services at the colleges you're considering. For a broader choice of scholarships, consider those that have nothing to do with your disability, but depend instead on your career goals, military experience, ethnic background, religious affiliation, extracurricular activities, and so forth. To search for current scholarships, see the section called "Funding Sources." You can also research scholarships on the Internet (see "Sources" for specific web sites) and in the many reference books at your local or school library.

Loans are a form of financial aid that must be repaid over an extended period of time after you finish college. Work-study allows you to work to earn money to cover your college expenses. One of the best sources of information about loans and work-study programs is the financial aid officer at each college to which you apply.

Other sources of financial assistance for students with disabilities include Supplemental Security Income (SSI), a federal program that provides assistance to people who are aged, blind, or disabled and have little or no income, and Social Security Disability Insurance (SSDI), which assists certain students who have been employed, who have a parent who has filed for Social Security, or who have a deceased parent. Discuss these options with your VR counselor or contact the Social Security administration office.

Here are some final thoughts about applying for financial aid: You'll be dealing with reams of paperwork. It's vital that you meet the deadlines and provide accurate information. Ask someone to proofread your forms and applications. During the application process, contact the colleges' financial aid offices to confirm that your data is being processed. It doesn't hurt to ask your VR counselor to stay in touch with the colleges, too.

Now You're in College!

The 1973 Rehabilitation Act and 1990 Americans with Disabilities Act states: "No otherwise qualified individual with a disability shall, solely by reason of his/her disability, be excluded from participation in, be denied the benefits of, or be subjected to discrimination under any program or activity of a public entity." But, as Jim Marks, Director of Disability Services for Students at the University of Montana, says, "As a college student, you have a civil right to access, but the responsibility to advocate is up to you. If you see discrimination, you have to fight it."

No matter how excellent a college or university is at providing accommodations for disabled students, you know better than anyone what your needs are. So it's up to you to make requests. Some accommodations are simple, such as a student with low vision asking to be seated in the front row. Other accommodations require creativity, like the student with a learning disability who asks a professor to incorporate tactile demonstrations into her instruction. Getting to know other students with disabilities on campus will give you a chance to share ideas and accommodation strategies.

Shifting into self-advocacy can be a dramatic change for students who have previously relied on counselors, parents, or teachers to handle matters for them. Kathy Cook says that the biggest adjustment for the disabled students she works with is learning to speak up for themselves. "In many instances the students have never talked about their disability and how it affects them academically," she says. "Students should start practicing these types of conversations before college so they'll be prepared."

Learning how to be a self-advocate is, in itself, a powerful skill, something you should aspire to gain from your time in college. You'll need to remind yourself of that occasionally when you face obstacles along the way to getting your degree. As Jim Marks says, however, "I can't think of a better way to prepare for the world of work."

Sources

Association on Higher Education and Disabilities (AHEAD)

University of Massachusetts, Boston
100 Morrissey Boulevard
Boston, MA 02125
617-287-3880
carol.desouza@umb.edu
http://www.ahead.org

AHEAD is an organization that addresses the need for upgrading the quality of services and support available to persons with disabilities in postsecondary education.

College and Career Programs for Deaf Students

http://gri.gallaudet.edu/ccg/index.html

At this site, you'll find excellent information that is intended for deaf students but is applicable to other disabilities as well.

DO-IT

University of Washington
PO Box 354842
Seattle, WA 98195-4842
206-685-DOIT
doit@u.washington.edu
http://www.washington.edu/doit

DO-IT (Disabilities, Opportunities, Internetworking, and Technology) works to increase the participation of individuals with disabilities in academic programs and careers.

FastWEB

http://www.fastweb.com

At this web site, you can set up a personalized profile that will match your specific skills, abilities, and interests to fastWEB's database of over 275,000 scholarships. You can also find information on other loan, work-study, and grant programs.

Financial Aid Information Page

http://www.finaid.org

This resource connects students with mailing lists, newsgroups, loan information, and scholarships for special-interest groups.

Funding Your Education

Federal Student Aid Programs
Box 84
Washington, DC 20044
800-433-3243
TDD/TTY: 800-730-8913

A free booklet from the U.S. Department of Education.

Heath Resource Center

1 Dupont Circle NW, Suite 800
Washington, DC 20036-1193
800-544-3284
http://www.acenet.edu/about/programs/Access&Equity/HEATH/home.html

The American Council on Education's national clearinghouse on postsecondary education for people with disabilities.

Talent Search and Educational Opportunity Centers

Division of Student Services
1250 Maryland Avenue, SW
Portals Building, Suite 600
Washington, DC 20202-5249

These programs provide counseling and other services to disadvantaged students and students with disabilities. The programs can help to negotiate financial assistance with postsecondary institutions.

Vocational Rehabilitation Offices

- To find one in your community:
- Look under the "State Government" pages of the phone book.
- Check with the local health and human services office.
- Call the local independent living center.
- Request a list from the National Rehabilitation Information Center, 8455 Colesville Road, Suite 935, Silver Spring, MD 20910. Phone: 800-346-2742.

Education Resources

Following is a list of funding resources for persons with disabilities who wish to pursue educational training. Included are grants, scholarships and loans.

Alabama Council of the Blind

1714 Vestawood Court, Suite A
Birmingham, AL 35216
205-967-5322
Disability Served: vision

Purpose: The Council provides grants to help defer postsecondary education expenses.
Eligibility: Residents of the state who are blind are eligible to apply.
Financial Details: The grant is in the amount of $200.
Number Awarded: Varies each year.
Deadline: Contact the Council for dates.

Alabama Department of Education

50 North Ripley
Montgomery, AL 36130
334-387-0555
http://www.alsde.edu/
Disability Served: vision

Purpose: To provide scholarships to help finance college study.
Eligibility: Residents of the state whose parents are blind may receive scholarship aid to attend a college or university in Alabama. Applicants must show that financial help is necessary to meet college expenses.
Financial Details: Award may cover tuition and required fees.
Number Awarded: Varies.
Deadline: Contact the Department for details.

Alabama Department of Veterans Affairs

770 Washington Avenue, Suite 530
Montgomery, AL 36104
334-242-5077
http://www.agencies.state.al.us
Disability Served: all

Purpose: To provide scholarships for the purpose of college study.
Eligibility: Children or spouses of Alabama military veterans who are disabled are eligible to apply. Recipients must attend a college or university in the state.
Financial Details: Amounts vary but benefits are limited to cost of tuition and fees. Awards are renewable for up to four years.
Number Awarded: Varies each year.
Deadline: Contact the Department for details.

Alabama State University

Office of Financial Aid
PO Box 271
Montgomery, AL 36101
334-229-4295
http://www.alasu.edu/
Disability Served: all

Purpose: To provide financial aid to help finance college study.
Eligibility: Students with disabilities attending the University are eligible to apply.
Financial Details: Amounts vary and depend on financial need.
Number Awarded: Varies each year.
Deadline: Contact the University for details.

Alexander Graham Bell Association for the Deaf and Hard of Hearing

3417 Volta Place, NW
Washington, DC 20007
202-337-5220
http://www.agbell.org
Disability Served: hearing

Purpose: To provide scholarships and financial aid awards for the purpose of college study.
Eligibility: Applicants must have a hearing loss and be able to communicate orally. Other specifications may apply, so contact the Association to learn more.
Financial Details: Scholarships range from $500 to $2,000. Financial aid awards are between $175 and $1,500.
Number Awarded: Approximately 150 scholarships and 400 awards are given each year.
Deadline: Applications must be requested between November 1 and December 1. Only the first 500 requests for applications will be accepted. Deadline for applications is March 15.

American Business Women's Association

9100 Ward Parkway
Kansas City, MO 64114
816-361-6621
Disability Served: all

Purpose: To provide financial aid for the purpose of financing college training.
Eligibility: Women with disabilities planning to attend college are eligible to apply.
Financial Details: Amounts vary. Write for details.
Number Awarded: Varies each year.
Deadline: Varies.

American Cancer Society Florida Division

3709 West Jetton Avenue
Tampa, FL 33629
813-253-0541
http://www.cancer.org
Disability Served: cancer patients and survivors

Purpose: Provides grants to help finance college training.
Eligibility: Florida residents who have had cancer before age twenty-one are eligible to apply.
Financial Details: Grants are for up to $2,000 plus $250 for textbooks.
Number Awarded: Varies each year.
Deadline: April 10 deadline for application for funding for the following academic year. Call Marilyn Westley at 813-253-0541 to request an application or e-mail her at mwestley@cancer.org.

American College of Healthcare Executives

One North Franklin Street, Suite 1700
Chicago, IL 60606
312-424-2800
Disability Served: all

Purpose: The Albert Dent Scholarship helps students with disabilities finance graduate training in a health care management field.
Eligibility: Applicants must be student members of the Association with a good undergraduate record
Financial Details: The scholarship is for $3,000.
Number Awarded: One per year.
Deadline: Application deadline is March 3.

American Council of the Blind

Scholarship Committee
1155 15th Street, NW, Suite 720
Washington, DC 20005
202-467-5081, 800-424-8666
http://acb.org/
Disability Served: vision

Purpose: The Council offers scholarships to help finance college study.
Eligibility: Students who are blind or visually impaired and admitted to an academic, vocational, technical, or professional training program are eligible to apply.
Financial Details: Awards range from $500 to $2,500.
Number Awarded: Fourteen scholarships are awarded each year.
Deadline: March 1.

American Foundation for the Blind

11 Penn Plaza South, Suite 300
New York, NY 10001
212-502-7600, 800-232-5463
Disability Served: vision

Purpose: The Foundation offers many scholarships for students who are legally blind and studying at the college level.
Eligibility: The Dillman Scholarship is open to undergraduate and graduate students preparing for the rehabilitation field. The Gillette Scholarship is open to an undergraduate woman studying music or literature. The Chinese American Scholarship Fund is open to Chinese American blind students who are pursuing a degree in higher education.
Financial Details: The Dillman Scholarship is for $2,500. The Gillette Scholarship is worth $1,000. The Chinese American Scholarship Fund awards up to $2,000.
Number Awarded: One each year.
Deadline: Varies. Contact the Foundation for details.

American Legion Auxiliary

720 Lyon Street
Des Moines, IA 50309
515-282-7987
Disability Served: all

Purpose: The Hoffman Memorial Scholarship is designed to help finance college training.
Eligibility: Descendants of a disabled veteran who are Iowa residents and who wish to pursue teaching careers are eligible.
Financial Details: The $200 grant is for use at the graduate level.
Number Awarded: Varies.
Deadline: Varies. Write for details.

American Legion, Maryland Auxiliary

Attn: Department Adjutant
War Memorial
Baltimore, MD 21202
410-752-3100
Disability Served: all

Purpose: Scholarships to finance college study are available.
Eligibility: Children of disabled veterans in Maryland are eligible to apply. Recipients must be no more than twenty years old.
Financial Details: Scholarships are for $500.
Number Awarded: Varies.
Deadline: Varies. Write for details.

American Legion, Mississippi Auxiliary

Attn: Department Secretary
PO Box 1682
Jackson, MS 39205
601-352-4986
Disability Served: all

Purpose: To provide scholarships for education.
Eligibility: State residents who are children of disabled veterans are eligible.
Financial Details: Scholarships are for $500 each.
Number Awarded: Varies each year.
Deadline: Contact the Legion for details.

American Legion, Nebraska Auxiliary

PO Box 880411
Lincoln, NE 68588
402-464-6338
Disability Served: all

Purpose: To provide grants to help finance college study.
Eligibility: Students who wish to prepare for careers to teach the handicapped and who plan to study at a Nebraska college or university are eligible to apply. Students must have some connection with a veteran but need not, themselves, be disabled.

American Legion, Oregon Auxiliary

PO Box 1730
Wilsonville, OR 97070
503-682-3162
Disability Served: all

Purpose: To provide a scholarship to help finance college study.
Eligibility: Oregon residents who are children of a disabled veteran and who plan to pursue post-secondary education at a school within the state are eligible.
Financial Details: Scholarships are for up to $1,000.
Number Awarded: Varies.
Deadline: Applications are due in March.

American Legion, Pennsylvania Auxiliary

PO Box 2643
Harrisburg, PA 17105
717-763-7545
Disability Served: all

Purpose: To provide grants to help finance college study at a state college or university.
Eligibility: Pennsylvania high school seniors who are sons or daughters of disabled veterans are eligible to apply. Candidates must demonstrate financial need.
Financial Details: Grants are for $600.
Number Awarded: One per year.
Deadline: Applications are due March 15.

American Legion, Washington Auxiliary

PO Box 3917
Lacey, WA 98503
360-491-4373
Disability Served: all

Purpose: To provide scholarships to help pay for college expenses.
Eligibility: Children of disabled veterans who live in Washington are eligible. Competition for the award includes writing an essay on educational goals.

Financial Details: The Scholarship is worth $300.
Number Awarded: One per year.
Deadline: Contact the organization for details.

American Nuclear Society

555 North Kensington Avenue
La Grange Park, IL 60526
708-352-6611
http://www.ans.org
Disability Served: all

Purpose: The Society offers the Robert Dannels Scholarship to help finance college study.
Eligibility: Students interested in graduate study in nuclear engineering or science are eligible. Candidates must have a strong undergraduate record and must be nominated by a faculty advisor or dean. Students with disabilities are particularly sought.
Financial Details: The Scholarship is for $4,000.
Number Awarded: One per year.
Deadline: Applications are due February 28.

American University

Office of Financial Aid
4400 Massachusetts Avenue, NW
Washington, DC 20016
202-885-3310
Disability Served: vision

Purpose: American University offers financial aid to students.
Eligibility: Students with disabilities are eligible to apply.
Financial Details: Amounts vary and depend on financial need.
Number Awarded: Varies.
Deadline: Varies. Contact the University for details.

Andalusia Health Services, Inc.

PO Box 667, 1208 Bypass West
Andalusia, AL 36420
205-222-2030
http://www.alaweb.com/~chamber/city.html
Disability Served: all

Purpose: To provide grants to help finance college study.
Eligibility: Residents of Covington County who are pursuing a degree in a medical field are eligible to apply.
Financial Details: Amounts vary.
Number Awarded: Varies.
Deadline: Contact the organization for details.

Aquinas College

Office of Financial Aid
1607 Robinson Road, SE
Grand Rapids, MI 49506
616-458-8281
http://www.aquinas.edu/home.html
Disability Served: all

Purpose: This liberal arts college provides financial aid to help finance college study.
Eligibility: Students with disabilities are eligible to apply.
Financial Details: Amounts vary and depend on financial need.
Number Awarded: Varies.
Deadline: Contact the College for dates.

Arizona Kidney Foundation

4019 North 44 Street, Suite 201
Phoenix, AZ 85018
602-840-1644
Disability Served: all

Purpose: The Foundation offers the Bidstrug Scholarship each year.
Eligibility: Arizona residents who are undergoing dialysis treatment or who have had a kidney transplant are eligible to apply.
Financial Details: Amount varies. Write for further information.
Number Awarded: Varies.
Deadline: Varies.

Arizona State University

Office of Financial Aid
Tempe, AZ 85287
520-965-4845
http://www.asu.edu/
Disability Served: communication

Purpose: The Sertoma Communicative Disorders Scholarship Program is available.
Eligibility: Full-time, graduate level students at the University studying speech language pathology or audiology are eligible to apply.

Financial Details: The award ranges from $2,500 to 5,000.
Number Awarded: Varies.
Deadline: Applications are available from December through April 1.

Arkansas Governor's Commission on People with Disabilities

1616 Brookwood Drive
Little Rock, AR 72202
501-296-1626
Disability Served: all

Purpose: To provide grants for higher education.
Eligibility: Graduate students with disabilities are eligible to apply. Recipients may attend any college in the country, but must have originally been a resident of Arkansas.
Financial Details: Grants start at $500.
Number Awarded: Varies each year.
Deadline: Applications are due in April.

Arkansas State University

Office of Financial Aid
PO Box 10
State University, AR 72467
501-972-2100
http://www.astate.edu/
Disability Served: all

Purpose: The University offers financial aid assistance.
Eligibility: Students with disabilities who require financial aid may apply.
Financial Details: Amounts vary and depend on need.
Number Awarded: Varies.
Deadline: Contact the University for details.

Art Institute of Philadelphia

1622 Chestnut Street
Philadelphia, PA 19103
215-246-3350
http://www.aiph.aii.edu
Disability Served: all

Purpose: This specialized art institute offers financial aid assistance.
Eligibility: Students with disabilities who require financial aid assistance may apply.
Financial Details: Amounts vary and depend on financial need.
Number Awarded: Varies.
Deadline: Contact the Institute for details.

Association for Education and Rehabilitation of the Blind and Visually Impaired

206 North Washington Street, Suite 320
Alexandria, VA 22314
703-548-1884
Disability Served: vision

Purpose: The Association awards the Ferrell Scholarship to help finance college study.
Eligibility: Visually impaired individuals who wish to prepare for work in the rehabilitation field are eligible.
Financial Details: Funds are limited and awards are made only in even-numbered years (1996, 1998, etc.).
Number Awarded: Varies.
Deadline: Applications are due April 15.

Association of Universities and Colleges of Canada

151 Slater Street
Ottawa, ON K1P 5N1 Canada
Disability Served: all

Purpose: The Imasco and Mattinson Scholarship is designed to help finance college training.
Eligibility: Canadian college students with disabilities are eligible to apply. There is no restriction on the field of study and it may be used at any undergraduate Canadian college or university.
Financial Details: Awards vary.
Number Awarded: One per year.
Deadline: Varies. Contact the Association for details.

Baptist General Convention of Texas

Attn: Ethnic Coordinator
333 North Washington
Dallas, TX 75246
214-828-5100
Disability Served: hearing

Purpose: The Ethnic Ministerial Scholarships to help finance training at a Baptist college or seminary are available.

Eligibility: Hearing impaired Texas residents who plan to attend a Baptist college or seminary are eligible. Hispanic students are particularly sought.
Financial Details: Scholarships are for $1,000 a year.
Number Awarded: Varies.
Deadline: Contact the Convention for details.

Bass Endowment Fund

200 North Main Street
Farmville, VA 23901
703-886-9450
Disability Served: vision

Purpose: The Fund offers grants to help finance graduate study.
Eligibility: Deaf graduates of the Virginia School for the Deaf and Blind pursuing additional training are eligible.
Financial Details: Grants of $600 to $1,000 are awarded.
Number Awarded: Varies.
Deadline: Call or write for details.

Bechtel Foundation

PO Box 193965
San Francisco, CA 94119-3965
415-768-5974
Disability Served: all

Purpose: The Foundation provides funds to support educational programs for the hearing impaired and the physically disabled for grades K through twelve.
Eligibility: Nonprofit organizations and educational institutions are eligible to apply. The Foundation is interested in supporting math, sciences, and technical educational programs. Preference is given to communities where Bechtel employees reside.
Financial Details: Amounts vary.
Number Awarded: Varies each year.
Deadline: Proposals are accepted throughout the year.

Blind Service Association

22 West Monroe Street, 22nd Floor
Chicago, IL 60603
312-236-0808
Disability Served: vision

Purpose: The Association awards scholarships to help finance college study.
Eligibility: Residents of the Greater Chicago area who are legally blind are eligible. Applicants must have a good academic record.
Financial Details: Scholarships of $100 to $2,500 are awarded.
Number Awarded: Varies.
Deadline: The deadline varies from year to year; call for details.

Blinded Veterans Association

477 H Street NW
Washington, DC 20001
202-371-8880, 800-669-7079
Disability Served: vision

Purpose: The Kathryn F. Gruber Scholarship helps finance undergraduate or graduate study.
Eligibility: Children or spouses of blind veterans are eligible.
Financial Details: Eight scholarships of $2000 and eight scholarships of $1000.
Number Awarded: One per year.
Deadline: Applications are due in May.

Boston Globe Foundation

135 Morrissey Boulevard, Box 2378
Boston, MA 02107
617-929-2895
http://www.bostonglobe/foundation
Disability Served: all

Purpose: To provide funds to nonprofit organizations.
Eligibility: Grants are limited to nonprofit organizations in Boston, Cambridge, Somerville, and Chelsea, Massachusetts.
Financial Details: Varies.
Number Awarded: Varies each year.
Deadline: None. Please contact the Foundation for guidelines.

Boston University

Attn: 504 Compliance Director
147 Bay Street
Boston, MA 02215
617-353-3568
http://web.bu.edu/
Disability Served: all

Bridge Endowment Fund

Scholarship Office, National FFA Office
PO Box 15160
Alexandria, VA 22309-0160
703-360-3600
Disability Served: all

Purpose: To provide scholarships to help finance college study.
Eligibility: Disabled students who are members of the Future Farmers of America may apply.
Financial Details: Amounts vary.
Number Awarded: Varies.
Deadline: Contact the organization for information.

Brigham Young University

1520 WSC
PO Box 27920
Provo, UT 84602
801-378-2767
http://www.byu.edu/home2.html
Disability Served: all

Purpose: This university offers a scholarship program for students with disabilities.
Eligibility: Disabled students who need financial assistance are eligible to apply.
Financial Details: Awards vary.
Number Awarded: Varies.
Deadline: Contact the University for details.

Calhoun Community College

PO Box 2216
Highway 31 North
Decatur, AL 35609
205-306-2500
http://calhoun.cc.al.us
Disability Served: all

Purpose: This two-year college offers financial aid for students with disabilities.
Eligibility: Disabled students who demonstrate financial need are eligible.
Financial Details: Awards vary according to need.
Number Awarded: Varies.
Deadline: Contact the College for details.

California Community Colleges

1107 Ninth Street
Sacramento, CA 95814
916-323-5953
Disability Served: all

Purpose: Extended Opportunity Grants to help finance college study are available.
Eligibility: Residents of the state with disabilities who are enrolled in a California two-year college with no more than seventy hours of course work completed are eligible.
Financial Details: Grants of up to $900 a year are awarded, based on expenses and financial need.
Number Awarded: Varies.
Deadline: Contact the financial aid office at institutions of interest.

California Council of the Bilnd

3919 West Magnolia Boulevard
Burbank, CA 91505
818-557-6378
Disability Served: vision

Purpose: The Council offers scholarships to help finance undergraduate or graduate training.
Eligibility: Residents of California who are legally blind may qualify for scholarships. Applicants must demonstrate financial need.
Financial Details: Scholarships of $300 to $3,000 are available.
Number Awarded: Varies.
Deadline: Contact the Council for details.

California Department of Veterans Affairs

PO Box 942895
Sacramento, CA 94295
916-653-2573
Disability Served: all

Purpose: The Department offers scholarships to help finance college training.
Eligibility: California children of veterans with a service-related disability are eligible for financial aid to attend a California state college, university, or community college. Applicants must have financial need.
Financial Details: Full scholarships for tuition and fees plus a stipend of $100 a month are awarded.
Number Awarded: Varies.
Deadline: Contact the Department for information.

California Governor's Committee for Employment of Disabled Persons

PO Box 972880
Sacramento, CA 94280
916-654-8055
Disability Served: all

Purpose: The Hal Connolly Scholarships are designed to help finance college study.
Eligibility: High school seniors who participated in varsity sports despite a handicap are eligible. Recipients need not plan to take part in sports while in college.
Financial Details: Awards of $250 to $1,000 are available.
Number Awarded: Varies.
Deadline: Write or call for more information.

California-Hawaii Elks Major Project, Inc.

5450 East Lamona Avenue
Fresno, CA 93727-2224
599-255-4531
http://www.cheo.org
Disability Served: all

Purpose: This program awards stipends to twenty residents of California and Hawaii with disabilities to help them finance college training.
Eligibility: California and Hawaii residents with disabilities are eligible. Applicants must be sponsored by an Elks member from one of the states.
Financial Details: Stipends are for $2,000 and are renewable for up to four years.
Number Awarded: Twenty per year.
Deadline: Contact a local Elks Lodge for information.

California State Polytechnic University

3801 West Temple Avenue
Pomona, CA 91768
909-869-2000
Disability Served: all

Purpose: This university offers a financial aid program for students with disabilities.
Eligibility: Disabled students who need financial assistance are eligible to apply.
Financial Details: Awards vary according to need.
Number Awarded: Varies.
Deadline: Contact the University for details.

California State University at Bakersfield

Office of Financial Aid
9001 Stockdale Highway
Bakersfield, CA 93311
805-664-3360
http://www.csubak.edu/
Disability Served: all

Purpose: This university offers a scholarship program for students with disabilities.
Eligibility: Disabled students who need financial assistance are eligible to apply.
Financial Details: Awards vary according to need.
Number Awarded: Varies.
Deadline: Contact the University for details.

California State University at Fresno

Office of Financial Aid
5241 North Maple Avenue
Fresno, CA 93740
209-278-2182
http://www.csufresno.edu/
Disability Served: all

Purpose: Among the financial aid awards at Cal State-Fresno is the Becky Honda Memorial Scholarship for students with disabilities.
Eligibility: Students with disabilities are eligible. Other restrictions may apply, so write for details.
Financial Details: Awards vary.
Number Awarded: Varies.
Deadline: Contact the University for details.

California State University at Fullerton

Services for Disabled Students
PO Box 34080
Fullerton, CA 92634
714-773-2011
http://www.fullerton.edu/
Disability Served: all

Purpose: This university offers a financial aid program for students with disabilities.
Eligibility: Disabled students who need financial assistance are eligible to apply.

Financial Details: Awards vary according to need.
Number Awarded: Varies.
Deadline: Contact the University for details.

California State University System

Office of the Chancellor
400 Golden Shore, Suite 222
Long Beach, CA 90802
562-985-2692
Disability Served: all

Purpose: The Forgivable Loan Program provides loans to help finance college training.
Eligibility: Women and persons with disabilities preparing for teaching careers in academic fields are eligible to apply.
Financial Details: Loans of $10,000 per year to a total of $30,000 are available. Twenty percent of the amount borrowed is forgiven for each year of college teaching.
Number Awarded: Varies.
Deadline: Write or call for additional information.

Calvin College

3201 Burton Street
Grand Rapids, MI 49546
616-957-6134
http://www.calvin.edu
Disability Served: all

Purpose: Several scholarships are available to finance college study.
Eligibility: First-year students with disabilities may apply.
Financial Details: Awards vary.
Number Awarded: Varies.
Deadline: Contact the College for details.

Candlelighters Childhood Cancer Foundation

PO Box 211
Vienna, VA 22183
703-803-7604
Disability Served: all

Purpose: The Candlelighters College Scholarship helps finance college study.
Eligibility: Persons who have had cancer before their twenty-first birthday are eligible.
Financial Details: Amounts vary.
Number Awarded: Varies.
Deadline: Write for details.

Central Intelligence Agency

Office of Student Programs
PO Box 12727
Arlington, VA 22209-8727
800-368-3886
http://www.odci.gov/cia/
Disability Served: all

Purpose: To provide scholarships for college study.
Eligibility: High school seniors with disabilities are eligible to apply. Other restrictions apply, so contact the CIA for additional information.
Financial Details: Scholars are awarded a yearly salary and up to $15,000 per school year for tuition, fees, books, and supplies.
Number Awarded: Varies each year.
Deadline: November 1.

Central Piedmont Community College

Office of Financial Aid
1201 Elizabeth Avenue
Charlotte, NC 28204
704-342-6739
Disability Served: all

Purpose: This two-year community college offers a financial aid program for students with disabilities.
Eligibility: Disabled students who need financial assistance are eligible to apply.
Financial Details: Awards vary according to need.
Number Awarded: Varies.
Deadline: Contact the College for details.

Central Texas College

Office of Financial Aid
PO Box 1800
Killeen, TX 76540
817-526-7161
Disability Served: all

Purpose: This college offers a financial aid program for students with disabilities.
Eligibility: Disabled students who need financial assistance are eligible to apply.

Financial Details: Awards vary according to need.
Number Awarded: Varies.
Deadline: Contact the College for details.

Central Washington University
400 E. Eighth Avenue.
Ellensburg, WA 98926-7431
509-963-2171
Disability Served: all

Cerritos College
Office of Admissions
11110 Alondra Boulevard
Norwalk, CA 90650
562-860-2451
Disability Served: all

Purpose: This two-year college offers a financial aid program for students with disabilities.
Eligibility: Disabled students who need financial assistance are eligible to apply.
Financial Details: Awards vary according to need.
Number Awarded: Varies.
Deadline: Contact the College for details.

Chairscholars Foundation, Inc.
16101 Carencia Lane
Odessa, FL 33556
813-920-2737
Disability Served: physically disabled

Purpose: To provide scholarships for college study.
Eligibility: High school seniors and college freshmen who are confined to wheelchairs are eligible.
Financial Details: Amounts vary.
Number Awarded: Varies.
Deadline: Contact the Foundation for details.

Cheff Center for the Handicapped
PO Box 368
Augusta, MI 49012
616-731-4471
Disability Served: all

Purpose: The Center was the first to teach therapeutic horseback riding to handicapped chil dren and adults. Graduates of the four-week program often become instructors of horseback riding for individuals with disabilities.
Eligibility: Handicapped children and adults who have an interest in horseback riding are eligible.
Financial Details: Half-tuition scholarships are available.
Number Awarded: Varies.
Deadline: Contact the Center for additional information.

Children of Deaf Adults Program
605 Commonwealth Avenue
Boston, MA 02215
Disability Served: hearing

Purpose: The Program provides scholarships to help finance college training.
Eligibility: High school seniors whose parents are deaf may apply.
Financial Details: Awards may range from $1,000 to $2,000.
Number Awarded: Two scholarships a year.
Deadline: Write for details.

Christian Heritage College
Office of Admissions
2100 Greenfield Drive
El Cajon, CA 92019
619-441-2200
http://www.christianheritage.edu
Disability Served: all

Purpose: This relatively small college has a scholarship to aid a student with disability.
Eligibility: Disabled students attending the College may apply.
Financial Details: Amounts vary.
Number Awarded: Varies.
Deadline: Contact the College for information.

Christian Record Services
4444 South 52nd Street
Lincoln, NE 68516
402-488-0981
Disability Served: vision

Purpose: This organization provides financial aid to help students finance course work toward a bachelor's degree.
Eligibility: Candidates who are legally blind are eligible to apply. Candidates must show financial need and how college will help them develop independence.
Financial Details: Amount of grant varies from year to year.
Number Awarded: Varies.
Deadline: Applications are accepted between November 1 and April 1.

College of DuPage

425 22nd Street
22nd Street and Lambert Road
Glen Ellyn, IL 60137
630-942-2380
http://www.cod.edu/
Disability Served: all

Purpose: This two-year college offers financial aid for students with disabilities.
Eligibility: Disabled students who demonstrate financial need are eligible.
Financial Details: Awards vary according to need.
Number Awarded: Varies.
Deadline: Contact the College for details.

College of Marin

Office of Financial Aid
Kentfield, CA 94904
510-457-8811
Disability Served: all

Purpose: The College offers scholarships to help pay for college study.
Eligibility: Students with disabilities may apply.
Financial Details: Grants of $150 per semester are awarded. Scholarships are renewable providing a 2.0 GPA is maintained.
Number Awarded: Varies.
Deadline: Apply by May 1.

College of Saint Elizabeth

Office of Financial Aid
Convent Station, NJ 07961
201-292-6300
Disability Served: all

Purpose: This women's college offers the Genevieve Walsh Scholarship to help finance schooling.
Eligibility: Entering freshmen with visual, mobility, or auditory impairment due to physical disability are eligible.
Financial Details: Awards range from $3,000 to $7,500.
Number Awarded: Varies each year.
Deadline: Applications are due June 1.

College of Southern Idaho

Office of Admissions
PO Box 1238
Twin Falls, ID 83303
208-733-9554
Disability Served: all

Purpose: This two-year college provides financial aid to students.
Eligibility: Students with disabilities who are attending the College and have financial need are eligible to apply.
Financial Details: Amounts vary and depend on need.
Number Awarded: Varies.
Deadline: Contact the College for details.

College of Staten Island

Department of Computer Science
2800 Victory Boulevard, IN-213
Staten Island, NY 10314
718-982-2850
http://www.csi.cuny.edu
Disability Served: vision

Purpose: To provide grants for the purpose of financing college education.
Eligibility: Blind and visually impaired students studying calculus and other mathematics and science courses are eligible to apply.
Financial Details: Amount varies and is funded

College of Staten Island

2800 Victory Boulevard, 2A-102
Staten Island, NY 10314
718-982-2030
http://www.csi.cuny.edu
Disability Served: all

Purpose: This college provides scholarships to help finance college study.

Eligibility: Students with disabilities who are attending the College are eligible to apply.
Financial Details: Amounts vary.
Number Awarded: Varies.
Deadline: Contact the College for details.

College of the Canyons

Office of Admissions
26455 North Rockwell Canyon Road
Santa Clarita, CA 91355
805-259-7800
Disability Served: all

Purpose: This two-year community college offers a financial aid program for students with disabilities.
Eligibility: Disabled students who need financial assistance are eligible to apply.
Financial Details: Awards vary according to need.
Number Awarded: Varies.
Deadline: Contact the College for details.

College of the Holy Cross

1 College Street
Worcester, MA 01610
508-793-2011
http://www.holycross.edu/
Disability Served: hearing

Purpose: The Mary Gammal Scholarship for students with a severe hearing disability is offered at Holy Cross.
Eligibility: Students with severe hearing disabilities are eligible. Priority is given to persons who live in the area of the college.

Columbia State Community College

Office of Admissions
PO Box 1315
Columbia, TN 38402
615-540-2572
Disability Served: all

Purpose: This two-year community college offers a scholarship program to help students with disabilities.
Eligibility: First-year students with disabilities are eligible.
Financial Details: Amounts vary.
Number Awarded: Varies.
Deadline: Contact the College for details.

Communications Disorders Foundation

PO Box 35653
Richmond, VA 23235
Disability Served: hearing

Purpose: The Foundation provides grants to help finance college study.
Eligibility: Persons who are studying to become an interpreter for the deaf or hard of hearing are eligible. Recipients may be enrolled in a Virginia school either full- or part-time.
Financial Details: Grants are for $250.
Number Awarded: Varies.
Deadline: Write for details.

Concordia University

Office of Financial Aid
1530 Concordia West
Irvine, CA 92715
714-854-8002
Disability Served: all

Purpose: This private four-year college offers financial aid to help students with disabilities.
Eligibility: Disabled students who need financial assistance are eligible to apply.
Financial Details: Amounts vary according to need.
Number Awarded: Varies.
Deadline: Write or call for additional details.

Conference of Educational Administrators

Department of Communications Disorders
San Diego State University
San Diego, CA 92182
Disability Served: hearing

Purpose: This organization offers a scholarship to help finance graduate study.
Eligibility: Minority students enrolled in an approved graduate program in the area of deafness are eligible.
Financial Details: The Scholarship is for $1,000.
Number Awarded: One per year.
Deadline: Contact the organization for further information.

Connecticut Department of Higher Education

Office of Student Financial Aid
Hartford, CT 06105
860-566-2618
Disability Served: all

Purpose: The Department awards grants to help finance undergraduate college study.
Eligibility: Connecticut residents who are dependents of a disabled Connecticut war veteran are eligible.
Financial Details: Grants of $400 are awarded.
Number Awarded: Varies.
Deadline: Varies. Call or write for information.

Council of Citizens with Low Vision

1400 North Drake Road, Suite 218
Kalamazoo, MI 49006
616-381-9566
Disability Served: vision

Purpose: To provide scholarships for education or training.
Eligibility: Persons preparing to work with those having low vision are eligible for the TeleSensory Systems Scholarship. Students who have low vision are eligible to apply for other scholarships.
Financial Details: Each scholarship is $1,000.
Number Awarded: One TeleSensory Systems Scholarship and three for those with low vision are awarded annually.
Deadline: March.

Crohn's & Colitis Foundation of America

386 Park Avenue South, 17th Floor
New York, NY 10016
800-932-2423
http://www.ccfa.org
Disability Served: all

Purpose: The Foundation awards the Brudnick Scholarship to help finance college study.
Eligibility: Undergraduate college students with Crohn's disease, colitis, or an ostomy are eligible. Applicants must be under twenty-four years of age, and priority is given to an individual who has demonstrated overcoming major obstacles in life.
Financial Details: The Scholarship is for $500.
Number Awarded: One per year.
Deadline: Applications are due in January.

Curry College

Learning Center
1071 Blue Hill Avenue
Milton, MA 02186
617-333-0500
Disability Served: learning disabled

Purpose: Several hundred students each year participate in the College's program for students with learning disabilities. Several awards are available, including the Phillips, Gordon, and Shapiro Scholarships.
Eligibility: Students with learning disabilities are eligible to apply.
Financial Details: Awards vary.
Number Awarded: Varies.
Deadline: Contact the College for information.

Cuyamaca College

900 Rancho San Diego Parkway
El Cajon, CA 92019
619-660-4275
http://www.cuyamaca.net
Disability Served: all

Purpose: This two-year community college offers a financial aid program for students with disabilities.
Eligibility: Disabled students who need financial assistance are eligible to apply.
Financial Details: Awards vary according to need.
Number Awarded: Varies.
Deadline: Contact the College for details.

David Lipscomb University

Office of Financial Aid
3901 Granny White Pike
Nashville, TN 37204
615-269-1791
Disability Served: all

Purpose: Among its other financial aid awards, the college offers a scholarship for students who have a parent with a disability.
Eligibility: Children of disabled parents are eligible to apply.
Financial Details: Amounts vary.

Number Awarded: One per year.
Deadline: Call or write for additional details.

Davis and Elkins College

Office of Admissions
100 Campus Drive
Elkins, WV 26241
304-636-1900
Disability Served: all

Purpose: This private four-year college offers a financial aid program for students with disabilities.
Eligibility: Disabled students who need financial assistance are eligible to apply.
Financial Details: Awards vary according to need.
Number Awarded: Varies.
Deadline: Contact the College for details.

Daytona Beach Community College

Office of Financial Aid
PO Box 2811
Daytona Beach, FL 32120
904-254-3328
Disability Served: all

Purpose: This two-year community college offers a financial aid program for students with disabilities.
Eligibility: Disabled students who need financial assistance are eligible to apply.
Financial Details: Awards vary according to need.
Number Awarded: Varies.
Deadline: Contact the College for details.

De Anza College

Office of Financial Aid
21250 Stevens Creek Boulevard
Cupertino, CA 95014
408-864-8567
Disability Served: all

Purpose: This large two-year college offers a financial aid program for students with disabilities.
Eligibility: Disabled students who need financial assistance are eligible to apply.
Financial Details: Awards vary according to need.
Number Awarded: Varies.
Deadline: Contact the College for details.

Defense Intelligence Agency

Civilian Personnel Division (DAH-2)
Washington, DC 20340
202-695-7353
Disability Served: all

Purpose: The Undergraduate Training Program is offered by the Agency.
Eligibility: High school seniors with disabilities who intend to study engineering, computer science, mathematics, geography, international relations, or political science in college are eligible.
Financial Details: The Program provides a paid summer job, financial aid during four years of college, and a job after graduation.
Number Awarded: Varies.
Deadline: Applications are due December 31.

Defiance College

Office of Financial Aid
701 North Clinton Street
Defiance, OH 43512
419-784-4010
Disability Served: all

Purpose: This four-year college offers a scholarship for students with disabilities.
Eligibility: Disabled students are eligible to apply.
Financial Details: Awards vary.
Number Awarded: Varies.
Deadline: Contact the College for details.

Delta Epsilon Sorority

c/o Daphne Cox McGregor
8619 Pin Oak Drive
Springfield, VA 22153
Disability Served: hearing

Purpose: The International Alumnae of Delta Epsilon offers a fellowship to help finance doctoral studies.
Eligibility: Deaf women enrolled in doctoral programs are eligible to apply. Candidates must have a strong GPA and financial need
Financial Details: The Fellowship is for $500.
Number Awarded: One per year.
Deadline: Applications are due April 1.

Delta Gamma Foundation

3250 Riverside Drive
Columbus, OH 43221
614-481-8169
http://www.deltagamma.org
Disability Served: vision

Purpose: Fellowships to help finance training are available.
Eligibility: Members of Delta Gamma who wish to prepare to work with the visually impaired are eligible to apply.
Financial Details: A Fellowship of $2,500 is awarded.
Number Awarded: One per year.
Deadline: Applications are due April 1.

Disabled American Veterans

PO Box 14301
Cincinnati, OH 45250
513-542-3281
Disability Served: physically disabled

Purpose: Scholarships to help finance college study are offered.
Eligibility: Children of veterans with a service-related disability are eligible. Interested students may apply when finishing high school or during any of the first three years of college. Scholarships are awarded based on financial need and strong academic record.
Financial Details: Scholarships range from $200 to $3,000.
Number Awarded: Varies.
Deadline: Write for information.

Disabled American Veterans Auxiliary

3725 Alexandria Pike
Cold Springs, KY 41076
606-441-7300
Disability Served: all

Purpose: The Auxiliary provides loans to help finance college study.
Eligibility: Children whose mothers were or are members of the DAV Auxiliary are eligible.
Financial Details: Loans of up to $1,000 are renewable for up to four years and must be repaid within seven years after graduating.
Number Awarded: Varies.
Deadline: Write or call for details.

Ear Foundation

2000 Church Street
Nashville, TN 37236
800-575-HEAR
http://www.earfoundation.org
Disability Served: hearing

Purpose: The Minnie Pearl Scholarship helps students meet college tuition.
Eligibility: Applicants must have a significant bilateral hearing loss, a 3.0 GPA, and have attended regular schools.
Financial Details: Scholarships are for up to $2,000 and are renewable.
Number Awarded: Varies.
Deadline: Call or write for further information.

East Central College

Highway 50 and Prairie Dell Road
PO Box 529
Union, MO 63084
314-583-5193
Disability Served: all

Purpose: Provides scholarships, grants, and loans to students of East Central College, a two-year public institution.
Eligibility: Funding is available to students who are deaf, blind, physically impaired, or learning disabled.
Financial Details: Amounts vary.
Number Awarded: Varies each year. In 1968, 252 scholarships, 800 grants, and 450 loans were awarded.
Deadline: Contact East Central College for dates.

East Los Angeles College

Office of Admissions
1301 Broken Avenue
Monterey Park, CA 91754
818-265-8787
Disability Served: all

Purpose: This two-year college offers financial aid for students with disabilities.
Eligibility: Disabled students who demonstrate financial need are eligible.
Financial Details: Awards vary according to need.
Number Awarded: Varies.
Deadline: Contact the College for details.

Easter Seal Society of Iowa, Inc.

Box 4002
Des Moines, IA 50333-4002
515-289-1933
Disability Served: all

Purpose: Provides scholarships for educational purposes.
Eligibility: Disabled Iowa residents attending or planning to attend an accredited college or university are eligible to apply.
Financial Details: Amounts vary.
Number Awarded: Eight per year.
Deadline: Apply after January 1. Contact the Easter Seal Society for application materials.

Easter Seals Iowa

401 NE 66th Street
Des Moines, IA 50313
515-289-1933
http://eastersealsia.org
Disability Served: all

Purpose: The Madden Mallory Scholarship is designed to help finance college training.
Eligibility: Iowa high school seniors with disabilities are eligible. Candidates must be in the top 40 percent of their class and plan to study full-time.
Financial Details: The Scholarship is for $1,000.
Number Awarded: One per year.
Deadline: Applications are due April 1.

Eastern Kentucky University

Office of Financial Aid
Richmond, KY 40475
606-622-2361
http://www.eku.edu/
Disability Served: all

Purpose: This university offers financial aid and scholarships for students with disabilities.
Eligibility: Disabled students who demonstrate financial need are eligible.
Financial Details: Awards vary according to need.
Number Awarded: Varies.
Deadline: Contact the University for details.

Edmonds Community College

Office of Financial Aid
20000 68th Avenue West
Lynnwood, WA 98536
425-640-1457
Disability Served: all

Purpose: This two-year college offers a scholarship program for students with disabilities.
Eligibility: Disabled students who demonstrate financial need are eligible.
Financial Details: Awards vary.
Number Awarded: Varies.
Deadline: Contact the College for details.

El Camino College

Office of Financial Aid
16007 Crenshaw Boulevard
Torrance, CA 90506
310-660-3296
Disability Served: all

Purpose: This two-year college offers financial aid for students with disabilities.
Eligibility: Disabled students who demonstrate financial need are eligible.
Financial Details: Awards vary according to need.
Number Awarded: Varies.
Deadline: Contact the College for details.

Electronic Industries Foundation

Scholarship Program Coordinator
919 18th Street, NW, Suite 900
Washington, DC 20016
202-955-5814
Disability Served: all

Purpose: Provides scholarships to help finance graduate studies in fields related to the electronics industry, including electrical engineering, industrial manufacturing, and physics.
Eligibility: Graduate students with documented disabilities who are studying fields related to the electronics industry may apply. Students must demonstrate financial need.
Financial Details: $5,000 is paid directly to the student's college or university.
Number Awarded: One per year.
Deadline: February 1.

Elizabeth City State University
Office of Financial Aid
Campus Box 914
Elizabeth City, NC 27909
919-335-3283
Disability Served: all

Purpose: This university offers financial aid and vocational rehabilitation scholarships for students with disabilities.
Eligibility: Disabled students who demonstrate financial need are eligible.
Financial Details: Awards vary according to need.
Number Awarded: Varies.
Deadline: Contact the University for details.

Emblem Club Scholarship Foundation
PO Box 712
San Luis Rey, CA 92068
619-757-0619
Disability Served: hearing

Purpose: The Foundation offers Emblem Club Scholarships to help finance college training.
Eligibility: Students who are studying for a master's degree preparing to teach the hard of hearing and deaf are eligible. Applicants must be in a program training special education teachers at one of a select number of schools: Gallaudet University, University of Nevada at Reno, Lewis and Clark College, the University of California, and the California State Universities at San Francisco, San Diego, and Los Angeles.
Financial Details: Scholarships average $4,000.
Number Awarded: Varies.
Deadline: Contact the Foundation for additional details.

Erskine College
Office of Financial Aid
PO Box 337
Due West, SC 29639
803-379-8838
Disability Served: all

Purpose: Among its other financial aid awards, the College offers a scholarship for students who have a parent with a disability.
Eligibility: Students who have a parent with a disability are eligible.
Financial Details: Amounts vary.
Number Awarded: One per year.
Deadline: Write for details.

Essex County Bar Foundation
One Newark Center, 7th Floor
Newark, NJ 07102-5497
201-622-6207
Disability Served: all

Purpose: The Foundation offers scholarships to help fund law school study for students with disabilities.
Eligibility: Law students in their second or third year who have a disability may apply. Candidates must have resided in Essex County at one time in their lives or have ties to Essex County.
Financial Details: Amounts vary.
Number Awarded: Varies.
Deadline: Apply by October 15.

Faulkner State Community College
1900 Highway 31 South
Bay Minette, AL 36507
334-520-2180
Disability Served: all

Purpose: This two-year community college offers financial aid for students with disabilities.
Eligibility: Disabled students who demonstrate financial need are eligible.
Financial Details: Awards vary according to need.
Number Awarded: Varies.
Deadline: Contact the College for details.

Fight for Sight Research Division of Prevent Blindness America
500 East Remington Road
Schaumburg, IL 60173
http://www.preventblindness.org
Disability Served: vision

Purpose: Fight for Sight offers summer research fellowships.
Eligibility: Undergraduate, graduate, and medical students from the United States or Canada who are interested in studying the eye from both its scientific and medical aspects are eligible to apply.

Financial Details: Awards up to $500 a month as a stipend for 60 to 90 days of full-time research.
Number Awarded: Varies.
Deadline: Contact the organization for details.

Florida Council of the Blind

PO Box 1229
Tallahassee, FL 32302
800-262-4448
http://www.fcb.org
Disability Served: vision

Purpose: The Academic Excellence Awards help students finance full-time college study.
Eligibility: Florida residents who are legally blind are eligible. Candidates must have a good prior academic record.
Financial Details: Awards are for $1,500.
Number Awarded: three.
Deadline: Applications are due in February.

Florida Department of Education

Office of Student Financial Assistance
State Programs
255 Collins
Tallahassee, FL 32399-0400
850-487-0049
http://www.firn.edu/doe/doehome.htm
Disability Served: all

Purpose: Provides scholarships covering tuition and fees at one of Florida's public colleges or universities.
Eligibility: Children of deceased or 100 percent disabled veterans pursuing or planning to pursue postsecondary education at one of Florida's public colleges or universities are eligible to apply.
Financial Details: Tuition and fees are covered.
Number Awarded: Approximately ninety scholarships are awarded per year.
Deadline: Apply by April 1.

Florida International University

Office of Financial Aid
University Park
Miami, FL 33199
305-348-3532
Disability Served: all

Purpose: The University offers a financial aid program to help students defer the costs of college training.
Eligibility: Students with disabilities who need financial assistance are eligible to apply.
Financial Details: Amounts vary and depend on need.
Number Awarded: Varies.
Deadline: Contact the University for details.

Florida Visual Aid Volunteers

2203 University Boulevard South
Jacksonville, FL 32216
Disability Served: vision

Purpose: This group awards a prize to recognize academic excellence.
Eligibility: Blind Florida high school seniors who have done well in school and are contemplating careers in science are eligible.
Financial Details: A prize of $75 is awarded.
Number Awarded: Varies.
Deadline: Applications are due in April. Write for further details.

Fordham University

Financial Aid Office
140 West 62nd Street, Room 125
New York, NY 10023
212-636-6815
http://www.fordham.edu/
Disability Served: vision

Purpose: The Amy Reiss Blind Student Scholarship is awarded to help finance law school.
Eligibility: Blind students at the Fordham University Law School with 2.3 GPAs are eligible.
Financial Details: The Scholarship covers partial tuition for three years.
Number Awarded: One per year.
Deadline: Contact the University for dates.

Foundation for Exceptional Children

1920 Association Drive
Reston, VA 20191-1589
703-620-3660
http://www.cec.sped.org
Disability Served: all

Purpose: Provides scholarships for full-time, postsecondary education or training (includes

two- and four-year undergraduate college programs or vocational, technical, or fine arts training programs).
Eligibility: The applicant must be disabled, enrolling in full-time, postsecondary education or training for the first time, and provide evidence of financial need. There are four categories for the Stanley E. Jackson Scholarship Awards: scholarship for students with disabilities, scholarship for ethnic minority students with disabilities, scholarship for talented and gifted students with disabilities, and scholarship for ethnic minority talented and gifted students with disabilities. Infitec Scholarships are eligible for students using an augmentative communication device or other technology-based alternative to oral communication.
Financial Details: Amounts vary. The Infitec Scholarship awards one $500 scholarship and one $1,000 scholarship.
Number Awarded: Varies each year. At least four Stanley E. Jackson Scholarships are awarded each year. Two Infitec Scholarships are awarded each year.
Deadline: Deadline to apply is February 1.

Foundation for Physical Therapy

1055 North Fairfax Street, Suite 350
Alexandria, VA 22314
703-684-5984
Disability Served: all

Purpose: The Sunrise Medical Scholarships help students finance college training.
Eligibility: Students with disabilities who wish to prepare for careers in physical therapy are eligible. Applicants must be preparing to work in a clinical setting.
Financial Details: $1,200 awards are given.
Number Awarded: Varies.
Deadline: Write or call for application materials and information.

Foundation for Science and Disability

Scholarship Committee
115 South Brainard Avenue
La Grange, IL 60525
708-352-1091
Disability Served: all

Purpose: The Foundation awards several grants each year to help finance graduate studies in a technical field.
Eligibility: Selection is based on need and the student's potential for a career in science or engineering.
Financial Details: Grants are for $1,000.
Number Awarded: Varies each year.
Deadline: December 1.

Foundation for Science and Disability

503 NW 89th Street
Gainesville, FL 32607-1400
352-374-5774
http://www.as.wvu.edu/~scidis/organizations/fsd_main.html
Disability Served: physically disabled

Purpose: Provides grants for the purpose of financing education.
Eligibility: Students working toward graduate degrees in the sciences or related fields are eligible to apply.
Financial Details: Grants are for the amount of $1,000.
Number Awarded: One to two per year.
Deadline: December 15.

Foundation Northwest

421 West Riverside, Suite 400
Spokane, WA 99201
509-624-2606
Disability Served: all

Purpose: The Foundation offers the Ren Riee Scholarship to help finance college study.
Eligibility: Spokane area residents with disabilities are eligible
Financial Details: The Scholarship covers tuition, fees, and books at a Washington state college or university. Scholarships are renewable.
Number Awarded: One per year.
Deadline: Applications are due in March.

Foust Educational Fund

c/o St. Andrews Episcopal Church
917 Lamar Street
Ft Worth, TX 76102
817-870-2649
Disability Served: all

Purpose: Financial assistance is given to help students finance college training.

Eligibility: Students with disabilities from Tarrant and Erath Counties in Texas who are attending a college or vocational school are eligible. Also eligible are nondisabled persons who are interested in preparing to serve persons with disabilities.
Financial Details: Amounts vary.
Number Awarded: Varies.
Deadline: Applications are due in March.

Friends of the Maryland State Library for the Blind and Handicapped

Scholarship Committee
1035 South Beechfield Avenue
Baltimore, MD 21229
410-247-6776
Disability Served: vision

Purpose: Scholarships for the purpose of financing college training are awarded.
Eligibility: Maryland residents who are preparing to use Braille to help the blind or who already work in the field are eligible. Recipients must agree to work for at least one year in Maryland in a job using Braille.
Financial Details: Scholarships are for $750.
Number Awarded: Two per year.
Deadline: Write or call for additional details.

Friends University

Office of Financial Aid
2100 University Avenue
Wichita, KS 67213
316-261-5846
http://www.friends.edu/
Disability Served: all

Purpose: Among the services for students with disabilities offered by this liberal arts college is financial aid.
Eligibility: Students with disabilities who need financial assistance are eligible.
Financial Details: Awards vary and depend on need.
Number Awarded: Varies.
Deadline: Varies. Contact the University for information.

Frostburg State University

Office of Financial Aid
Frostburg, MD 21532
301-689-4301
Disability Served: all

Purpose: The University offers Governor's Handicapped Aware Scholarships to students with disabilities.
Eligibility: Students with disabilities are eligible to apply.
Financial Details: Amounts vary.
Number Awarded: Varies.
Deadline: Contact the University for details.

Gallaudet University

Office of Financial Aid
800 Florida Avenue, NE
Washington, DC 20002
202-651-5290, 800-451-1073
http://www.gallaudet.edu/
Disability Served: hearing

Purpose: This is the only general college established exclusively to serve the deaf. It offers a full liberal arts program and financial aid to needy students. Among its offerings is a master's program in sign language interpreting.
Eligibility: Deaf students in need of financial assistance are eligible to apply.
Financial Details: Awards vary and depend on need.
Number Awarded: Varies.
Deadline: Contact the University for details.

Gallaudet University Alumni Association

800 Florida Avenue NE
Washington, DC 20002
202-651-5061
http://www.gallaudet.edu/~alumweb/
Disability Served: hearing

Purpose: The Alumni Association offers scholarships to help deaf and hard of hearing people finance graduate training.
Eligibility: Graduates of Gallaudet and others who are deaf and are pursuing doctoral studies are eligible.
Financial Details: Amounts vary.
Number Awarded: Varies.
Deadline: Applications are due April 20.

Galveston College
4015 Avenue Q
Galveston, TX 77550
409-763-6551
http://www.gc.edu
Disability Served: all

Purpose: This two-year community college offers a financial aid program for students with disabilities.
Eligibility: Disabled students who need financial assistance are eligible to apply.
Financial Details: Awards vary according to need.
Number Awarded: Varies.
Deadline: Contact the College for details.

Gardner-Webb University
PO Box 274
Boiling Springs, NC 28017
704-434-2371
Disability Served: all

Purpose: This private university offers a financial aid program for students with disabilities.
Eligibility: Disabled students who need financial assistance are eligible to apply.
Financial Details: Awards vary according to need.
Number Awarded: Varies.
Deadline: Contact the University for details.

Gateway Community College
108 North 40th Street
Phoenix, AZ 85034
602-392-5027
Disability Served: all

Purpose: This two-year community college offers a financial aid program for students with disabilities.
Eligibility: Disabled students who need financial assistance are eligible to apply.
Financial Details: Awards vary according to need.
Number Awarded: Varies.
Deadline: Contact the College for details.

Gateway Community-Technical College
60 Sargent Drive
New Haven, CT 06511
203-789-7058
http://www.gctc.commnet.edu/
Disability Served: all

Purpose: This two-year community college offers a financial aid program for students with disabilities.
Eligibility: Disabled students who need financial assistance are eligible to apply.
Financial Details: Awards vary according to need.
Number Awarded: Varies.
Deadline: Contact the College for details.

Geoffrey Foundation
PO Box 1112
Ocean Avenue
Kennebunkport, ME 04046
207-967-5798
Disability Served: hearing

Purpose: The Foundation awards grants to help finance education. It offers financial aid to help with the expenses of an auditory-verbal program.
Eligibility: Students with severe hearing impairments who intend to enroll in an auditory-verbal program are eligible.
Financial Details: Up to $5,000 may be awarded..
Number Awarded: Varies.
Deadline: Contact the Foundation for details.

Geological Society of America
PO Box 9140
Boulder, CO 80301
303-447-2020
http://www.geosociety.org/
Disability Served: all

Purpose: The Society awards research grants to students.
Eligibility: Geology students with disabilities who are studying at a university in the southeastern, south central, or northeastern states are eligible.

Financial Details: Research grants of $400 to $2,500 are awarded.
Number Awarded: Varies.
Deadline: Write for details.

George Washington University

Office of Financial Aid
Washington, DC 20052
202-994-8250
http://www.gwu.edu/
Disability Served: all

Purpose: This university offers a scholarship for students with disabilities.
Eligibility: Disabled students attending the University are eligible to apply.
Financial Details: Awards vary.
Number Awarded: Varies.
Deadline: Contact the University for details.

Georgia Council of the Blind

PO Box 682
Milledgeville, GA 21060
912-453-2128
Disability Served: vision

Purpose: The Council awards a scholarship to help pay for college.
Eligibility: Georgia students with a visual impairment or whose parents have a severe loss of vision are eligible. Students may apply as a high school senior or during the first year of college. Selection is based on academic record, with financial need as a secondary factor.
Financial Details: Scholarship is for approximately $8,500.
Number Awarded: One per year.
Deadline: Contact the Council for information.

Georgia Southwestern University

Office of Financial Aid
800 Wheatley Street
America, GA 31709
912-928-1378
Disability Served: all

Purpose: This university offers a financial aid program for students with disabilities.
Eligibility: Disabled students who need financial assistance are eligible to apply.
Financial Details: Awards vary according to need.
Number Awarded: Varies.
Deadline: Contact the University for details.

Georgia Student Finance Authority

2082 East Exchange Place, Suite 200
Tucker, GA 30084
770-414-3000
Disability Served: all

Purpose: The Georgia Law Enforcement Personnel Dependents Grant helps students meet college expenses.
Eligibility: Children of disabled police, fire, and other law enforcement staffs in Georgia are eligible. Applicants must be long-term residents of Georgia and must be attending college in Georgia.
Financial Details: The grant is for $2,000 a year and is renewable.
Number Awarded: One per year.
Deadline: Write for information.

Glendale Community College

1500 North Verdugord
Glendale, CA 91208
626-270-1000
Disability Served: all

Purpose: This large, two-year community college offers a financial aid program for students with disabilities.
Eligibility: Disabled students who need financial assistance are eligible to apply.
Financial Details: Awards vary according to need.
Number Awarded: Varies.
Deadline: Contact the College for details.

Gordon College

Office of Financial Aid
255 Grapevine Road
Wenham, MA 01984
508-927-2300
Disability Served: all

Purpose: This private four-year college offers a scholarship program for students with disabilities.
Eligibility: Disabled students are eligible to apply.

Financial Details: Awards vary.
Number Awarded: Varies.
Deadline: Contact the College for details.

Gordon West College

15744 Gordon West Street
Huntington Beach, CA 92647
714-892-8721
Disability Served: all

Purpose: This college offers financial aid to students with disabilities.
Eligibility: Disabled students who demonstrate financial need are eligible.
Financial Details: Awards vary according to need.
Number Awarded: Varies.
Deadline: Contact the College for details.

Gore Family Memorial Foundation

c/o Sun Bank Trust Department
PO Box 14728
Ft Lauderdale, FL 33302
Disability Served: all

Purpose: The Foundation provides grants to help with college costs.
Eligibility: Residents of Broward County, Florida, with disabilities, or persons with severe disabilities from anywhere in the country, are eligible to apply. Financial need is taken into consideration.
Financial Details: Scholarship amount in a recent year was up to $6,000, but most average $1,000 to $2,000.
Number Awarded: Varies.
Deadline: Write for additional information.

Grand Valley State University

Office of Financial Aid
Allendale, MI 49401
616-895-3234
Disability Served: all

Purpose: The University offers scholarships for students with disabilities.
Eligibility: Students with disabilities attending the University are eligible.
Financial Details: Amounts vary.
Number Awarded: Two per year.
Deadline: Write for details.

Grays Harbor College

Office of Financial Aid
1620 Edward Smith Drive
Aberdeen, WA 98520
360-538-4000
Disability Served: all

Purpose: This two-year college offers financial aid and a scholarship program for students with disabilities.
Eligibility: Disabled students who demonstrate financial need are eligible.
Financial Details: Awards vary according to need.
Number Awarded: Varies.
Deadline: Contact the College for details.

Guilead College

Office of Financial Aid
5800 West Friendly Avenue
Greensboro, NC 27410
910-316-2200
Disability Served: all

Purpose: This private four-year college offers financial aid for students with disabilities.
Eligibility: Disabled students who demonstrate financial need are eligible.
Financial Details: Awards vary according to need.
Number Awarded: Varies.
Deadline: Contact the College for details.

Hannibal-La Grange College

Office of Financial Aid
2800 Palmyra Road
Hannibal, MO 63401
314-221-3670
Disability Served: all

Purpose: This small four-year liberal arts college offers financial aid for students with disabilities.
Eligibility: Disabled students who demonstrate financial need are eligible.
Financial Details: Awards vary according to need.
Number Awarded: Varies.
Deadline: Contact the College for details.

Harding University
Office of Financial Aid
PO Box 2282
Searcy, AR 72149
501-279-4257
http://www.harding.edu/
Disability Served: all

Purpose: This university offers scholarships to help with college expenses.
Eligibility: Students whose parents have disabilities are eligible.
Financial Details: Awards vary.
Number Awarded: Varies.
Deadline: Contact the University for details.

Harry Alan Gregg Foundation
1 Verney Drive
Greenfield, NH 03047
603-547-3311, ext. 401
http://www.hag.org
Disability Served: all

Purpose: Funds may be requested for broad purposes but must specifically benefit the individual for whom funds are sought.
Eligibility: Residents of New Hampshire with physical, emotional, or intellectual disabilities are eligible to apply
Financial Details: Awards range from $300 to $500.
Number Awarded: 250 grants are awarded each year.
Deadline: Trustees meet quarterly, and applications should be received at least one month prior to the meeting date to be reviewed. Contact the Foundation for meeting dates.

Hawaii Community Foundation
900 Fort Street Mall, Suite 1300
Honolulu, HI 96813
808-537-6333
Disability Served: all

Purpose: The Foundation offers several awards to help Hawaiians with disabilities.
Eligibility: Public employees injured in the line of duty, persons over fifty with disabilities, and Native Hawaiian children with a learning disability are eligible for support.
Financial Details: Amounts vary and depend on need.
Number Awarded: Varies.
Deadline: Contact the Foundation for specifics.

Hawkeye Community College
Office of Financial Aid
1501 East Orange Road
Waterloo, IA 50704
319-296-4014
Disability Served: all

Purpose: This two-year college offers a financial aid program for students with disabilities.
Eligibility: Disabled students who demonstrate financial need are eligible.
Financial Details: Awards vary according to need.
Number Awarded: Varies.
Deadline: Contact the College for details.

Hofstra University
Office of Financial Aid
Hempstead, NY 11549
516-463-5840
http://www.hofstra.edu/
Disability Served: all

Purpose: In addition to its regular financial aid offerings, Hofstra also has a scholarship reserved for students with disabilities.
Eligibility: Students with disabilities are eligible to apply for the scholarship.
Financial Details: Amounts vary.
Number Awarded: One per year.
Deadline: Varies. Contact the University for information.

Home Mission Board
1350 Spring Street, NW
Atlanta, GA 30367
404-898-7000
Disability Served: hearing

Purpose: Language Missions Scholarships help finance college study.
Eligibility: Hearing impaired students who are interested in work as Christian workers are eligible. Applicants must be members of the Southern Baptist Church and plan to enroll full time in an academic program.

Financial Details: Up to $300 a school year is awarded.
Number Awarded: Varies.
Deadline: Write or call for information.

Houston Community College System

22 Waugh Drive
PO Box 7849
Houston, TX 77007
713-718-8550
http://www.hccs.cc.tx.us/
Disability Served: all

Purpose: This public two-year college offers financial aid for students with disabilities.
Eligibility: Disabled students who demonstrate financial need are eligible.
Financial Details: Awards vary according to need.
Number Awarded: Varies.
Deadline: Contact the College for details.

Humboldt State University

Office of Financial Aid
Arcata, CA 95521
707-826-4678
http://www.humboldt.edu/
Disability Served: all

Purpose: This public university offers financial aid for students with disabilities.
Eligibility: Disabled students who demonstrate financial need are eligible.
Financial Details: Awards vary according to need.
Number Awarded: Varies.
Deadline: Contact the University for details.

Idaho State Board of Education

Len B Jordan Office Building
650 West State Street, Room 307
Boise, ID 83720
208-334-2270
Disability Served: all

Purpose: The Board offers At Risk grants to help meet college expenses.
Eligibility: Residents of Idaho with disabilities who need financial help are eligible. Applicants must use the funds to attend a college within the state
Financial Details: Grants of $2,500 are awarded.
Number Awarded: Varies.
Deadline: Apply through the financial aid officer at the institution of interest.

Idaho State University

Office of Financial Aid
Campus Box 8077
Pocatello, ID 83209
208-236-2981
http://www.isu.edu/
Disability Served: all

Purpose: The University provides scholarships to help finance college study.
Eligibility: Students with disabilities may apply.
Financial Details: Amounts vary.
Number Awarded: Two scholarships are awarded each year.
Deadline: Call or write for details.

Illinois Department of Veterans Affairs

PO Box 19432
Springfield, IL 62794
217-524-4645
Disability Served: all

Purpose: The Department offers grants to help finance college training.
Eligibility: Children of disabled military service veterans whose disability occurred as the result of active service are eligible. In addition, the Department offers the Honorary Scholarship to children of disabled veterans.
Financial Details: Grants of up to $250 are offered. The Honorary Scholarship offers a tuition waiver at any branch of the University of Illinois.
Number Awarded: Grant numbers vary. One student from each county in Illinois is awarded the Honorary Scholarship.
Deadline: Write for details.

Illinois State University

Office of Financial Aid
Normal, IL 61790
309-438-2231
http://www.ilstu.edu/
Disability Served: all

Purpose: The University offers awards to help finance college study.
Eligibility: Students with disabilities enrolled in vocational rehabilitation programs are eligible.
Financial Details: Amounts vary.
Number Awarded: Several each year.
Deadline: Write or call for details.

Immune Deficiency Foundation

25 West Chesapeake Avenue, Suite 206
Towson, MD 21204
410-321-6647, 800-296-4433
http://primaryimmune.org
Disability Served: AIDS

Purpose: Scholarships help finance college study.
Eligibility: Students with a diagnosed primary immune deficiency disease are eligible to apply. Selection is based on financial need.
Financial Details: Amounts vary.
Number Awarded: Varies.
Deadline: Contact the Foundation for information.

Indiana State University

Office of Financial Aid
Reeve Hall
Terre Haute, IN 47809
812-237-2211
http://www-isu.indstate.edu/
Disability Served: all

Purpose: Among the other financial aid awards at the University are scholarships to help students finance college training.
Eligibility: Students whose parents have disabilities are eligible.
Financial Details: Amounts vary.
Number Awarded: Varies.
Deadline: Write or call for details.

Indiana-Purdue University at Fort Wayne

Office of Financial Aid
32010 East Coliseum Boulevard
Ft Wayne, IN 46805
219-481-6820
Disability Served: all

Purpose: Fort Wayne Street Rod Association Scholarships are available to help finance college study.
Eligibility: High school students with disabilities are eligible.
Financial Details: Amounts vary.
Number Awarded: Varies.
Deadline: Contact the University for information.

Indiana-Purdue University at Indianapolis

Office of Financial Aid
355 North Lansing Street
Indianapolis, IN 46202
317-274-5555
Disability Served: all

Purpose: This joint university venture offers degrees in a variety of fields through the doctorate. It offers financial aid to help students with disabilities.
Eligibility: Students with disabilities who need financial assistance are eligible
Financial Details: Amounts depend on need.
Number Awarded: Varies.
Deadline: Contact the University for more information.

International Christian Youth Exchange

134 West 26th Street
New York, NY 10001
212-206-7307
Disability Served: physically disabled

Purpose: Scholarships to help finance the International Christian Youth Exchange's school year abroad program are offered.
Eligibility: Students with disabilities, in high school or college, who have been selected to take part in the program are eligible.
Financial Details: Amounts vary.
Number Awarded: Varies.
Deadline: Contact the organization for more information.

Iowa Division of Vocational Rehabilitation Services

Department of Education
Des Moines, IA 50319
515-281-4311
Disability Served: all

Purpose: Financial aid is offered to help finance college training.
Eligibility: Students with disabilities from Iowa are eligible for financial aid to help defer college tuition, fees, and supplies.
Financial Details: Amounts vary according to need.
Number Awarded: Varies.
Deadline: Contact the agency for details.

Iowa State University

Office of Financial Aid
Ames, IA 50011
515-294-1020
http://www.iastate.edu/
Disability Served: all

Purpose: In addition to its regular financial aid awards, Iowa State offers scholarship assistance to students with disabilities.
Eligibility: Students with disabilities are eligible to apply.
Financial Details: Amounts vary.
Number Awarded: Varies.
Deadline: Call or write for details.

Iowa Western Community College

Office of Financial Aid
2700 College Road
Council Bluffs, IA 51502
712-325-3282
Disability Served: all

Purpose: This public two-year college aids approximately 100 students with disabilities each year through a variety of services. It also has a financial aid program to assist them.
Eligibility: Disabled students in need of financial assistance are eligible.
Financial Details: Awards vary according to need.
Number Awarded: Varies.
Deadline: Call or write for application materials and information.

Irvine Valley College

Office of Financial Aid
5500 Irvine Center Drive
Irvine, CA 92720
714-559-3243
Disability Served: all

Purpose: This public two-year college offers scholarships to help finance college study.
Eligibility: Students attending the College who have disabilities may apply.
Financial Details: Amounts vary.
Number Awarded: Varies.
Deadline: Contact the College for information.

Jewish Braille Institute of America

110 East 30th Street
New York, NY 10016
212-889-2525
Disability Served: vision

Purpose: To provide scholarships to help finance training.
Eligibility: Visually impaired students who wish to train to become Jewish educators or rabbis may apply. Students must demonstrate financial need.
Financial Details: Varies.
Number Awarded: Varies.
Deadline: Applications are accepted throughout the year.

Jim Smith Scholarship Fund

241 John Knox Road, Suite 200
Tallahassee, FL 32303
Disability Served: chemical dependency

Purpose: To provide loans for the purpose of financing college training.
Eligibility: Florida residents who have successfully completed a drug rehabilitation program are eligible to apply.
Financial Details: Loans are for up to $1,000 for each of two years to finance college training.
Number Awarded: Varies each year.
Deadline: Write for application materials and further information.

John Milton Society for the Blind

475 Riverside Drive, Room 455
New York, NY 10115
212-870-3335
http://www.jmsblind.org
Disability Served: vision

Purpose: Provides free Christian publications in Braille, large print, and on cassette tape to those who cannot see to read regular print.It also provides scholarships for education.

Eligibility: Funds are limited to students in particular programs at the Perkins School for the blind in Massachusetts and the Overbrook School for the Blind in Pennsylvania, as well as students recommended from the New York State Commission for the Blind and Visually Impaired.
Financial Details: Scholarships totalling $15,000 are awarded.
Number Awarded: Approximately 5.

Kappa Kappa Gamma

PO Box 2079
Columbus, OH 43216
614-291-3922
http://www.kappa.org
Disability Served: all

Purpose: Kappa Kappa Gamma Foundation Scholarships/Grants are available only to members of Kappa Kappa Gamma. For complete information and application materials, please send a self-addressed, stamped envelope to Kappa Kappa Gamma Foundation, PO Box 38, Columbus, OH 43216-0038. Please note your chapter membership on your request.

Kendall College of Art and Design

11 North Division Avenue
Grand Rapids, MI 49503
616-451-2787
http://www.kcad.edu
Disability Served: physically disabled

Purpose: The College offers the Berkowitz Scholarship to help finance college study.
Eligibility: Students attending the College who have physical disabilities are eligible.
Financial Details: Amounts vary.
Number Awarded: Varies.
Deadline: Contact the College for information.

Kent State University

Office of Financial Aid
Kent, OH 44242
216-672-3391
http://www.kent.edu/
Disability Served: all

Purpose: To provide a scholarship to help finance college training.
Eligibility: Students with disabilities may apply.
Financial Details: Amounts vary.
Number Awarded: One per year.
Deadline: Contact the University for information.

Kentucky Department of Veteran Affairs

525 South Third Street
Louisville, KY 40202
502-595-4447
Disability Served: all

Purpose: The Center offers tuition waivers at public colleges and universities in the state of Kentucky.
Eligibility: Kentucky residents who are children of disabled veterans are eligible.
Financial Details: Tuition waivers are awarded.
Number Awarded: Varies.
Deadline: Contact the Center for details.

Kentucky State University

Office of Financial Aid
East Main Street
Frankfort, KY 40601
502-227-5960
http://www.kysu.edu/
Disability Served: all

Purpose: This public university offers financial aid assistance.
Eligibility: Students whose parents have a disability are eligible for financial aid.
Financial Details: Amounts vary according to need.
Number Awarded: Varies.
Deadline: Contact the University for details.

La Sertoma International

1912 East Meyer Boulevard
Kansas City, MO 64312
816-492-3116
Disability Served: vision

Purpose: This organization provides scholarships for college training.
Eligibility: Graduate students planning to earn degrees to assist the blind may apply

Financial Details: Amounts vary.
Number Awarded: Varies.
Deadline: Contact the organization for information.

Lake-Sumter Community College

9501 US Highway 441
Leesburg, FL 34788
352-787-3747
http://lscc.cc.fl.us
Disability Served: all

Purpose: This two-year community college offers a financial aid program to help finance college study.
Eligibility: Disabled students who demonstrate financial need may apply.
Financial Details: Amounts depend on need.
Number Awarded: Varies.
Deadline: Contact the College for dates.

Lamar University

Communication Disorders
PO Box 10076
Beaumont, TX 77710
409-880-8170
http://www.lamar.edu/
Disability Served: hearing

Purpose: The University offers scholarships to help finance college study.
Eligibility: Doctoral candidates, who already hold a master's degree and who have three years of classroom experience with deaf children or in youth or clinical work are eligible. Applicants must know American Sign Language.
Financial Details: Amounts vary.
Number Awarded: Varies.
Deadline: Write or call for details.

Landmark College

Rural Route 1, Box 1000
Putney, VT 05346
802-387-4779
Disability Served: learning disabled

Purpose: This is the nation's only college designed exclusively for dyslexic students and students with learning disabilities. It has approximately 200 students enrolled and offers several scholarships to help those with financial need.
Eligibility: Students attending the College who demonstrate financial need are eligible.
Financial Details: Amounts vary according to need.
Number Awarded: Varies.
Deadline: Contact the College for information.

Landscape Architecture Foundation

4401 Connecticut Avenue, NW, Suite 500
Washington, DC 20008
202-686-0068
Disability Served: all

Purpose: The Lester Walls Scholarship is available for a student with a disability studying landscape architecture.
Eligibility: Students with disabilities who are studying landscape architecture may apply. Applicants must submit samples of work as a part of the application process.
Financial Details: The Scholarship is worth $500.
Number Awarded: One per year.
Deadline: Apply by May 1.

Las Positas College

Office of Financial Aid
3033 Collier Canyon Road
Livermore, CA 94550
510-373-4908
Disability Served: all

Purpose: This two-year college offers financial aid to its students with disabilities.
Eligibility: Financially needy students with disabilities are eligible to apply.
Financial Details: Awards vary according to need.
Number Awarded: Varies.
Deadline: Contact the College for details.

Lewis-Clark State College

500 Eighth Street
Lewiston, ID 83501
208-799-2269
Disability Served: all

Purpose: This public four-year institution offers financial aid to its students with disabilities.
Eligibility: Financially needy students with disabilities are eligible to apply.

Financial Details: Awards vary according to need.
Number Awarded: Varies.
Deadline: Contact the College for details.

Lighthouse, Inc. (The)

111 East 59th Street
New York, NY 10022
212-821-9200, 800-334-5497
http://www.lighthouse.org
Disability Served: vision

Purpose: To provide scholarships to students who are legally blind.
Eligibility: Legally blind students who reside and attend school in the Greater New York area and New England states are eligible to apply.
Financial Details: $5,000 scholarships are available.
Number Awarded: Five per year.
Deadline: Contact the organization for details.

Lions Club International

300 22nd Street
Oak Brook, IL 60521
630-571-5466
Disability Served: vision

Purpose: Local Lions Clubs often sponsor scholarships or other forms of assistance to aid blind persons in their area.
Eligibility: Requirements vary from chapter to chapter, so call or write for details.
Financial Details: Amounts vary.
Number Awarded: Varies.
Deadline: For details on programs in your area, contact your local Lions Club.

Loma Linda University

Office of Financial Aid
Loma Linda, CA 92350
909-724-4577
http://www.llu.edu/
Disability Served: all

Purpose: This public four-year university offers a financial aid program to help students with disabilities.
Eligibility: Disabled students in need of financial assistance are eligible to apply.
Financial Details: Amounts vary and depend on need.
Number Awarded: Varies.
Deadline: Varies. Write or call for details.

Los Medanos College

2700 East Leland Road
Pittsburg, CA 94565
510-439-2181
Disability Served: all

Purpose: This public two-year institution offers financial aid to its students with disabilities.
Eligibility: Financially needy students with disabilities are eligible to apply.
Financial Details: Awards vary according to need.
Number Awarded: Varies.
Deadline: Contact the College for details.

Louisiana Department of Veterans Affairs

PO Box 94095
Capitol Station
Baton Rouge, LA 70804
504-922-0500
Disability Served: all

Purpose: The Department helps students pay for college training.
Eligibility: Children of Louisiana veterans who are 100 percent disabled as a result of wartime active duty service are eligible to apply.
Financial Details: Free tuition and fees at one of the state's public colleges and universities are awarded.
Number Awarded: Varies.
Deadline: Contact the agency for information.

Louisiana State University

Office of Financial Aid
Baton Rouge, LA 70803
504-388-3103
Disability Served: all

Purpose: The University offers a financial aid program.
Eligibility: Students whose parents have a disability are eligible for financial aid.

Financial Details: Amounts vary and depend on need.
Number Awarded: Varies.
Deadline: Varies. Write or call for details.

Madonna University

Office of Financial Aid
36660 Schoolcraft Road
Livonia, MI 48150
313-591-5132
http://www.munet.edu/
Disability Served: all

Purpose: This private four-year university offers financial aid to its students with disabilities.
Eligibility: Financially needy students with disabilities are eligible to apply.
Financial Details: Awards vary according to need.
Number Awarded: Varies.
Deadline: Contact the University for details.

Maharishi University of Management

1000 North Fourth Street
PO Box 1132
Fairfield, IA 52556
515-472-1156
http://www.mum.edu/
Disability Served: cerebral palsy

Purpose: The University offers the Shelley Hoffman Scholarship to help finance college training.
Eligibility: Students with cerebral palsy and/or creative writing skills may apply. Recipients must maintain a 2.0 GPA to retain the award.
Financial Details: Awards vary.
Number Awarded: One to four per year.
Deadline: Applications are due June 1.

Maine Division of Veterans Services

State House Station 11
35 Anthony Avenue
Augusta, ME 04333
207-626-4464
Disability Served: physically disabled

Purpose: This agency offers grants and tuition waivers to help with the costs of college training.
Eligibility: Maine residents who are children of a severely disabled veteran are eligible.
Financial Details: Free tuition at one of the state's public colleges or $300 to be applied toward the cost at a private college of choice is awarded.
Number Awarded: Varies.
Deadline: Call or write for information.

Maple Woods Community College

2601 Northeast Barry Road
Kansas City, MO 64156
816-437-3000
Disability Served: all

Purpose: This two-year community college offers financial aid to its students with disabilities.
Eligibility: Financially needy students with disabilities are eligible to apply.
Financial Details: Awards vary according to need.
Number Awarded: Varies.
Deadline: Contact the College for details.

Marine Corps Scholarship

PO Box 3008
Princeton, NJ 08543
609-921-3534
Disability Served: all

Purpose: Scholarships are awarded to help with the costs of college.
Eligibility: Children of a Marine, either on active duty or discharged, are eligible. Candidates must come from a family with a total annual income under $45,000.
Financial Details: Scholarships of $500 to $2,500 are awarded.
Number Awarded: Varies.
Deadline: April 1. Contact the Foundation for information.

Marquette University

Office of Disability Services
PO Box 1881
615 North 11th Street
Milwaukee, WI 53233
414-288-1645
Disability Served: all

Purpose: This private four-year university offers financial aid and scholarships to its students with disabilities.
Eligibility: Financially needy students with disabilities are eligible to apply.
Financial Details: Awards vary according to need.
Number Awarded: Varies.
Deadline: Contact the University for details.

Marshalltown Community College

Office of Financial Aid
3700 South Center Street
Marshalltown, IA 50158
515-752-7106
Disability Served: all

Purpose: This two-year community college offers financial aid to its students with disabilities.
Eligibility: Financially needy students with disabilities are eligible to apply.
Financial Details: Awards vary according to need.
Number Awarded: Varies.
Deadline: Contact the College for details.

Maryland Higher Education Commission

Attn: State Scholarship Administration
16 Francis Street
Annapolis, MD 21401
410-974-5370
http://www.mhec.state.md.us/
Disability Served: all

Purpose: The Edward Conroy Scholarship helps finance college study at a state college.
Eligibility: Children of a Maryland permanently disabled veteran are eligible.
Financial Details: Up to full tuition and fees at a state college are awarded.
Number Awarded: One per year.
Deadline: Applications are due in July.

Maryland State Grange

Attn: Michael L. Guessford
Deaf Activities Committee
815 Frederick Street
Hagerstown, MD 21740
Disability Served: hearing

Purpose: The Grange offers scholarships to help finance college training.
Eligibility: Deaf students who are residents of Maryland, who graduated from a high school in the state, and who plan to attend college in Maryland are eligible for a scholarship for either undergraduate or graduate training. Also available is an award for persons who are preparing to work with the deaf or hard of hearing.
Financial Details: Amounts vary. Write for details.
Number Awarded: One of each.
Deadline: Contact the Grange for information.

Massachusetts Epilepsy Association

59 Temple Place, Suite 550
Boston, MA 02111
617-542-2292
Disability Served: all

Purpose: To provide scholarships to help finance college training.
Eligibility: Massachusetts residents with epilepsy are eligible. Priority is given to a student preparing for a career in the human services.
Financial Details: Scholarships are for $500 or more. These are one-time awards and may not be renewed.
Number Awarded: One per year.
Deadline: Applications are due in July.

Massachusetts Office of Student Financial Assistance

330 Stuart Street, Room 300
Boston, MA 02116
617-727-9420
Disability Served: all

Purpose: The Christian Herter Scholarship is designed to help fund college training.
Eligibility: Massachusetts residents who are in their second or third year of high school are eligible.
Financial Details: Amount varies.
Number Awarded: One per year.
Deadline: Write or call for details.

Massachusetts State Scholarship Office

330 Stuart Street, Room 300
Boston, MA 02116
617-727-9420
Disability Served: all

Purpose: The Office provides tuition waivers for disabled veterans.
Eligibility: Massachusetts residents who are disabled veterans of the Vietnam War and attending any public college or university in the state are eligible.
Financial Details: Full tuition waivers are awarded.
Number Awarded: Varies.
Deadline: Contact the Office for information.

McLennan Community College

1400 College Drive
Waco, TX 76708
817-756-6551
Disability Served: all

Purpose: This two-year community college offers a financial aid program to help finance college study.
Eligibility: Disabled students who demonstrate financial need may apply.
Financial Details: Amounts depend on need.
Number Awarded: Varies.
Deadline: Contact the College for dates.

Michigan Association for Deaf, Hearing, and Speech Services

724 Abbott Road
East Lansing, MI 48823
517-337-1646
Disability Served: hearing

Purpose: The Association awards scholarships to help students finance college training.
Eligibility: Michigan residents with hearing or speech impairments may apply. Awards are given to those completing high school.
Financial Details: Scholarships are for $500.
Number Awarded: Two scholarships per year.
Deadline: Applications are due March 1.

Michigan Commission for the Blind

201 North Washington, Victor Building, 2nd Floor
PO Box 30652
Lansing, MI 48909
517-373-2062, 800-292-4200
Disability Served: vision

Purpose: The Fund offers the Roy Johnson Scholarship to help finance graduate study at a college or university in Michigan.
Eligibility: Blind students who hold a bachelor's degree from any college in the country who plan to pursue graduate study at a college or university in Michigan may apply.
Financial Details: Awards range from $250 to $1,000.
Number Awarded: Varies.
Deadline: Applications are due in May.

Michigan Trust Fund

611 West Ottawa
Lansing, MI 48909
517-373-3130
Disability Served: physically disabled

Purpose: To provide grants to help finance college study.
Eligibility: Children of Michigan veterans who are totally disabled are eligible for Trust Fund tuition grants. Candidates must be between the ages of sixteen and twenty-two and have lived in Michigan for at least one year.
Financial Details: Grants are for up to the cost of tuition at a public college or university in the state.
Number Awarded: Varies.
Deadline: Contact the organization for details.

Midlands Technical College

Office of Financial Aid
PO Box 2408
Columbia, SC 29202
803-822-3508
Disability Served: all

Purpose: To provide financial aid to students with disabilities.
Eligibility: Disabled individuals who attend Midlands Technical College, a two-year community college, are eligible to apply.
Financial Details: Amounts vary.

Number Awarded: Varies.
Deadline: Contact the College for dates.

Minnesota Department of Veterans Affairs

Department of Education
20 West 12th Street
St Paul, MN 55155
612-296-2562
http://www.mdva.state.mn.us/
Disability Served: all

Purpose: The Department offers grants to help finance college training.
Eligibility: Disabled Minnesota veterans are eligible.
Financial Details: Grants of up to $350 are available.
Number Awarded: Varies.
Deadline: Contact the Department for details.

Miss Deaf America Award

804 SW Sixth Avenue
Faribault, MN 55021
507-334-2422
Disability Served: hearing

Purpose: This competition selects Miss Deaf America.
Eligibility: Deaf women between the ages of 18 and 28 are eligible to compete for the title of Miss Deaf America. Women compete first at the state level and later at the national competition.
Financial Details: Winners receive transportation to the national and small cash grants.
Number Awarded: Varies.
Deadline: Contact the organization for information. The competition is held only in even-numbered years (1998, 2000, etc.).

Mississippi Association for Education and Rehabilitation of the Blind and Visually Impaired

Scholarship Committee
1860 Meadowbrook Road
Jackson, MS 39211
Disability Served: vision

Purpose: To provide scholarships to help finance college study.
Eligibility: High school seniors who have at least one legally blind parent are eligible to apply. Academic record plays a major part in determining the winner of this award
Financial Details: Scholarship is for $400 to help finance college study.
Number Awarded: One per year.
Deadline: Write for details.

Missouri Council of the Blind

8206-A Gravois Road
St Louis, MO 63123
314-832-7172
Disability Served: vision

Purpose: The Council offers grants to help finance undergraduate or graduate study.
Eligibility: College students from Missouri who are blind may apply.
Financial Details: Grants are for several hundred dollars.
Number Awarded: Varies.
Deadline: Contact the Council for dates.

Molloy College

1000 Hempstead Avenue
Rockville Centre, NY 11570
516-678-5000
http://www.molloy.edu
Disability Served: all

Purpose: This private four-year college on Long Island offers a scholarship to a student with a disability to finance college.
Eligibility: Students attending the College who have documented disabilities may apply.
Financial Details: Amount varies.
Number Awarded: One per year.
Deadline: Contact the College for information.

Mount Vernon College

Office of Financial Aid
2100 Foxhall Road, NW
Washington, DC 20007
202-625-4682
Disability Served: all

Purpose: This private, four-year college offers financial aid to help finance college study.
Eligibility: Students with disabilities may apply for financial assistance.
Financial Details: Amounts vary and depend on financial need.

Number Awarded: Varies.
Deadline: Contact the College for deadline dates.

Ms. Wheelchair America

1598 Richards Street
Salt Lake City, UT 84115
801-484-5098
Disability Served: physically disabled

Purpose: Not a scholarship as such but a state and national competition for outstanding women who use wheelchairs on a regular basis.
Eligibility: Women who use wheelchairs may compete.
Financial Details: Winners at the state level receive approximately $100 and the national winner, $250.
Number Awarded: Varies.
Deadline: Contact the organization for additional details.

NASA

Office of Education, Mail Stop 400-GSRP/UMDF
NASA Langley Research Center
Hampton, VA 23681-0001
757-864-5209, 757-864-9701
http://ednet.gsfc.nasa.gov/gsrp
Disability Served: all

Purpose: NASA awards grants to students pursuing advanced degrees in science and engineering while making significant contributions to aerospace efforts.
Eligibility: Disabled graduate students attending accredited U.S. universities on a full-time basis may apply.
Financial Details: The maximum yearly award is for $22,000. Awards are renewable for up to three years.
Number Awarded: Varies.
Deadline: February 1.

National AMBUCS Inc.

3315 North Main Street
PO Box 5127
High Point, NC 27262
336-869-2166
http://www.ambucs.com/ambucs/
Disability Served: all

Purpose: AMBUCS is a national nonprofit service organization dedicated to creating independence for people with disabilities by performing community service, providing scholarships to therapists, and by providing AmTrykes, the therapeutic bicycle, to children with disabilities.

National Amputation Foundation

38-40 Church Street
Malverne, NY 11565
516-887-3600
Disability Served: physically disabled

Purpose: To provide scholarships for postsecondary education.
Eligibility: Major limb amputees who are attending undergraduate college on a full-time basis are eligible to apply.
Financial Details: Scholarships are for $125.
Number Awarded: Twenty-four scholarships are awarded each year.
Deadline: Contact the Foundation for information.

National Amputee Golf Association

PO Box 4801
Coralville, IA 52241
603-673-1135
Disability Served: physically disabled

Purpose: The Association offers a scholarship to help finance college study.
Eligibility: Persons who have lost a limb or their dependents are eligible to apply. Applicants must be members of the Association but need not be serious golfers.
Financial Details: The award is for $1,000 a year, which may be renewed.
Number Awarded: One per year.
Deadline: Applications are due in May.

National Association of the Deaf

814 Thayer Avenue, Suite 250
Silver Spring, MD 20910
301-587-1788
http://www.nad.org
Disability Served: hearing

Purpose: To provide the Stokoe Scholarship to help finance graduate study.
Eligibility: Deaf graduates students pursuing full- or part-time studies in a field related to

sign language or the deaf community may apply.
Financial Details: $1,000 scholarship.
Number Awarded: One per year.
Deadline: March 15.

National Captioning Institute, Inc.
1900 Gallows Road, Suite 3000
Vienna, VA 22182
703-917-7600
http://www.us.net/nci/
Disability Served: hearing

Purpose: The Malcolm Norwood Awards are intended to help finance college training.
Eligibility: Students with hearing impairments who wish to prepare for careers serving the deaf or hard of hearing may apply.
Financial Details: Awards are for $2,000 and may be used for tuition, room, or board. Funds are awarded directly to the college.
Number Awarded: Varies.
Deadline: April 1.

National Easter Seal Society
Media Access Office
8121 Van Nuys Boulevard, Suite 214
Van Nuys, CA 91402
818-781-1093
http://seals.com
Disability Served: all

Purpose: To provide Easter Seal Society Acting Scholarships.
Eligibility: Los Angeles area residents with disabilities who are under age eighteen may apply. Selection is based on an audition.
Financial Details: Amounts vary.
Number Awarded: Varies.
Deadline: Contact the Society for details.

National Federation of Music Clubs
c/o Mr. B. E. Walsh
905 Dial Drive
Kennett, MO 63857
314-888-3347
Disability Served: all

Purpose: The Joyce Walsh Scholarship is intended to help finance musical studies.
Eligibility: Vocal or instrumental musicians with disabilities who are under the age of nineteen are eligible to apply. Applicants must be junior members of the National Federation of Music Clubs.
Financial Details: Award amount varies.
Number Awarded: One per year.
Deadline: Contact the Federation for details.

National Federation of Music Clubs
c/o Mrs. Gus Paris, Chair, Music for the Blind
1115 Scherm Road
Owensboro, KY 42301
Disability Served: vision

Purpose: Regional scholarships are offered to blind musicians in each area in which the National Federation has affiliates.
Eligibility: Applicants must submit a recommendation from a teacher as well as an audiotape presenting at least three different selections performed by the musician.
Financial Details: Awards are for $200.
Number Awarded: Varies.
Deadline: Contact the Federation for details.

National Federation of Music Clubs
c/o Mrs. Wendell Heiny, Chair
2768 South Ivan Way
Denver, CO 80227
303-986-8022
Disability Served: vision

Purpose: The Vivian Menees Scholarship is available to help finance college study.
Eligibility: Vocalist or instrumentalists who are blind or who have another disability are eligible to apply.
Financial Details: Award is for $1,000.
Number Awarded: One per year.
Deadline: Applications are due shortly after the first of the year.

National Federation of the Blind
1800 Johnson Street
Baltimore, MD 21230
410-659-9314
http://www.nfb.org
Disability Served: vision

Purpose: The NFB offers scholarships for full-time, postsecondary education.
Eligibility: Legally blind students pursuing or planning to pursue full-time, postsecondary education are eligible to apply. Other restric-

tions may apply, so contact the federation for further information.
Financial Details: Scholarships from $3,000 to $10,000 are available.
Number Awarded: One for $10,000, three for $4,000 each, and twenty-two for $3,000 each, are awarded annually.
Deadline: March 31.

National Federation of the Blind of California

3934 Kern Court
Pleasanton, CA 94588
925-846-6086
Disability Served: vision

Purpose: To provide academic scholarships for educational purposes.
Eligibility: Visually impaired students pursuing or planning to pursue postsecondary education in California are eligible to apply.
Financial Details: A total of $4,250 to $5,000 is awarded each year.
Number Awarded: Four or five scholarships are awarded each year.
Deadline: Contact the Federation for deadline information.

National Federation of the Blind of Colorado

1830 South Acoma
Denver, CO 80223
303-778-1130
Disability Served: vision

Purpose: The Federation provides grants to help finance college training.
Eligibility: Visually impaired students from Colorado are eligible to apply. Selection is based on academic record, need, and community involvement.
Financial Details: Grants are for up to $1,500.
Number Awarded: Varies each year.
Deadline: Applications are due in May.

National Federation of the Blind of Indiana

1707 North Arbogast, Suite #O-L
Griffith, IN 46319
219-923-7517
Disability Served: vision

Purpose: To provide grants to help finance college study.
Eligibility: Legally blind residents of Indiana planning to pursue college educations are eligible to apply
Financial Details: A grant of $400 is available.
Number Awarded: Varies.
Deadline: Contact the Federation for details.

National Federation of the Blind of Maryland

5843 Blue Sky Street
Elkridge, MD 21075
410-379-6130
Disability Served: vision

Purpose: To provide scholarships for higher education.
Eligibility: Legally blind residents of Maryland pursuing college educations are eligible to apply.
Financial Details: Scholarships of $1,800 and $1,200 are available.
Number Awarded: Two scholarships are awarded annually.
Deadline: Contact the Federation for deadline information.

National Federation of the Blind of Michigan

Scholarship Committee
15688 Woodland Drive
Dearborn, MI 48120
313-271-8700
Disability Served: vision

Purpose: The Palmer-Mallin Scholarship helps to finance postsecondary education.
Eligibility: Blind residents of Michigan may apply.
Financial Details: Scholarships range from $250 to $1,500.
Number Awarded: Varies.
Deadline: Applications are due in May.

National Federation of the Blind of New Hampshire

Division of Vocational Rehabilitation
361 Lincoln Street
Manchester, NH 03103
603-669-8733

Disability Served: vision

Purpose: The Floyd Callward Scholarship is designed to help finance postsecondary study.
Eligibility: Blind residents or students in the state may apply
Financial Details: Scholarship is for $1,000.
Number Awarded: One per year.
Deadline: Applications are due in early July.

National Federation of the Blind of New Mexico

PO Box 37110
Albuquerque, NM 87176
505-883-1941
Disability Served: vision

Purpose: The Federation offers a scholarship to help finance college study.
Eligibility: Legally blind students from the state are eligible to apply. Applicants must demonstrate financial need.
Financial Details: The award is for $500.
Number Awarded: One per year.
Deadline: Contact the Federation for specifics.

National Federation of the Blind of North Carolina

Scholarship Committee
705 Northcliff Drive
Raleigh, NC 27609
919-847-8470
Disability Served: vision

Purpose: The Robert Stanley Scholarships help students finance college training.
Eligibility: North Carolina blind residents who plan to attend a college or university in North Carolina may apply. Selection is based on community service, academic record, and financial need.
Financial Details: Scholarships are for $1,000.
Number Awarded: Two per year.
Deadline: Contact the Federation for dates.

National Federation of the Blind of Vermont

200 Berlin Street
Montpelier, VT 05602
802-229-1230
Disability Served: vision

Purpose: To provide scholarships to help defer postsecondary education expenses.
Eligibility: Blind students from Vermont are eligible to apply
Financial Details: The award is for $500.
Number Awarded: One per year.
Deadline: Applications are due in March.

National Four-H Council

7100 Connecticut Avenue
Chevy Chase, MD 20815
301-961-2800
http://www.fourhcouncil.edu/
Disability Served: all

Purpose: The Council offers scholarships for college study.
Eligibility: Students with disabilities who are in 4-H Clubs may apply.
Financial Details: Amounts vary.
Number Awarded: Varies.
Deadline: Contact the Council for details.

National Fraternal Society of the Deaf

1300 West Northwest Highway
Mount Prospect, IL 60056
847-392-9282
Disability Served: hearing

Purpose: Scholarships to help finance college training are offered by the Society.
Eligibility: Persons who have been a member of the Society for at least one year and who hold an insurance policy issued by it are eligible to apply. Applicants must be hearing impaired.
Financial Details: Scholarships are for $1,000.
Number Awarded: Varies.
Deadline: Applications are due July 1.

National Italian American Foundation

1860 19th Street, NW
Washington, DC 20009
202-387-0600
Disability Served: all

Purpose: The Deniel Stella Scholarship helps finance college study.
Eligibility: Members of the Foundation who have Cooley's Anemia are eligible to apply. Applicants must show financial need and be working toward a bachelor's degree.

Financial Details: The Scholarship is for $1,000.
Number Awarded: One per year.
Deadline: Contact Dr. Maria Lombardo at NIAF.

National Research Council

2101 Constitution Avenue
Washington, DC 20418
202-334-2125
Disability Served: all

Purpose: The Council administers the National Science Foundation Graduate Fellowship Program.
Eligibility: Graduate students and students with disabilities in the mathematical, physical, biological, engineering, and social sciences are eligible.
Financial Details: Awards are for $14,000 per year for three years.
Number Awarded: Approximately 700 awards are given each year.
Deadline: Write for details.

National Science Foundation

4201 Wilson Boulevard
Arlington, VA 22230
703-306-1637
Disability Served: all

Purpose: Doctoral Dissertation Research Grants are available to help students with funding for the research phase of their graduate studies.
Eligibility: Disabled students at the doctoral dissertation phase of their studies are eligible
Financial Details: Awards vary.
Number Awarded: Varies.
Deadline: Write for details on the current program.

National Society of Daughters of the Revolution-Office of Committees

1776 D Street, NW
Washington, DC 20006-5392
202-879-3293
Disability Served: learning disabled

Purpose: Margaret Howard Hamilton Scholarships help finance college study.
Eligibility: High school students who plan to enroll in the jones Learning for the Learning Disabled program at the University of the Ozarks are eligible. Candidates must be sponsored by a local DAR chapter.
Financial Details: Scholarships are for $1,000 a year.
Number Awarded: Varies.

Nazareth College of Rochester

Office of Admissions
4145 East Avenue
Rochester, NY 14610
716-586-2525
Disability Served: all

Purpose: This private four-year college offers financial aid to students with disabilities.
Eligibility: Disabled students who are in need of financial assistance are eligible.
Financial Details: Amounts vary according to need.
Number Awarded: Varies.
Deadline: Contact the College for details.

New England Hemophilia Association

180 Rustcraft Road
Dedham, MA 02026
617-326-7645
Disability Served: inherited bleeding disorders

Purpose: This organization provides information and referral, support, and advocacy for families with inherited bleeding disorders.

New Hampshire Charitable Fund

PO Box 1334
Concord, NH 03302
603-225-6641
Disability Served: all

Purpose: The Allen Ring Awards are designed to help finance college training.
Eligibility: New Hampshire residents with disabilities may apply. Applicants must pay a $6 application fee and testify that they do not drink alcoholic beverages or smoke.
Financial Details: Awards range from $500 to $2,500.
Number Awarded: Varies.
Deadline: Applications are due in April.

New Jersey Commission for the Blind and Visually Impaired

153 Halsey Street, 6th Floor
Newark, NJ 07102
973-648-2324
Disability Served: vision

Purpose: To provide scholarships for the purpose of financing schooling.
Eligibility: Visually impaired residents of New Jersey are eligible for financial aid to help them meet needed resources to attend a public college in the state

Nicholls State University

Office of Financial Aid
PO Box 20005
Thibodeaux, LA 70310
504-448-4048
Disability Served: all

Purpose: To provide financial aid to help with the costs of a college education.
Eligibility: Students whose parents have a disability may apply. Applicants must demonstrate financial need.
Financial Details: Awards vary, depending on need.
Number Awarded: Varies.
Deadline: Contact the University for information.

North Carolina Department of Health and Human Services, Division of Vocational Rehabilitation Services

2810 Mail Service Center
PO Box 26053
Raleigh, NC 27699-2801
919-733-3364
Disability Served: all

Purpose: The North Carolina Division of Vocational Rehabilitation Services can provide assistance with tuition and fees for postsecondary training.
Eligibility: Residents of North Carolina who have a mental or physical disability may apply. Interested parties may apply at any of the thirty-two local Vocational Rehabilitation unit offices or can contact the state office.
Financial Details: Amounts vary according to need.
Number Awarded: Varies.
Deadline: Contact the Department for information.

North Carolina Division of Services for the Blind

Rehabilitation Services
309 Ashe Avenue
Raleigh, NC 27606
919-733-9700
http://www.dhhs.state.nc.us
Disability Served: vision

Purpose: To provide financial aid to help cover college tuition and fees.
Eligibility: Legally blind residents of the state who demonstrate financial need are eligible.
Financial Details: Amounts vary and depend on need.
Number Awarded: Varies.
Deadline: Contact the office for information.

North Dakota State College of Science

Office of Admissions
800 North Sixth Street
Wahpeton, ND 48076
701-671-2327
Disability Served: all

Purpose: This public two-year community college offers financial aid to students with disabilities.
Eligibility: Students with disabilities who demonstrate financial need may apply.
Financial Details: Awards vary according to need.
Number Awarded: Varies.
Deadline: Contact the College for details.

North Harris College

2700 W.W. Thorne Drive
250 North Sam Houston Parkway
Houston, TX 77073-3499
281-618-5400
http://www.nhmccd.edu
Disability Served: all

Purpose: This two-year community college provides financial aid to students.
Eligibility: Financially needy students with disabilities who are attending the College are eligible to apply.

Financial Details: Amounts vary and depend on need.
Number Awarded: Varies.
Deadline: Contact the College for details.

North Lake College

Office of Admissions
5001 North MacArthur Boulevard
Irving, TX 75038
972-659-5237
Disability Served: all

Purpose: This public two-year college has a financial aid program to help with the costs of college training.
Eligibility: Disabled students who need financial assistance are eligible.
Financial Details: Amounts vary according to need.
Number Awarded: Varies.
Deadline: Contact the College for information.

Northampton Community College

Office of Admissions
3835 Green Pond Road
Bethlehem, PA 18017
610-861-5342
Disability Served: all

Purpose: This two-year community college has student support services and a financial aid program open to students with disabilities.
Eligibility: Disabled students who need financial assistance are eligible.
Financial Details: Amounts vary according to need.
Number Awarded: Varies.
Deadline: Contact the College for information.

Northern Arizona State University

Office of Financial Aid
Box 4108
Flagstaff, AZ 86011
520-523-4951
http://www.nau.edu/
Disability Served: all

Purpose: The University offers a scholarship to help finance college study.
Eligibility: First-year students with disabilities are eligible.
Financial Details: Amounts vary.
Number Awarded: Varies.
Deadline: Write for application materials and further information.

Northwest Nazarene College

Office of Admissions
623 Holly Street
Nampa, ID 83686
208-467-8644
Disability Served: all

Purpose: This is a private four-year college that has a financial aid program open to students with disabilities.
Eligibility: Disabled students who need financial assistance are eligible.
Financial Details: Amounts vary according to need.
Number Awarded: Varies.
Deadline: Contact the College for information.

Northwestern University

Office of Disability Services
720 University Place
Evanston, IL 60208
847-491-7458
http://www.nwu.edu/
Disability Served: all

Purpose: This private four-year university provides financial aid to students.
Eligibility: Financially needy students with disabilities who are attending the University are eligible to apply.
Financial Details: Amounts vary and depend on need.
Number Awarded: Varies.
Deadline: Contact the University for details.

Norwalk Community-Technical College

188 Richards Avenue
Norwalk, CT 06854
203-857-7192
http://www.nctc.commnet.edu
Disability Served: all

Purpose: NCTC is a public, two-year, commuter college offering associate-degree programs in the following areas of study: accounting, architectural engineering technology, business administration, business office technology/

office administration, communications technology, computer information systems, construction technology, criminal justice, drug and alcohol rehabilitation counselor, early childhood education, electrical engineering technology, engineering pathway, environmental technology, finance and banking, fire technology and administration, general studies, hotel/motel management, human services, legal assistant, liberal arts and sciences, management, marketing, mass communication, nursing, recreation and leisure studies, respiratory care, restaurant/food service management, archaeology as an avocation, culinary arts, English as a second language, medical assistant, mental health, and paramedic. Services are available to students with disabilities that have been diagnosed and documented by a professional who is qualified to make such a diagnosis. Services are determined on a case-by-case basis. Students are advised to call for an appointment at least six weeks prior to the beginning of classes to allow for documentation review, consultation, and accommodation planning.

NSF Graduate Research Fellowship Program

PO Box 3010
Oak Ridge, TN 37831
615-483-3344
Disability Served: all

Purpose: The National Science Foundation Graduate Research Fellowship helps with the costs of graduate study.
Eligibility: Students with disabilities enrolled in any university with an appropriate program in science or engineering are eligible.
Financial Details: Awards of up to $14,000 a year plus tuition are offered.
Number Awarded: One per year.
Deadline: Write for details.

Oakland City College

Office of Admissions
143 North Lucretia Street
Oakland City, IN 47660
812-749-4781
Disability Served: all

Purpose: This private four-year college provides financial aid to students.
Eligibility: Financially needy students with disabilities attending the College are eligible to apply.
Financial Details: Amounts vary and depend on need.

Oakland Community College

Office of Admissions
2480 Ondyke Road
Bloomfield Hills, MI 48304
313-540-1500
Disability Served: all

Purpose: This two-year college provides financial aid to students.
Eligibility: Financially needy students with disabilities attending the College are eligible to apply.
Financial Details: Amounts vary and depend on need.
Number Awarded: Varies.
Deadline: Contact the College for details.

Odessa College

Office of Admissions
201 West University Boulevard
Odessa, TX 79764
915-335-6433
Disability Served: all

Purpose: This two-year college provides financial aid to students.
Eligibility: Financially needy students with disabilities attending the College are eligible to apply.
Financial Details: Amounts vary and depend on need.
Number Awarded: Varies.
Deadline: Contact the College for details.

Office for Equal Opportunity Programs

State University System of Florida
325 Gaines Street, Suite 1454
Tallahassee, FL 32399
850-487-1896
http://www.bor.state.fl.us/
Disability Served: all

Purpose: To provide scholarships for attending a Florida state university.
Eligibility: Florida students with disabilities working toward bachelor's degrees at a state university are eligible to apply.
Financial Details: The Johnson Scholarship provides up to $3,500 a year.
Number Awarded: A limited number of awards are available each year.
Deadline: Application materials are available in February. Deadline to apply is mid-May.

Ohio State University

Office of Financial Aid
1760 Nell Avenue
Columbus, OH 43210
614-292-4190
http://www.ohio-state.edu/
Disability Served: all

Purpose: This public four-year university provides financial aid to students.
Eligibility: Financially needy students with disabilities attending the University are eligible to apply.
Financial Details: Amounts vary and depend on need.
Number Awarded: Varies.
Deadline: Contact the University for details.

Oklahoma Department of Veterans Affairs

2311 North Central
PO Box 53067
Oklahoma City, OK 73152
405-521-3684
Disability Served: all

Purpose: The Department provides tuition waivers.
Eligibility: Oklahoma veterans who have a service-related disability and are planning to attend an Oklahoma vocational or technical school are eligible.
Financial Details: Free tuition for up to thirty-six months is awarded.
Number Awarded: Varies.
Deadline: Write for information.

Oklahoma State University

Office of Disability Services
326 Student Union
Stillwater, OK 74078
918-744-7116
Disability Served: all

Purpose: This four-year university provides financial aid to students.
Eligibility: Financially needy students with disabilities attending the University are eligible to apply.
Financial Details: Amounts vary and depend on need.

Old Dominion University

2228 Webb Center
108 Administration Building
Norfolk, VA 23529
804-683-4655
http://www.odu.edu/
Disability Served: all

Purpose: This four-year university provides a scholarship to students with disabilities.
Eligibility: Students with disabilities attending the University are eligible to apply.
Financial Details: Amount varies.
Number Awarded: Varies.
Deadline: Contact the University for details.

Olivet Nazarene University

Office of Financial Aid
PO Box 592
Kankakee, IL 60901
815-939-5249
http://www.olivet.edu/
Disability Served: all

Purpose: The University offers awards to help students with disabilities.
Eligibility: Students with disabilities in a vocational rehabilitation program may apply.
Financial Details: Amounts vary.
Number Awarded: Varies.
Deadline: Write or call for details.

Opportunities for the Blind, Inc.

PO Box 510
Leonardtown, MD 20650
301-862-1990
Disability Served: vision

Purpose: This organization offers grants to help blind persons meet college expenses, establish a business, or obtain needed equipment.

Eligibility: Blind persons in need of assistance may apply.
Financial Details: Grants of $1,000 to $5,000 are available.
Number Awarded: Varies.
Deadline: Contact the organization for information.

Oregon Council of the Blind

4730 Auburn Road NE, Suite 52
Salem, OR 97301
503-362-4151
Disability Served: vision

Purpose: The Council awards scholarships to help finance college study.
Eligibility: High school seniors who are blind are eligible.
Financial Details: Scholarships of $2,500 are given.
Number Awarded: Two.
Deadline: Varies. Write or call for information.

Paducah Community College

Office of Admissions
PO Box 7380
Paducah, KY 92002
502-554-9200
Disability Served: all

Purpose: This two-year college has a financial aid program to help entering students with disabilities.
Eligibility: Disabled students who demonstrate financial need may apply.
Financial Details: Amounts vary and depend on need.
Number Awarded: Varies.
Deadline: Contact the College for details.

Paralyzed Veterans of America

801 18th Street, NW
Washington, DC 20006
800-424-8200
http://www.pva.org
Disability Served: physically disabled

Purpose: To provide scholarships to finance education.
Eligibility: PVA members and their dependents 23 years of age or younger pursuing college degrees are eligible to apply.
Financial Details: Awards are for $2,500.
Number Awarded: Varies each year. In 1997, twenty scholarships were awarded.
Deadline: Applications are due by June 30.

Parke-Davis Epilepsy Scholarship Award

c/o Intramed Educational Group
1180 Avenue of the Americas
New York, NY 10036
800-972-7503
Disability Served: epilepsy

Purpose: Scholarships are awarded to help finance college study.
Eligibility: Students undergoing treatment for epilepsy who are college freshmen, sophomores, or juniors are eligible. Selection is based on academic and extracurricular records and recommendations.
Financial Details: Scholarships are for $3,000.
Number Awarded: Two per year.
Deadline: Applications are due March 1.

Pennsylvania State University

Office of Financial Aid
105 Booker Building
University Park, PA 16802
814-863-1807
http://www.psu.edu/
Disability Served: all

Purpose: This four-year university provides financial aid to students.
Eligibility: Financially needy students with disabilities who are attending the University are eligible to apply.
Financial Details: Amounts vary and depend on need.
Number Awarded: Varies.
Deadline: Contact the University for details.

Pennsylvania State University at Harrisburg

Office of Financial Aid
Route 230
Middletown, PA 17057
717-948-6025
http://www.hbg.psu.edu/studaf/cac.htm
Disability Served: all

Purpose: This four-year university provides financial aid to students.
Eligibility: Financially needy students with disabilities who are attending the University are eligible to apply.
Financial Details: Amounts vary and depend on need.
Number Awarded: Varies.
Deadline: Contact the University for details.

Pilot International Foundation

PO Box 5600
Macon, GA 31208
912-743-7403
Disability Served: all

Purpose: To provide grants for the purpose of financing education.
Eligibility: Students preparing to work with individuals with disabilities are eligible to apply. Candidates must be sponsored by a local Pilot Club.
Financial Details: Grants of up to $1,500 a year are available. Grants may be renewed.
Number Awarded: Varies each year.
Deadline: Applications are due April 1.

Portland State University

Office of Graduate Studies and Research
105 Neuberger Hall
Portland, OR 97207
503-725-3000
http://www.pdx.edu/
Disability Served: physically disabled

Purpose: The Robert and Rosemary Law Memorial Scholarship is reserved for full-time graduate students.
Eligibility: Full-time graduate students with physical disabilities and good academic records are eligible to apply.
Financial Details: Amounts vary.
Number Awarded: One per year. Scholarships may not be awarded every year.
Deadline: Applications are due April 15.

Potomac State College of West Virginia

Office of Financial Aid
Keyser, WV 26726
304-788-6856
Disability Served: all

Purpose: This two-year community college provides financial aid to students.
Eligibility: Financially needy students with disabilities who are attending the College are eligible to apply.
Financial Details: Amounts vary and depend on need.
Number Awarded: Varies.
Deadline: Contact the College for details.

President's Committee on Employment of People with Disabilities

1331 F Street, NW, Suite 300
Washington, DC 20004
202-376-6200
http://www.pcepd.gov
Disability Served: all

Purpose: To provide scholarships to undergraduate students with disabilities who wish to pursue courses in higher education.
Eligibility: United States citizens with documented disabilities who are planning to attend classes at a four-year, accredited college or university are eligible to apply.
Financial Details: Awards vary.
Number Awarded: Varies each year.
Deadline: Deadlines vary and are announced annually. Contact the organization for details.

Purdue University

Department of Chemical Engineering
Freshman Engineering
West Lafayette, IN 47907
765-494-3886
http://www.purdue.edu/
Disability Served: hearing

Purpose: To provide funding to help students finance college educations in engineering.
Eligibility: Deaf and hard-of-hearing students in engineering are eligible to apply.
Financial Details: Amounts vary. Funds are from the National Science Foundation.
Number Awarded: Varies each year.
Deadline: Contact the University for details.

Quota Club of Flint

PO Box 39
Flint, MI 48502
Disability Served: hearing

Purpose: This chapter of Quota offers a scholarship for students preparing to work in the field of deafness.
Eligibility: College juniors or seniors who are either deaf or hard of hearing or who are hearing students preparing to work in the field of deafness are eligible to apply. Applicants must be residents of the Flint area.
Financial Details: Write the Club for details.
Number Awarded: Varies each year.
Deadline: Contact the Club for details.

Quota International Fellowship Fund

1420 21st Street, NW
Washington, DC 20036
202-331-9694
Disability Served: hearing

Purpose: To provide fellowships for the purpose of studying to become a teacher or other worker with deaf students.
Eligibility: Deaf or hearing students interested in studying to become a teacher or other worker with deaf students are eligible to apply.
Financial Details: Fellowships range from $500 to $3,000.
Number Awarded: Varies each year.
Deadline: Write for further information.

Randolph Community College

Office of Financial Aid
PO Box 1009
Asheboro, NC 27203
910-629-1471
Disability Served: all

Purpose: This two-year community college provides financial aid to students.
Eligibility: Financially needy students with disabilities who are attending the College are eligible to apply.
Financial Details: Amounts vary and depend on need.
Number Awarded: Varies.
Deadline: Contact the College for details.

Rask Family Memorial Fund

c/o West One Bank
PO Box 2882
Portland, OR 97208
503-248-6644
Disability Served: all

Purpose: Provides scholarships to help finance higher education.
Eligibility: Students with disabilities who plan to pursue college degrees may apply.
Financial Details: Scholarships range from $500 to $1,800.
Number Awarded: Varies each year.
Deadline: Contact the Fund fro details.

Recording for the Blind & Dyslexic

20 Roszel Road
Princeton, NJ 08540
800-221-4792
http://www.rfbd.org
Disability Served: vision

Purpose: This organization provides recorded and computerized textbooks at all academic levels to people who cannot read standard print effectively because of a visual impairment, learning disability, or physical disability.

Rehabilitation Research and Training Center on Blindness & Low Vision

Mississippi State University
PO Box 6189
Mississippi State, MS 39762
601-325-2001
http://www.msstate.edu/dept/rrtc/blind.html
Disability Served: vision

Purpose: The Jennings Randolph Research Awards program offers awards for basic field-initiated research or to assist in the implementation of applied research projects related to blindness or low vision at Mississippi State University.
Eligibility: Rehabilitation agency staff or graduate students at Mississippi State University are eligible to apply.
Financial Details: $500 awards are available.
Number Awarded: Two awards per year.
Deadline: Contact the University for deadline dates.

Rickard Scholarship Committee

Rural Route 1
West Willington, CT 06279
Disability Served: vision

Purpose: To provide the Howard Rickard Scholarship for the Blind to help finance college study.

Eligibility: Legally blind students are eligible to apply.
Financial Details: The award is for $1,200.
Number Awarded: One per year.
Deadline: Applications are due May 1.

Roane State Community College

276 Patton Lane
Harriman, TN 37748
615-882-4545
http://www.rscc.cc.tn.us
Disability Served: all

Purpose: To provide financial aid to help finance college study.
Eligibility: Students with disabilities attending this two-year college are eligible to apply.
Financial Details: Amounts vary and are based on financial need.
Number Awarded: Varies.
Deadline: Contact the College for information.

Roosevelt University

430 South Michigan Avenue
Chicago, IL 60608
312-341-3810
http://www.roosevelt.edu/
Disability Served: all

Purpose: This private four-year university provides financial aid to students.
Eligibility: Financially needy students with disabilities who are attending the University are eligible to apply.
Financial Details: Amounts vary and depend on need.
Number Awarded: Varies.
Deadline: Contact the University for details.

Ruth Cantrall Trust

c/o Bank IV Olathe
PO Box 400
Olathe, KS 66051
913-752-5434
Disability Served: hearing

Purpose: The Ruth Cantrall Trust offers scholarships to help finance college study.
Eligibility: Hearing impaired students may apply for scholarships to help finance study at the Kansas State School for the Deaf.
Financial Details: Scholarships of up to $325 are available.
Number Awarded: Varies.
Deadline: Write for details.

Saint Anselm College

100 Saint Anselm Drive
Manchester, NH 03102
603-641-7000
http://www.anselm.edu
Disability Served: all

Purpose: This private four-year college provides financial aid to students.
Eligibility: Financially needy students with disabilities who are attending the college are eligible to apply.
Financial Details: Amounts vary and depend on need.
Number Awarded: Varies.
Deadline: Contact the college for details.

Saint Cloud State University

Atwood Center
St Cloud, MN 56301
320-255-3111
Disability Served: all

Purpose: This public four-year university provides financial aid to students.
Eligibility: Financially needy students with disabilities who are attending the University are eligible to apply.
Financial Details: Amounts vary and depend on need.
Number Awarded: Varies.
Deadline: Contact the University for details.

San Diego City College

1313 12th Avenue
San Diego, CA 92101
619-230-2400
http://www.sdccd.cc.ca.us/campuses/city/index.html
Disability Served: all

Purpose: This public two-year college enrolls several hundred students with disabilities. It has a scholarship program to aid them.
Eligibility: Students with disabilities are eligible.
Financial Details: Awards vary.

Number Awarded: Varies each year.
Deadline: Contact the College for details.

San Diego Epilepsy Society

2247 San Diego Avenue, Suite 234
San Diego, CA 92110
619-296-0161
Disability Served: physically disabled

Purpose: To provide grants to help finance college study.
Eligibility: Students from the area with epilepsy are eligible for grants to help finance attendance at a San Diego County college or university.
Financial Details: Grants of up to $1,000 are available.
Number Awarded: Varies each year.
Deadline: Applications are due in December.

San Jose State University

One Washington Square
San Jose, CA 95192
408-924-1000
Disability Served: all

Purpose: This four-year university provides financial aid to students.
Eligibility: Financially needy students with disabilities who are attending the University are eligible to apply.
Financial Details: Amounts vary and depend on need.
Number Awarded: Varies.
Deadline: Contact the University for details.

Santa Barbara Elks Lodge

PO Box 6720
Santa Barbara, CA 93160
805-967-2188
Disability Served: physically disabled

Purpose: To provide renewable scholarships for the purpose of financing college study.
Eligibility: Students with physical disabilities from the Santa Barbara area are eligible to apply for the Elks Club scholarships. Students must demonstrate financial need.
Financial Details: Scholarships are for $2,000 a year.
Number Awarded: Varies.
Deadline: Applications are due in March.

Schenectady County Community College

Office of Financial Aid
78 Washington Avenue
Schenectady, NY 12308
518-346-6211
Disability Served: all

Purpose: This public two-year college has a financial aid program to help students finance college training.
Eligibility: Students with disabilities who need financial assistance are eligible.
Financial Details: Amounts vary and depend on need.
Number Awarded: Varies.
Deadline: Contact the College for details.

Scripps College

Office of Financial Aid
Claremont, CA 91711
909-621-8000
Disability Served: all

Purpose: To provide a scholarship to help finance college study.
Eligibility: Students with disabilities attending the College are eligible to apply.
Financial Details: Amount varies.
Number Awarded: One per year.
Deadline: Contact the College for details.

Shawnee State University

940 Second Street
Portsmouth, OH 45662
740-354-3205
http://www.shawnee.edu/
Disability Served: all

Purpose: This public university has a financial aid program to help students pay for their college education.
Eligibility: Students with disabilities who need financial assistance are eligible.
Financial Details: Amounts vary and depend on need.
Number Awarded: Varies.
Deadline: Contact the University for details.

Shenandoah University

Office of Financial Aid
1460 University Drive
Winchester, VA 22601

540-665-4538
http://www.su.edu/
Disability Served: vision

Purpose: The University offers a scholarship to students from Virginia with visual disabilities.
Eligibility: First-year students with disabilities are eligible
Financial Details: Awards vary.
Number Awarded: One per year.
Deadline: Write for application materials and further information.

Sickle Cell Foundation

PO Box 55017
Orlando, FL 32805
407-293-9555
Disability Served: all

Purpose: The Foundation offers scholarships to help finance college training.
Eligibility: Residents of Orange, Osceola, or Seminole counties in Florida who have sickle cell disease are eligible. Selection is based on financial need and prior academic record.
Financial Details: The Scholarship awards $2,500 per year.
Number Awarded: One per year.
Deadline: Write for details.

Sierra College

Office of Admissions
5000 Rocklin Road
Rocklin, CA 95677
916-624-3333
Disability Served: all

Purpose: This public two-year college has a financial aid program.
Eligibility: Students with disabilities who need financial assistance are eligible.
Financial Details: Amounts vary and depend on need.
Number Awarded: Varies.
Deadline: Contact the College for details.

Soroptomist International of the Americas

1616 Walnut Street
Philadelphia, PA 19103
215-732-0512
Disability Served: physically disabled

Purpose: The Venture Clubs Scholarships help finance college study.
Eligibility: Students with physical disabilities between the ages of fifteen and thirty-five are eligible. Applicants must demonstrate how college training will contribute to development.
Financial Details: Amounts vary.
Number Awarded: Varies.
Deadline: Write or call for information.

South Dakota Board of Regents

207 East Capitol Avenue
Pierre, SD 57501
605-773-3455
Disability Served: vision

Purpose: The Board provides tuition waivers.
Eligibility: Visually impaired residents of South Dakota attending any public college or university in the state may apply.
Financial Details: Waivers of tuition, fees, and other expenses are given.
Number Awarded: Varies.
Deadline: Varies. Write or call for information.

South Dakota School of Mines and Technology

Office of Financial Aid
Rapid City, SD 57701
605-394-2274
Disability Served: all

Purpose: This technical school provides financial aid to students.
Eligibility: Financially needy students with disabilities who are attending the School are eligible to apply.
Financial Details: Amounts vary and depend on need.

South Dakota State University

Office of Financial Aid
PO Box 2201
Brookings, SD 57000
605-688-4496
http://www.sdstate.edu/
Disability Served: all

Purpose: This four-year university provides financial aid to students.
Eligibility: Financially needy students with disabilities who are attending the University are eligible to apply.

Financial Details: Amounts vary and depend on need.
Number Awarded: Varies.
Deadline: Contact the University for details.

South Mountain Community College

7050 South 24th Street
Phoenix, AZ 85040
602-243-8000
http://www.smc.maricopa.edu
Disability Served: all

Purpose: This two-year community college provides financial aid to students.
Eligibility: Financially needy students with disabilities who are attending the College are eligible to apply.
Financial Details: Amounts vary and depend on need.
Number Awarded: Varies.
Deadline: Contact the College for details.

Southern Illinois University at Carbondale

Office of Financial Aid
Carbondale, IL 62901
618-453-8738
Disability Served: all

Purpose: This four-year university provides financial aid to students.
Eligibility: Financially needy students with disabilities who are attending the University are eligible to apply.
Financial Details: Amounts vary and depend on need.
Number Awarded: Varies.
Deadline: Contact the University for details.

Southern Vermont College

982 Mansion Drive
Bennington, VT 05201
802-447-3604
http://www.sc.edu
Disability Served: all

Purpose: This private four-year college provides financial aid to students.
Eligibility: Financially needy students with disabilities who are attending the College are eligible to apply.
Financial Details: Amounts vary and depend on need.
Number Awarded: Varies.
Deadline: Contact the College for details.

Southwest Missouri State University

Office of Financial Aid
901 South National
Springfield, MO 65804
417-836-5262
http://www.smsu.edu
Disability Served: all

Purpose: This university provides financial aid to students.
Eligibility: Financially needy students with disabilities who are enrolled in a vocational rehabilitation program are eligible to apply.
Financial Details: Amounts vary and depend on need.
Number Awarded: Varies.
Deadline: Contact the University for details.

Spina Bifida Association of America

4590 MacArthur Boulevard, NW, Suite 250
Washington, DC 20007
202-944-3285, 800-621-3141
http://www.sbaa.org/
Disability Served: physically disabled

Purpose: To provide grants for the purpose of financing college education.
Eligibility: College students who were born with spina bifida and who are members of the Association are eligible to apply.
Financial Details: Grants range up to $1,000 based on prior academic record, financial need, and community involvement.
Number Awarded: Varies each year.
Deadline: Contact the Association for details.

Spoon River College

Office of Admissions
Rural Route 1
Canton, OH 61520
330-647-4645
Disability Served: all

Purpose: This two-year institution provides financial aid to students.
Eligibility: Financially needy students with disabilities who are attending the College are eligible to apply.

Financial Details: Amounts vary and depend on need.

Sterling College
Office of Financial Aid
Sterling, KS 67579
316-278-2173
http://sterling.edu
Disability Served: all

Purpose: This private four-year college provides scholarships to students.
Eligibility: Students with disabilities who are attending the College are eligible to apply.
Financial Details: Amounts vary.
Number Awarded: Varies.
Deadline: Contact the College for details.

Stony Wold-Herbert Fund
136 East 57th Street, Room 1705
New York, NY 10022
212-753-6565
Disability Served: all

Purpose: This organization offers financial aid to help students pay for college costs.
Eligibility: Students with respiratory diseases from the Greater New York area are eligible to apply.
Financial Details: Awards are approximately $1,500 each.
Number Awarded: Varies.
Deadline: Call or write for information.

Sussex County Community College
Office of Admissions
One College Hill
Newton, NJ 07860
201-300-2153
Disability Served: all

Purpose: This public two-year community college provides financial aid to students.
Eligibility: Financially needy students with disabilities are eligible to apply.
Financial Details: Amounts vary and depend on need.
Number Awarded: Varies.
Deadline: Contact the College for details.

Syracuse University
Office of Disability Services
Syracuse, NY 13244
315-443-4357
http://www.syr.edu/
Disability Served: all

Purpose: This four-year university has a scholarship program for students with disabilities.
Eligibility: Students with disabilities who are attending the University are eligible to apply.
Financial Details: Amounts vary.
Number Awarded: Varies.
Deadline: Contact the University for details.

Tarrant County Junior College
Office of Financial Aid
828 Harwood Road
Hurst, TX 76054
817-788-6333
Disability Served: all

Purpose: This two-year institution provides financial aid to students.
Eligibility: Financially needy students with disabilities are eligible to apply.
Financial Details: Amounts vary and depend on need.
Number Awarded: Varies.
Deadline: Contact the College for details.

Temple University
Office of Financial Aid
1300 Cecile Moore Avenue
Philadelphia, PA 19122
215-204-1280
http://www.temple.edu/
Disability Served: all

Purpose: This four-year university provides financial aid to students.
Eligibility: Financially needy students with disabilities are eligible to apply.
Financial Details: Amounts vary and depend on need.
Number Awarded: Varies.
Deadline: Contact the University for details.

Texas A&M University
Office of Financial Aid
College Station, TX 77843
409-845-1247
http://www.tamu.edu/
Disability Served: all

Purpose: This four-year university provides scholarships to students, including one for a student with disabilities.
Eligibility: Students with disabilities who are attending the University are eligible to apply.
Financial Details: Amounts vary.
Number Awarded: Varies.
Deadline: Contact the University for details.

Texas Higher Education Coordinating Board

PO Box 12788, Capitol Station
Austin, TX 78711
512-483-6340
Disability Served: vision

Purpose: The Board offers tuition waivers to students.
Eligibility: Blind students from Texas attending state colleges and universities are eligible. Applicants must otherwise qualify for admission.
Financial Details: Tuition and fees are waived.
Number Awarded: Varies.
Deadline: Write or call for details.

Texas Woman's University

304 Administration Drive
Denton, TX 76204
940-898-3835
http://www.twu.edu/
Disability Served: all

Purpose: This four-year university provides financial aid to students.
Eligibility: Financially needy students with disabilities who are attending the University are eligible to apply.
Financial Details: Amounts vary and depend on need.
Number Awarded: Varies.
Deadline: Contact the University for details.

The Charlotte W. Newcombe Foundation

35 Park Place
Princeton, NJ 08542
609-924-7022
Disability Served: all

Purpose: To provide grants to colleges and universities for scholarship support.
Eligibility: The Foundation does not aid individual students but awards grants to colleges and universities in Pennsylvania, New York, New Jersey, Delaware, Maryland, and Washington, DC, which, in turn, offer scholarships of up to $700 a year to students with disabilities.
Financial Details: A total of $300,000 was awarded to nine colleges and universities for the 1998-99 academic year.
Number Awarded: Varies each year.
Deadline: Contact the Foundation for additional information.

Twitty, Milsap, Sterban Foundation

PO Box 43517
Detroit, MI 48243
Disability Served: vision

Purpose: The Foundation offers scholarships to help finance undergraduate or graduate training.
Eligibility: Blind or visually impaired students with strong academic records and achievements are eligible.
Financial Details: $500 or more is awarded.
Number Awarded: Varies.
Deadline: Applications are due September 1.

UCB Pharma, Inc.

Marketing Department
1950 Lake Park Drive
Atlanta, GA 30080
404-437-5500
Disability Served: all

Purpose: This company offers the Asthma Athlete of the Year Awards.
Eligibility: Persons with outstanding athletic records who have asthma are eligible. Candidates must be nominated by a physician.
Financial Details: The Award is for $2,500.
Number Awarded: One per year.
Deadline: Write or call for information.

UCP Research and Educational Foundation

1660 L Street NW, Suite 700
Washington, DC 20036
202-776-0406, 800-872-5827
http://www.ucpa.org
Disability Served: cerebral palsy

Purpose: To provide grants for the research of cerebral palsy, its treatment, diagnosis, and prevention.
Eligibility: Eligibility requirements vary. Contact the Foundation for application materials.
Financial Details: Awards vary.

United Cerebral Palsy Association
Human Resources
1522 K Street, NW, Suite 112
Washington, DC 20005
202-842-1266
http://www.ucpa.org/
Disability Served: cerebral palsy

Purpose: The Association offers a scholarship for a student with a disability.
Eligibility: Students with disabilities are eligible. Other restrictions may apply, so write for details.
Financial Details: Amounts vary.
Number Awarded: Varies.
Deadline: Contact the Association for information.

United States National Institutes of Health
Division of Research Grants
6701 Rockledge Drive, MSC 7762
Bethesda, MD 20892
301-435-0714
Disability Served: all

Purpose: To provide grants to support summer or school-year research projects.
Eligibility: High school and college undergraduate students with disabilities are eligible. They are expected to spend approximately three months of full-time effort on the research, and it must be done under the supervision of a principal investigator, usually a teacher.
Financial Details: Amounts vary.
Number Awarded: Varies.
Deadline: Write or call for details.

University of Arizona
Old Main, Room 235
Tucson, AZ 85721
520-621-2483
http://w3.arizona.edu/~finaid/finaid.html
Disability Served: all

Purpose: The University offers a scholarship to students with disabilities.
Eligibility: Students at the University with documented disabilities are eligible to apply.
Financial Details: Amounts vary.
Number Awarded: One per year.
Deadline: Contact the University for dates.

University of California at Los Angeles
Project YES
3820 Del Amo Boulevard, Suite 201
Torrance, CA 90503
310-825-4321
http://www.ucla.edu/
Disability Served: all

Purpose: Project YES helps students with a disability participate in college programs in the sciences and engineering.
Eligibility: Disabled students interested in science and engineering are eligible.
Financial Details: Amounts vary.
Number Awarded: Varies.
Deadline: Applications are due June 1.

University of California at Santa Cruz
1156 High Street
Santa Cruz, CA 95064
831-459-4008
http://www2.ucsc.edu/
Disability Served: all

Purpose: This university offers a financial aid program for students with disabilities.
Eligibility: Disabled students who need financial assistance are eligible to apply.
Financial Details: Awards vary according to need.
Number Awarded: Varies.
Deadline: Contact the University for details.

University of Central Arkansas
Office of Financial Aid
201 Bernard Hall
Conway, AR 72035
501-450-3140
Disability Served: all

Purpose: This university offers a financial aid program for students with disabilities.
Eligibility: Disabled students enrolled in voca-

tional rehabilitation programs who need financial assistance are eligible to apply.
Financial Details: Awards vary according to need.
Number Awarded: Varies.
Deadline: Contact the University for details.

University of Cincinnati

Office of Financial Aid
2624 Clifton Avenue
Cincinnati, OH 45221
513-556-6816
Disability Served: all

Purpose: This large four-year university offers a financial aid program for students with disabilities.
Eligibility: Disabled students who need financial assistance are eligible to apply.
Financial Details: Awards vary according to need.
Number Awarded: Varies.
Deadline: Contact the University for details.

University of Colorado at Boulder

Office of Financial Aid
Campus Box 106
Boulder, CO 80309-0106
303-492-5091
http://www.colorado.edu
Disability Served: all

Purpose: To provide funds for disabled students at the University of Colorado at Boulder.

University of Florida at Gainesville

Office of Financial Aid
PO Box 114075
Gainesville, FL 32611
352-392-1261
Disability Served: all

Purpose: This major state university offers financial aid for students with disabilities.
Eligibility: Disabled students who demonstrate financial need are eligible.
Financial Details: Awards vary according to need.
Number Awarded: Varies.
Deadline: Contact the University for details.

University of Georgia

Office of Financial Aid
Athens, GA 30602
706-542-8719
http://www.uga.edu/
Disability Served: all

Purpose: This major university offers a financial aid program for students with disabilities.
Eligibility: Disabled students who need financial assistance are eligible to apply.
Financial Details: Awards vary according to need.

University of Hartford

Office of Financial Aid
200 Bloomfield Avenue
West Hartford, CT 06117
860-768-4312
Disability Served: all

Purpose: This university offers a scholarship for students with disabilities.
Eligibility: Disabled students attending the University are eligible to apply.
Financial Details: Awards vary.
Number Awarded: Varies.
Deadline: Contact the University for details.

University of Houston

Office of Financial Aid
Houston, TX 77204
713-743-5400
Disability Served: all

Purpose: This university offers a scholarship for students with disabilities.
Eligibility: Disabled students attending the University are eligible to apply.
Financial Details: Awards vary.
Number Awarded: Varies.
Deadline: Contact the University for details.

University of Idaho

Students Advisory Services
Moscow, ID 83943
208-885-6757
http://www.uidaho.edu/
Disability Served: all

Purposc: This public university offers a financial aid program to help students with disabilities.

Eligibility: Disabled students who need financial assistance are eligible.
Financial Details: Awards vary according to need.

University of Iowa
Office of Financial Aid
Iowa City, IA 52242
319-353-6967
Disability Served: physically disabled

Purpose: The David Braverman Scholarship helps finance graduate or professional studies.
Eligibility: Students with physical disabilities may apply. Selection is based on need, prior academic record, and intention to serve the community.
Financial Details: An award of $1,000 is offered.
Number Awarded: Varies.
Deadline: Contact the University for deadlines.

University of Maine at Augusta
46 University Drive
Augusta, ME 04330
207-877-1234
http://www.uma.maine.edu
Disability Served: all

Purpose: The University offers financial aid to its students with disabilities.
Eligibility: Financially needy students with disabilities are eligible to apply.
Financial Details: Awards vary according to need.
Number Awarded: Varies.
Deadline: Contact the University for details.

University of Maryland at College Park
Office of Financial Aid
College Park, MD 20740
Disability Served: all

Purpose: The University offers many scholarships.
Eligibility: Students with disabilities are eligible.
Financial Details: Amounts vary.
Number Awarded: Varies.
Deadline: Call or write for details.

University of Maryland, Eastern Shore
Office of Financial Aid
Princess Anne, MD 21853
410-651-6261
Disability Served: all

Purpose: This branch of the university system offers financial aid assistance to help its students with disabilities.
Eligibility: Students with disabilities who are in need of financial assistance may apply.
Financial Details: Awards depend on need.
Number Awarded: Varies.
Deadline: Contact the University for details.

University of Michigan
Services for Students with Disabilities
G-625 Haven Hall
Ann Arbor, MI 48109-1045
313-763-3000
http://www.umich.edu/
Disability Served: all

Purpose: The Ridley Scholarship is awarded to students attending the University of Michigan.
Eligibility: Michigan residents with permanent disabilities who demonstrate financial need may apply for tuition assistance.
Financial Details: Awards range from $500 to $2,000.
Number Awarded: Varies.
Deadline: November 14.

University of Minnesota at Morris
Office of Financial Aid
600 Fourth Street
Morris, MN 56267
612-589-6179
Disability Served: all

Purpose: The University offers financial aid to help students pay for college study.
Eligibility: Students with disabilities who demonstrate financial need may apply.
Financial Details: Awards vary according to need.
Number Awarded: Varies.
Deadline: Contact the University for details.

University of Minnesota, Twin Cities
Office of Financial Aid
101 Pleasant Street
Minneapolis, MN 55455

612-624-4037
Disability Served: all

Purpose: Financial aid is available to help students finance college training.
Eligibility: Students with disabilities who demonstrate financial need may apply
Financial Details: Awards vary according to need.
Number Awarded: Varies.
Deadline: Contact the University for details.

University of Mississippi

Office of Financial Aid
University, MS 38677
601-232-5972
Disability Served: all

Purpose: The University offers financial aid to help finance college study.
Eligibility: Students with disabilities may apply for financial assistance.
Financial Details: Amounts vary and depend on financial need.
Number Awarded: Varies.
Deadline: Contact the University for deadline dates.

University of Nevada, Las Vegas

4505 South Maryland Parkway
Las Vegas, NV 89154
702-895-3011
http://www.unlv.edu/
Disability Served: all

Purpose: The University offers a financial aid program to help finance college training.
Eligibility: Disabled students who demonstrate financial need are eligible.
Financial Details: Amounts vary and depend on need.
Number Awarded: Varies.
Deadline: Contact the University for information.

University of North Carolina at Charlotte

South University City Boulevard
Charlotte, NC 28223
704-547-4354
Disability Served: all

Purpose: The University offers financial aid to assist with the financing of college study.
Eligibility: Disabled students who demonstrate financial need may apply.
Financial Details: Amounts vary according to need.
Number Awarded: Varies.
Deadline: Contact the University for details.

University of Pennsylvania

Office of Financial Aid
418 Services Drive
Philadelphia, PA 19104
215-898-6993
Disability Served: all

Purpose: This private four-year university provides financial aid to students.
Eligibility: Financially needy students with disabilities who are attending the university are eligible to apply.
Financial Details: Amounts vary and depend on need.
Number Awarded: Varies.
Deadline: Contact the University for details.

University of Rhode Island

Office of Financial Aid
Kingston, RI 02881
401-792-2314
Disability Served: all

Purpose: Provides a scholarship to help finance a college education.
Eligibility: Students with disabilities attending the University are eligible to apply for the Paul DePace Scholarship.
Financial Details: The amount varies.

University of San Francisco

McLarne Graduate School of Management
EMMDS Program
2130 Fulton Street
San Francisco, CA 94117-1045
415-422-2531
http://www.usfca.edu/
Disability Served: all

Purpose: Provides scholarships to help finance graduate study in management and disability services.
Eligibility: Students with disabilities who wish to participate in the University's master's pro-

gram in management and disability services are eligible to apply.
Financial Details: Awards vary.
Number Awarded: Varies.
Deadline: Contact the University for details.

University of Southern Indiana

8600 University Boulevard
Evansville, IN 47712
812-464-1767
http://www.usi.edu
Disability Served: all

Purpose: Provides scholarships to help finance college study.
Eligibility: Children of eligible disabled veterans attending college are eligible to apply.
Financial Details: Amounts vary but average approximately $1,200.
Number Awarded: Varies.
Deadline: Contact the University for details.

University of Texas at Arlington

Office of Financial Aid
PO Box 19199
Arlington, TX 76019
817-273-3566
Disability Served: all

Purpose: This four-year university provides scholarships to students.
Eligibility: Students with disabilities who are attending the University are eligible to apply
Financial Details: Amounts vary.
Number Awarded: Varies.
Deadline: Contact the University for details.

University of Toledo

Office of Accessibility
2801 West Bancroft
Toledo, OH 43606
419-537-4981
http://www.utoledo.edu/
Disability Served: all

Purpose: This public four-year university provides financial aid to students.
Eligibility: Financially needy students with disabilities who are attending the University are eligible to apply.
Financial Details: Amounts vary and depend on need.
Number Awarded: Varies.
Deadline: Contact the University for details.

University of Utah

Financial Aid & Scholarships
201 South 1480 East, Room 105
Salt Lake City, UT 84112-9055
801-581-6211, 800-868-5618
http://www.saff.utah.edu/finance
Disability Served: all

Purpose: Provides funding to students at the University of Utah.
Eligibility: Disabled individuals attending the University of Utah are eligible to apply for any and all financial aid. The Louise Snow scholarship is the only scholarship open to disabled students only. The student must have at least a 2.5 GPA to be eligible.
Financial Details: Amounts vary.
Number Awarded: Varies each year.
Deadline: March 1.

University of Washington

School of Public Health and
Community Medicine
Seattle, WA 98195
206-685-3057
Disability Served: all

Purpose: Students with a disability are eligible for financial aid via a program administered by the Office of Minority Affairs.
Eligibility: Students with disabilities who need financial assistance are eligible to apply.
Financial Details: Awards vary according to need.
Number Awarded: Varies.
Deadline: Applications are due January 1.

University of Wisconsin at Madison

Office of Financial Aid
905 University Avenue
Madison, WI 53715
608-263-2741
Disability Served: all

Purpose: This major state university enrolls several hundred students with disabilities. A scholarship has been established for students with disabilities.
Eligibility: Students with disabilities are eligible to apply.

Financial Details: Amounts vary.
Number Awarded: Varies.
Deadline: Call or write for additional information.

University of Wyoming

Disability Services
Box 3808, University Station
Laramie, WY 82071
307-766-6189
http://www.uwyo.edu/
Disability Served: all

Purpose: The University offers scholarships, such as the Bernadette Smith Memorial Scholarship, to assist students with disabilities.
Eligibility: Disabled students attending the University may apply.
Financial Details: Amounts vary.
Number Awarded: Varies.
Deadline: Contact the University for more information.

University of Wyoming

Office of Financial Aid
Box 3335
Laramie, WY 82071
307-766-2118
http://www.uwyo.edu/
Disability Served: all

Purpose: Among the other financial aid programs administered by the University is the Wyoming War Orphans Scholarship.
Eligibility: Children of disabled veterans are eligible to apply.
Financial Details: Amounts vary.
Number Awarded: One scholarship is awarded each year.
Deadline: Write for details.

Utah Valley State College

Office of Financial Aid
800 West 1200 South Street
Orem, UT 84058
801-222-8806
Disability Served: all

Purpose: This public four-year college enrolls approximately 400 students with disabilities each year and has a financial aid program to help those with need.
Eligibility: Students with disabilities who demonstrate financial need are eligible
Financial Details: Amounts vary and depend on need.
Number Awarded: Varies.
Deadline: Contact the College for details.

Venture Clubs of the Americas

2 Penn Center Plaza, Suite 1000
Philadelphia, PA 19102
215-557-9300
Disability Served: physically disabled

Purpose: Local Venture Clubs offer scholarships to help fund college training.
Eligibility: Persons between the ages of 15 and 40 with physical disabilities are eligible. Applicants must compete for awards at the local and national level
Financial Details: First Place, $5000; Second Place, $2500.
Number Awarded: Two.
Deadline: December 31. Send a self-addressed, stamped envelope with a request for an application to address above.

Very Special Arts

1300 Connecticut Avenue, NW, Suite 700
Washington, DC 20036
202-628-2800, 800-933-8721
http://www.vsarts.org
Disability Served: all

Purpose: Provides scholarships to finance the study of music and playwriting.
Eligibility: Students of music and playwriting are eligible to apply.
Financial Details: Award amounts vary.
Number Awarded: Four scholarships are given in music (two in the United States and two internationally), and two scholarships are given in playwriting.
Deadline: Contact Very Special Arts for dates.

Virgin Islands Board of Education

PO Box 11900
St Thomas, VI 00801
809-774-4546
Disability Served: all

Purpose: The Exceptional Children Scholarship helps finance college study of subjects not available in the Islands.

Eligibility: Residents of the Virgin Islands who suffer from a physical or mental disability are eligible.
Financial Details: A $2,000 award is offered.
Number Awarded: One per year.
Deadline: Applications are due in March.

Virginia State University

Student Support Services
PO Box 9003
Blacksburg, VA 23806
804-524-5811
http://www.vsu.edu/
Disability Served: all

Purpose: This federally-funded program provides support for students with disabilities.
Eligibility: Priority is given to students from low-income families. Among those served are blind and deaf students and students with cerebral palsy.
Financial Details: Awards vary.
Number Awarded: Varies.
Deadline: Write or call for additional details.

Visually Impaired Data Processors International

c/o American Council for the Blind
1155 15th Street, NW, Suite 720
Washington, DC 20005
800-424-8666
Disability Served: vision

Purpose: The Kelly Cannon Scholarship is offered by this organization.
Eligibility: Students with a visual impairment who wish to prepare for a career in the computer field are eligible.
Financial Details: Amount varies.
Number Awarded: One per year.
Deadline: Write for details.

Wal-Mart Foundation

708 Southwest Eighth Street
Bentonville, AR 72716
501-273-4000
Disability Served: all

Purpose: Provides scholarships to help fund college education.
Eligibility: High school seniors who live in communities where Wal-Mart stores are located and are planning to attend colleges or universities are eligible to apply.
Financial Details: Scholarships are for $1,000.
Number Awarded: Varies each year.
Deadline: Contact the Foundation for dates.

Washington State Higher Education Coordinating Board

917 Lakeridge Way, GV-11
Olympia, WA 98504
360-753-3571
Disability Served: vision

Purpose: The Board offers small grants to help students purchase educational equipment.
Eligibility: Blind students from the state are eligible. The goal is to help pay for any equipment needed because of visual impairment.
Financial Details: Funds of up to $200 per quarter or $300 per semester are available.
Number Awarded: Varies.
Deadline: Contact the Board for information.

Waubonsee Community College

Access Center for Students with Disabilities
Route 47 at Harter Road
Sugar Grove, IL 60554-9799
630-466-7900
http://www.wcc.cc.il.us
Disability Served: all

Purpose: This large public community college offers a financial aid program to help students finance college training.
Eligibility: Students with disabilities who need financial assistance are eligible to apply.
Financial Details: Awards vary according to need.
Number Awarded: Varies.
Deadline: Contact the College for details.

Wayne State University

Office of Financial Aid
Detroit, MI 48202
313-993-3416
http://www.wayne.edu/
Disability Served: all

Purpose: The Dorothy Begun Memorial Endowment fund provides financial aid for students with disabilities.

Eligibility: Disabled students attending the University are eligible.
Financial Details: Amounts vary.
Number Awarded: Varies.
Deadline: Write for details.

Wayne State University

Handicapped Educational Services
5221 Gullen Mall, MS 579
Detroit, MI 48202
313-577-1851
http://www.wayne.edu/
Disability Served: all

Purpose: This university offers a financial aid program to help students finance college training.
Eligibility: Students with disabilities who need financial assistance are eligible to apply.
Financial Details: Awards vary according to need.
Number Awarded: Varies.
Deadline: Contact the University for details.

West Texas A&M University

Office of Financial Aid
PO Box 999
Canyon, TX 79016
806-656-2000
Disability Served: all

Purpose: This public university offers a financial aid program to help students finance college training.
Eligibility: Students with disabilities who need financial assistance are eligible to apply.
Financial Details: Awards vary according to need.
Number Awarded: Varies.
Deadline: Contact the University for details.

West Virginia State College

Po Box 1000,
Campus Box 187
Institute, WV 25112
304-766-3131
Disability Served: all

Purpose: This four-year college offers a financial aid program to help students finance college training.
Eligibility: Students with disabilities who need financial assistance are eligible to apply.
Financial Details: Awards vary according to need.
Number Awarded: Varies.
Deadline: Contact the College for details.

Western Connecticut State University

Office of Financial Aid
181 White Street
Danbury, CT 06810
203-797-4347
Disability Served: all

Purpose: This university offers a financial aid program to help students finance college training.
Eligibility: Students with disabilities who need financial assistance are eligible to apply.
Financial Details: Awards vary according to need.
Number Awarded: Varies.
Deadline: Contact the University for details.

Western Michigan University

Office of Financial Aid
Kalamazoo, MI 49008
616-387-1000
http://www.wmich.edu/
Disability Served: all

Purpose: This public four-year university provides financial aid to students.
Eligibility: Financially needy students with disabilities attending the University are eligible to apply.
Financial Details: Amounts vary and depend on need.
Number Awarded: Varies.
Deadline: Contact the University for details.

Western New Mexico University

Office of Financial Aid
1000 West College Avenue
Silver City, NM 88061
505-538-6400
Disability Served: all

Purpose: This four-year university provides financial aid to students.
Eligibility: Financially needy students with disabilities attending the University are eligible to apply.

Financial Details: Amounts vary and depend on need.

William Rainey Harper College

1200 West Algonquin Road
Palatine, IL 60067-7398
847-925-6266
http://www.harper.cc.il.us
Disability Served: all

Purpose: Provides scholarships to currently enrolled students with disabilities.
Eligibility: Students with disabilities at William Rainey Harper College are eligible to apply.
Financial Details: Awards range from $500 to $2,000.
Number Awarded: Seven per year.
Deadline: Contact the College for deadline information.

Winston-Salem Foundation

329 First Union National Bank Building
Winston-Salem, NC 27101
919-725-3282
Disability Served: all

Purpose: The Foundation offers the Zimmerman Scholarships to help finance college study.
Eligibility: Students with disabilities from Forsyth County, North Carolina, are eligible. In some cases, candidates for the award are nominated by the colleges they attend. Nondisabled persons who wish to prepare for careers serving persons with disabilities are also eligible.
Financial Details: Up to $1,000 awards are available.
Number Awarded: Varies.
Deadline: Contact the Foundation for information.

Wisconsin Higher Education Aid Board

PO Box 7885
Madison, WI 53707
608-266-0888
Disability Served: vision

Purpose: The Visual and Hearing Impaired Program awards grants to help defer college expenses.
Eligibility: Wisconsin residents with disabilities may apply. Candidates must complete a form to be signed by a physician.
Financial Details: Awards are for up to $1,800.
Number Awarded: Varies.
Deadline: Write or call for details.

Women's National Farm and Garden Association

c/o Treadwell Schaedel
Farmstead Lane
West Simsbury, CT 05092
Disability Served: all

Purpose: The Association offers a scholarship to help with college expenses.
Eligibility: Students with disabilities who wish to study agriculture or a related field at an advanced level are eligible.
Financial Details: A scholarship of $500 is awarded.
Number Awarded: One per year.
Deadline: Write for details.

Woodrow Wilson National Fellowship Foundation

5 Vaughn Drive, Suite 300
CN5281
Princeton, NJ 08543-5281
609-452-7007
http://www.Woodrow.org/
Disability Served: all

Purpose: The Charlotte Newcome Doctoral Dissertation Fellowships help finance doctoral studies.
Eligibility: Disabled students pursuing doctoral degrees in the humanities and social sciences may apply.
Financial Details: Fellowship is worth approximately $15,500.
Number Awarded: Varies.
Deadline: Request an application by December 6.

Wright State University

Office of Disability Services
Colonel Glenn Highway
Dayton, OH 45435
937-873-5680
http://www.wright.edu/
Disability Served: all

Purpose: The University offers scholarships to assist students with disabilities.
Eligibility: Disabled students attending the University may apply.
Financial Details: Amounts vary.
Number Awarded: Varies.
Deadline: Contact the University for more information.

York Technical College
452 South Anderson Road
Rock Hill, SC 29730
803-327-8000
http://www.yorktech.com
Disability Served: all

Purpose: This two-year institution offers financial aid to help finance college study.
Eligibility: Students with disabilities may apply for financial assistance.
Financial Details: Amounts vary and depend on financial need.

Nonprofits

The following organizations and foundations provide funding to nonprofit organizations to support charitable projects and programs. Eligibility requirements vary widely.

Adolph Coors Foundation
350-C Clayton Street
Denver, CO 80206
303-388-1636
Disability Served: all

Purpose: Provides grants in the areas of health, education, youth, and community services.
Eligibility: Charitable organizations are eligible to apply.
Financial Details: Awards vary.
Number Awarded: Varies.
Deadline: Contact the Foundation for additional details.

Agnes M Lindsay Trust
95 Market Street
Manchester, NH 03101
603-669-4140
Disability Served: all

Purpose: The Trust offers grants to fund cultural programs for the mentally ill, blind, and deaf.
Eligibility: Charitable organizations in Maine, Massachusetts, New Hampshire, and Vermont are eligible to apply.
Financial Details: Amounts vary.
Number Awarded: Varies.
Deadline: Contact the Trust for details.

Ahmanson Foundation
9215 Wilshire Boulevard
Beverly Hills, CA 90210
310-278-0770
Disability Served: all

Purpose: Provides grants for the improvement of the quality of life of Southern California and Los Angeles County.
Eligibility: Charitable organizations in Southern California working in arts and humanities, education, mental health, or other social welfare programs are eligible to apply.
Financial Details: Awards vary.
Number Awarded: Varies.
Deadline: Contact the Foundation for details.

Alabama Power Foundation
600 North 18th Street, 17th Floor
Birmingham, AL 35291
205-250-2508
Disability Served: all

Purpose: Provides grants for charitable purposes.
Eligibility: Nonprofit organizations in Alabama are eligible to apply. Funding is not given to political or religious organizations.
Financial Details: Amounts vary.
Number Awarded: Varies each year.
Deadline: Contact the Foundation for details.

Alexander and Margaret Stewart Trust
88817th Street NW, Suite 210
Washington, DC 20006
202-785-9892
Disability Served: physically disabled

Purpose: The Trust provides funds for cancer treatment.
Eligibility: Facilities that provide care and treatment of cancer patients in the Washington, DC, area may apply.
Financial Details: Amounts vary.
Number Awarded: Varies.
Deadline: Varies. Write for details.

Alfred Bersted Foundation

231 South LaSalle Street
Chicago, IL 60697
312-828-1785
Disability Served: all

Purpose: The Foundation supports projects for the mentally and physically disabled.
Eligibility: Nonprofit organizations in the counties of DuPage, Kane, McHenry, and DeKalb may apply. Other restrictions may apply, so contact the Foundation for details.
Financial Details: Amounts vary.
Number Awarded: Varies.
Deadline: Varies.

Alice Tweed Tuohy Foundation

205 East Carillo Street, Suite 219
Santa Barbara, CA 93101
805-962-6430
Disability Served: all

Purpose: Provides grants for the purpose of rehabilitation, recreation, or constructing new buildings in Santa Barbara county.
Eligibility: Charitable organizations in the Santa Barbara area are eligible to apply.
Financial Details: Amounts vary.
Number Awarded: Varies.
Deadline: Varies. Contact the Foundation for additional details.

Amax Foundation, Inc.

Amax Center
Greenwich, CT 06836
203-629-6901
Disability Served: all

Purpose: Provides grants to finance programs in education, health and welfare, the arts, and civic services.
Eligibility: Nonprofit organizations are eligible to apply.
Financial Details: Amounts vary.
Number Awarded: Varies.
Deadline: Contact the Foundation for details.

American Express Philanthropic Program

American Express Company
200 Vessey Street
New York, NY 10285
212-640-5661
http://www.americanexpress.com/corp/philanthropy/
Disability Served: all

Purpose: The Foundation supports programs in a variety of fields, including community service, cultural heritage, and economic independence.
Eligibility: Charitable organizations in Arizona, California, Colorado, Florida, Georgia, Illinois, Minnesota, North Carolina, Nebraska, New York, Texas, Utah, Massachusetts, and Pennsylvania are eligible to apply.
Financial Details: Amounts vary widely.
Number Awarded: Varies.
Deadline: Contact the Foundation for information.

American National Bank and Trust Company

33 North LaSalle Street
Chicago, IL 60690
312-661-6115
Disability Served: all

Purpose: Provides grants in the areas of health, education, arts and culture, social services, community affairs, and economic development.
Eligibility: Nonprofit organizations in the Chicago metropolitan area are eligible.
Financial Details: Amounts vary.
Number Awarded: Varies.
Deadline: Varies.

Amerock Charities Trust

PO Box 1537
Rockford, IL 61110
815-963-9631
Disability Served: all

Purpose: The Trust supports projects that promote wellness, health, and rehabilitation of those with physical or visual impairments.

Eligibility: Charitable organizations involved in projects in the areas mentioned above may apply.
Financial Details: Amounts vary and depend on need.
Number Awarded: Varies.
Deadline: Varies. Write for information.

Anheuser-Busch Foundation

One Busch Place
St Louis, MO 63118
314-577-7368
Disability Served: all

Purpose: The Foundation provides grants in the areas of the environment, conservation, community affairs, and more.
Eligibility: Nonprofit organizations are eligible.
Financial Details: Amounts vary depending on project need.

Ann Arbor Area Community Foundation

201 South Main, Suite 400
Ann Arbor, MI 48104
313-663-0401
http://www.aaacf.org
Disability Served: all

Purpose: The Foundation provides financial support for projects designed to improve the quality of life for residents of the Ann Arbor area.
Eligibility: Charitable organizations serving the Ann Arbor area may apply.
Financial Details: Amounts vary and depend on project need.
Number Awarded: Varies.
Deadline: Contact the Foundation for details.

Annuziata Sanguinetti Foundation

420 Montgomery Street, 5th Floor
San Francisco, CA 94163
Disability Served: all

Purpose: Provides grants to help finance projects designed to help San Francisco Bay area residents who are hearing impaired or speech impaired. Grants are also available to support recreational projects.
Eligibility: Charitable organizations in the San Francisco Bay area devoted to helping the hearing impaired or the speech impaired are eligible to apply.
Financial Details: Varies.
Number Awarded: Varies.
Deadline: Contact the Foundation for details.

Anschutz Family Foundation

2400 Anaconda Tower
555 17th Street
Denver, CO 80202
303-293-2338
Disability Served: all

Purpose: Provides grants for the purpose of improving conditions for the elderly, young, and economically disadvantaged.
Eligibility: Charitable organizations dedicated to helping the elderly, young, and economically disadvantaged are eligible to apply.
Financial Details: Awards vary.
Number Awarded: Varies.
Deadline: Contact the Foundation for details.

Apple Computer, Inc.

20525 Mariani Avenue
Cupertino, CA 95014
Disability Served: all

Purpose: Provides grants and computer equipment in the areas of education, health, or company operations.
Eligibility: Organizations or schools with project proposals in education, health, or company operations are eligible to apply.
Financial Details: Awards vary.
Number Awarded: Varies.
Deadline: Varies.

Archstone Foundation

401 East Ocean Boulevard, Suite 1000
Long Beach, CA 90802
562-590-8655
http://www2.Archstone.com/Archstone/
Disability Served: elderly

Purpose: The Foundation offers grants for projects dealing with the health and welfare of the elderly.
Eligibility: Nonprofit organizations dedicated to helping the elderly are eligible.
Financial Details: Amounts vary according to project need.

Number Awarded: Varies each year.
Deadline: Applications are accepted throughout the year. Funding decisions are made in March, June, September, and December by the Board of Directors.

Argyros Foundation

950 South Coast Drive, Suite 200
Costa Mesa, CA 92626
Disability Served: all

Purpose: The Foundation provides grants to support a number of projects in the Southern California area.
Eligibility: Charitable organizations dedicated to helping the physically disabled, speech impaired, and hearing impaired are eligible to apply.
Financial Details: Amounts vary.
Number Awarded: Varies each year.
Deadline: Contact the Foundation for details.

AT&T Foundation

32 Avenue of the Americas, 24th Floor
New York, NY 10013
212-387-4801
http://www.att.com/foundation/
Disability Served: all

Purpose: The Foundation supports projects in the areas of education, arts and culture, and civic and community service.
Eligibility: Nonprofit organizations involved in the areas mentioned above are eligible.
Financial Details: Amounts vary according to project need. In 1995 and 1996, the Foundation contributed $75 million.
Number Awarded: Varies each year.
Deadline: Applications and proposals are accepted throughout the year.

Atherton Family Foundation

111 South King Street
Honolulu, HI 96813
Disability Served: all

Purpose: This private foundation provides funds for charitable purposes. Areas of interest include education, health and welfare, social services, and religious concerns.
Eligibility: Nonprofit organizations in Hawaii are eligible to apply.
Financial Details: Amounts vary and depend on the project.
Number Awarded: Varies.
Deadline: Contact the Foundation for dates.

Atkinson Foundation

1100 Grundy Lane, Suite 140
San Bruno, CA 94066
650-876-0222
Disability Served: all

Purpose: Provides grants for community service, education, and civic organizations in San Mateo County.
Eligibility: Charitable organizations in San Mateo County dedicated to helping the elderly, youth, the disadvantaged, and persons needing rehabilitation are eligible to apply.
Financial Details: Amounts vary but average $5,000 each. A total of approximately $750,000 is awarded each year.
Number Awarded: Varies.
Deadline: Contact the Foundation for details.

Autry Foundation

5858 Sunset Boulevard
PO Box 710
Los Angeles, CA 90078
Disability Served: all

Purpose: The Foundation supports charitable projects in Los Angeles, Riverside, and Orange Counties in Southern California.
Eligibility: Nonprofit organizations serving the counties listed above may apply.
Financial Details: Amounts vary and depend on financial need.
Number Awarded: Varies.
Deadline: Contact the Foundation for information.

Ball Brothers Foundation

PO Box 1408
Muncie, IN 47308
765-741-5500
Disability Served: all

Purpose: Provides grants for charitable, religious, or educational purposes.
Eligibility: Organizations in the state of Indiana

are eligible to apply. Grants are not given to individuals.
Financial Details: A total amount of $3,200,000 was awarded in a recent year.
Number Awarded: Varies. In a recent year, thirty-nine were awarded.
Deadline: Contact the Foundation for deadline information.

Bank of Boston Corporation Charitable Foundation

100 Federal Street
Boston, MA 02110
617-434-2171
Disability Served: all

Purpose: Provides grants for charitable purposes.
Eligibility: Nonprofit organizations in the New England area are eligible.
Financial Details: Amounts vary according to project need.
Number Awarded: Varies each year.
Deadline: Contact the Foundation for details.

BankAmerica Foundation

PO Box 37000
Department 3246
San Francisco, CA 94137
415-953-3175
Disability Served: all

Purpose: The Foundation offers grants in the areas of arts and culture, health and human services, community investment, education, and conservation and environment.
Eligibility: Charitable organizations involved in the areas listed above are eligible to apply.
Financial Details: Amounts vary and depend on project need.
Number Awarded: Varies.
Deadline: Contact the Foundation for details.

Bell Atlantic Foundation

1095 Avenue of the Americas, Room 3200
New York, NY 10036
800-360-7955
http://www.bellatlanticfoundation.com/
Disability Served: all

Purpose: The Foundation supports projects designed to improve the education of science, math, and technology in secondary schools.
Eligibility: Schools and organizations working on programs to improve education are eligible to apply.
Financial Details: Amounts vary.
Number Awarded: Varies.
Deadline: Proposals are accepted throughout the year.

Bertha Russ Foundation

PO Box 893
Ferndale, CA 95536
Disability Served: all

Purpose: The Foundation supports the Easter Seal Society, the Association for Retarded Citizens, and building and equipment funds.
Eligibility: Charitable organizations such as those listed above may apply.
Financial Details: Awards vary and depend on need.
Number Awarded: Varies.
Deadline: Contact the Foundation for details.

Blount Foundation, Inc.

4520 Executive Park Drive
Montgomery, AL 36116
334-244-4000
Disability Served: all

Purpose: The Foundation provides grants for a variety of charitable projects.
Eligibility: Charitable organizations dedicated to improving the quality of life of society are eligible to apply.
Financial Details: Amounts vary.
Number Awarded: Varies.
Deadline: Contact the Foundation for details.

Blowitz-Ridgeway Foundation

2700 River Road, Suite 211
Des Plaines, IL 60018
847-298-2378
Disability Served: all

Purpose: The Foundation provides grants designed to support projects for the physically or mentally disabled in Illinois.
Eligibility: Organizations serving the disabled or children and youth in Illinois are eligible to apply.
Financial Details: Amounts vary.

Number Awarded: Varies.
Deadline: Contact the Foundation for dates.

Booth Ferris Foundation

60 Wall Street, 46th Floor
New York, NY 10260
212-809-1630
Disability Served: all

Purpose: The Foundation provides grants for charitable purposes.
Eligibility: Nonprofit organizations serving the New York metropolitan area are eligible.
Financial Details: Amounts vary according to need.
Number Awarded: Varies each year.
Deadline: Contact the Foundation for additional details.

Bothin Foundation

PO Box 29906
San Francisco, CA 94129
415-561-6540
Disability Served: all

Purpose: The Foundation provides grants to charitable organizations in the counties of San Francisco, Marin, Sonoma, San Mateo, and Santa Barbara. The areas of interest include health services, community concerns, the environment, and education.
Eligibility: Charitable organizations serving the counties listed above are eligible. Priority is given to organizations concerned with the elderly, youth, and the disabled.
Financial Details: Amounts vary.
Number Awarded: Varies.
Deadline: Contact the Foundation for information.

Broward Community Foundation, Inc.

2601 East Oakland Park Boulevard, Suite 202
Ft Lauderdale, FL 33306
954-761-9503
Disability Served: all

Purpose: Provides grants in order to improve the quality of life for citizens of Broward County. Areas of interest include health, education, the environment, the arts, social concerns, and animal welfare.
Eligibility: Charitable organizations serving the Broward County area may apply.
Financial Details: Amounts vary.
Number Awarded: Varies.
Deadline: Contact the Foundation for information.

Brown Foundation, Inc.

2217 Welch Avenue
PO Box 130646
Houston, TX 77219-0646
713-523-6867
Disability Served: all

Purpose: This foundation offers grants in primary and secondary education.
Eligibility: Nonprofit organizations and schools in Texas are eligible.
Financial Details: Grants range from $10,000 to $100,000.
Number Awarded: Varies.
Deadline: Contact the Foundation for details.

Burlington Northern Foundation

3800 Colonial Plaza
777 Main Street
Ft Worth, TX 76102
Disability Served: all

Purpose: The Foundation provides grants in the arts, civic service, education, and more.
Eligibility: Charitable organizations and universities are eligible to apply.
Financial Details: Amounts vary.
Number Awarded: Varies.
Deadline: Contact the Foundation for details.

Burlington Resources Foundation

999 Third Avenue, 45th Floor
Seattle, WA 98104-4097
206-728-8625
Disability Served: all

Purpose: The Foundation provides funding in the areas of community affairs, education, youth organizations, medical facilities, arts and culture, and human services.
Eligibility: Nonprofit organizations are eligible to apply.
Financial Details: Amounts vary.
Number Awarded: Varies.
Deadline: Contact the Foundation for application forms and deadlines.

Bush Foundation

E-900 First National Bank Building
332 Minnesota Street
St Paul, MN 55101
612-227-0891
Disability Served: all

Purpose: Provides grants to those interested in the arts, education, health, human services, and the development of leadership.
Eligibility: Grants are limited to nonprofit organizations in Minnesota, North Dakota, and South Dakota.
Financial Details: Amounts vary.
Number Awarded: Varies.
Deadline: Varies. Contact the Foundation for additional details.

Bushrod H Campbell and Adah F Hall Charity Fund

c/o Palmer and Dodge LLP
One Beacon Street, Suite 2100
Boston, MA 02108
617-573-0328
Disability Served: all

Purpose: The Fund provides grants in the areas of health care, population control, and the aged.
Eligibility: Nonprofit organizations in the Greater Boston Area, Massachusetts, are eligible to apply.
Financial Details: Amounts vary.
Number Awarded: Varies.
Deadline: January 15 for review in February, April 15 for review in May, August 15 for review in September, and October 15 for review in December. Contact the Fund for information.

California Community Foundation

445 South Figueroa, Suite 3400
Los Angeles, CA 90071-1638
213-413-4130
http://www.calfund.org/index.html
Disability Served: all

Purpose: Provides grants to support programs dedicated to improving the lives of the residents of Los Angeles County.
Eligibility: Nonprofit organizations serving Los Angeles County are eligible.
Financial Details: Amounts vary depending on program need.
Number Awarded: Varies.
Deadline: Contact the Foundation for application materials. Deadline dates vary.

California Wellness Foundation

6320 Canoga Avenue, Suite 1700
Woodland Hills, CA 91367-7111
818-593-6600
http://www.tcwf.org
Disability Served: all

Purpose: This private foundation awards grants in the areas of community health, population health improvement, teenage pregnancy prevention, violence prevention, and work and health.
Eligibility: Nonprofit organizations with a focus on the areas listed above are eligible to apply.
Financial Details: Amounts vary according to program need. Each year approximately $40 million is given.
Number Awarded: Varies.
Deadline: Proposals are accepted throughout the year.

Campbell Soup Foundation

Campbell Place
Camden, NJ 08103
609-342-6431
Disability Served: all

Purpose: The Foundation supports projects in the areas of education, health and nutrition, arts and culture, and youth.
Eligibility: Nonprofit organizations devoted to community service in the areas listed above are eligible to apply. Priority is given to organizations in the New Jersey area.
Financial Details: Amounts vary.
Number Awarded: Varies.
Deadline: Varies. Contact the Foundation for further details.

Cannon Foundation, Inc.

PO Box 548
Concord, NC 28026
704-786-8216
Disability Served: all

Purpose: The Foundation supports projects that serve the residents of North Carolina.
Eligibility: Charitable organizations in the

North Carolina area are eligible.
Financial Details: Amounts vary.
Number Awarded: Varies each year.
Deadline: Write or call for information.

Capital Cities/ABC Foundation, Inc.

77 West 66th Street
New York, NY 10023
212-456-7777
Disability Served: all

Purpose: The Foundation supports higher education, including medical education and building funds, hospitals and medical research, youth programs, civic and community affairs, and programs benefiting minorities.
Eligibility: Nonprofit organizations involved in the areas listed above are eligible to apply.
Financial Details: Awards vary according to project need.
Number Awarded: Varies.
Deadline: Applications are accepted throughout the year and reviewed quarterly.

Champlin Foundations

410 South Main Street
Providence, RI 02903
401-736-0370
Disability Served: all

Purpose: Provides grants for charitable purposes.
Eligibility: Nonprofit organizations serving the Rhode Island area are eligible.
Financial Details: Amounts vary according to need.
Number Awarded: Varies each year.
Deadline: Write or call for details.

Charles Bloom Foundation, Inc.

240 Eucalyptus Hill Drive
Santa Barbara, CA 93108
805-966-1793
Disability Served: all

Purpose: The Foundation offers grants in the areas of health, education, and community services.
Eligibility: Charitable organizations may apply.
Financial Details: Amounts vary according to project needs.
Number Awarded: Varies.
Deadline: Write for details.

Chatlos Foundation, Inc.

PO Box 915048
Longwood, FL 32791-5048
407-862-5077
Disability Served: all

Purpose: The Foundation provides grants in the areas of higher education, social causes, and medical issues.
Eligibility: Nonprofit organizations and universities may apply. Emphasis is placed on overall mission statements rather than individual projects.
Financial Details: Amounts vary.
Number Awarded: Varies.
Deadline: Varies.

Chicago Community Trust

222 North LaSalle Street, Suite 1400
Chicago, IL 60601
312-372-3356
Disability Served: all

Purpose: The Trust disseminates grants on behalf of organizations or individuals wishing to provide funds for charitable purposes.
Eligibility: Nonprofit organizations serving Illinois are eligible to apply. Other requirements may apply so contact the Trust for information.
Financial Details: Amounts vary.
Number Awarded: Varies.
Deadline: Contact the Trust for details.

Chichester DuPont Foundation

3120 Kennett Pike
Wilmington, DE 19807
302-658-5244
Disability Served: all

Purpose: Provides grants in the areas of culture, education, and health.
Eligibility: Nonprofit organizations may apply.
Financial Details: Amounts vary.
Number Awarded: Varies.
Deadline: Please contact the Foundation for details.

Children's Fresh Air Society Fund

Baltimore Community Foundation
2 East Read Street
Bethesda, MD 21202
301-332-4171
Disability Served: all

Purpose: Provides grants for the purpose of financing tuition to summer camp for Maryland youth who are disadvantaged and disabled.
Eligibility: Nonprofit camps are eligible to apply.
Financial Details: Amounts vary.

Clark-Winchcole Foundation

4550 Montgomery Avenue
Bethesda, MD 20814
301-654-3607
Disability Served: all

Purpose: The Foundation provides grants to programs for the deaf, physically disabled, and higher education.
Eligibility: Charitable organizations in the Washington, DC, area may apply.
Financial Details: Amounts vary.

Clipper Ship Foundation, Inc.

Hartford Insurance Group
Hartford Plaza
Hartford, CT 06115
860-547-5000
Disability Served: all

Purpose: Provides financial assistance to organizations dedicated to helping the homeless, the poor, the sick, the handicapped, children, the elderly, or those with special needs.
Eligibility: Charitable organizations serving the people of the Boston area are eligible.
Financial Details: Amounts vary and depend on program need.
Number Awarded: Varies each year.
Deadline: Varies. Contact the Foundation for information.

Clorox Company Foundation

PO Box 24305
Oakland, CA 94623-1305
510-271-2199, 510-271-7751
http://www.clorox.com/community.html
Disability Served: all

Purpose: Provides grants for the purpose of improving the quality of life in communities where Clorox employees live and work.
Eligibility: Charitable organizations serving a community where Clorox has an operating facility or where its employees reside are eligible to apply.
Financial Details: Grants range from $1,000 to $10,000.
Number Awarded: Varies.
Deadline: July 1, October 1, January 1, and April 1.

Cockrell Foundation, Inc.

1600 Smith Street, Suite 3900
Houston, TX 77002
713-209-7300
Disability Served: all

Purpose: The Foundation provides grants for charitable purposes.
Eligibility: Nonprofit organizations serving the Houston area may apply.
Financial Details: Amounts vary.
Number Awarded: Varies each year.
Deadline: Contact the Foundation for details.

Commonwealth Fund

1 East 75th Street
New York, NY 10021
212-535-0400
http://www.cmwf.org/
Disability Served: all

Purpose: The Fund supports programs in health care, elderly issues, children and youth, and minority concerns.
Eligibility: Nonprofit organizations involved in the areas listed above are eligible to apply.
Financial Details: Amounts vary.
Number Awarded: Varies.
Deadline: Letters of inquiry are accepted throughout the year.

Communities Foundation of Texas

4605 Live Oak Street
Dallas, TX 75204-8019
214-826-5231
Disability Served: all

Purpose: This foundation provides grants for charitable purposes.

Eligibility: Nonprofit organizations serving Texas residents are eligible.
Financial Details: Amounts vary.
Number Awarded: Varies.
Deadline: Contact the Foundation for additional details.

Community Foundation of New Jersey

PO Box 317
35 Knox Hill Road
Morristown, NJ 07963
201-267-5533
Disability Served: all

Purpose: The Foundation provides funds in the areas of health care, education, youth programs, human services, community development, and public affairs.
Eligibility: Nonprofit organizations serving New Jersey are eligible.
Financial Details: Amounts vary.
Number Awarded: Varies.
Deadline: December 31, March 31, and June 30.

Community Foundation of Santa Clara County

960 West Hedding, #220
San Jose, CA 95126
408-278-0270
Disability Served: all

Purpose: The Foundation provides grants in the areas of arts and humanities, community and social services, education, environment, and health.
Eligibility: Nonprofit organizations serving Santa Clara County and southern San Mateo County may apply.
Financial Details: Amounts vary.
Number Awarded: Varies each year.
Deadline: January 13.

Connecticut Mutual Life Foundation, Inc.

140 Garden Street
Hartford, CT 06154
860-987-6500
Disability Served: all

Purpose: Provides grants to help fund charitable programs.
Eligibility: Nonprofit organizations are eligible to apply.
Financial Details: Amounts vary.
Number Awarded: Varies.
Deadline: Contact the Foundation for details.

Conrad N Hilton Foundation

100 West Liberty Street, Suite 840
Reno, NV 89501
702-323-4221
Disability Served: all

Purpose: The Foundation develops long-term charitable projects and looks for organizations to carry them out.
Eligibility: Nonprofit organizations involved in areas of interest to the Foundation may contact the Foundation for information.
Financial Details: Amounts vary, depending on the project.
Number Awarded: Varies.
Deadline: Contact the Foundation for information.

Crail-Johnson Foundation

222 West 6th Street, #1010
San Pedro, CA 90731
310-519-7413
http://www.crail-johnson.org/
Disability Served: all

Purpose: The Foundation funds projects that benefit children in the areas of education, health, and social services.
Eligibility: Charitable organizations dedicated to helping children are eligible.
Financial Details: Awards vary.

Crescent Porter Hale Foundation

220 Bush Street, Suite 1069
San Francisco, CA 94104
415-986-5177
Disability Served: all

Purpose: The Foundation supports projects that benefit the residents of the San Francisco Bay area, primarily in the areas of education, youth concerns, human services, and capital funding.
Eligibility: Nonprofit organizations involved in projects that serve the San Francisco Bay area community are eligible.
Financial Details: Amounts vary.

Number Awarded: Varies.
Deadline: None.

Cullen Foundation

601 Jefferson, 40th Floor
Houston, TX 77002
713-651-8837
Disability Served: all

Purpose: Provides funds for charitable projects in Texas.
Eligibility: Nonprofit organizations in Texas are eligible.
Financial Details: Amounts vary and depend on program need.
Number Awarded: Varies.
Deadline: Varies. Contact the Foundation for details.

David and Lucile Packard Foundation

300 Second Street, Suite 200
Los Altos, CA 94022
650-948-7658
http://www.packfound.org/packhome.htm
Disability Served: all

Purpose: The Foundation provides funding in the areas of science, children, conservation, film and arts preservation, education, community services, and children.
Eligibility: Charitable organizations are eligible. Other restrictions may apply, so contact the Foundation for details.
Financial Details: Amounts vary.
Number Awarded: Varies.
Deadline: Deadlines for proposals are March 16, June 15, September 15, and December 15.

Deutsch Foundation

2444 Wilshire Boulevard, Suite 600
Santa Monica, CA 90403
310-453-0055
Disability Served: all

Purpose: The Foundation supports projects that serve the residents of California.
Eligibility: Nonprofit organizations in California are eligible.
Financial Details: Amounts vary according to project need.
Number Awarded: Varies each year.
Deadline: Contact the Foundation for information.

DeWitt Wallace-Reader's Digest Fund

2 Park Avenue, 23rd Floor
New York, NY 10016
212-251-9700
http://www.wallacefunds.org
Disability Served: all

Purpose: This private foundation provides grants to improve the quality of educational opportunities for school-age youth, especially those in low-income communities.
Eligibility: Nonprofit organizations are eligible.
Financial Details: Awards vary, but in general, the Fund does not make grants of less than $100,000.
Number Awarded: Varies.
Deadline: Letters of inquiry are accepted throughout the year, but the Fund rarely, if ever, makes grants to unsolicited projects.

Dole Foundation

1819 H Street, NW, Suite 340
Washington, DC 20006
202-457-0318
Disability Served: all

Purpose: The Foundation offers grants to support the employment of persons with disabilities.
Eligibility: Nonprofit organizations dedicated to helping persons with disabilities gain employment, whether it is through training, employment programs, or assistive technology assessment, may apply.
Financial Details: Amounts vary and depend on program need.
Number Awarded: Varies.
Deadline: Varies.

Duchossois Foundation

845 Larch Avenue
Elmhurst, IL 60126
630-279-3600
Disability Served: all

Purpose: Provides grants for community services in areas where Duchossois operates.
Eligibility: Nonprofit organizations dedicated to

improving the quality of life in Illinois may apply.
Financial Details: Amounts vary.

Duke Endowment

100 North Tryon Street, Suite 3500
Charlotte, NC 28202-4012
704-376-0291
http://www.dukeendowment.org/
Disability Served: all

Purpose: This charitable trust provides support in the areas of education, health care organizations, child care institutions, and rural churches.
Eligibility: Nonprofit organizations serving North and South Carolina are eligible. Other restrictions may apply, so contact the Endowment for details.
Financial Details: Amounts vary. In 1996 more than $65 million was bestowed.
Number Awarded: Varies.
Deadline: Letters of inquiry are accepted throughout the year.

East Bay Community Foundation

501 Wickson Avenue
Oakland, CA 94610
510-836-3223
Disability Served: all

Purpose: The foundation provides grants to support programs designed to better the lives of the residents of the East Bay of the San Francisco Bay area.
Eligibility: Nonprofit organizations in Alameda and Contra Costa Counties are eligible.
Financial Details: Awards vary.
Number Awarded: Varies.
Deadline: Call or write for details.

Eckerd Corporation Foundation

8333 Bryan Dairy Road
Largo, FL 33758
727-395-6000
http://www.eckerd.com
Disability Served: all

Purpose: The Foundation offers funds to support projects in areas where Eckerd operates stores.
Eligibility: Nonprofit organizations with SOIC3 status, primarily health organizations, pharmaceutical colleges, and organizations benefiting women and children, are eligible.
Financial Details: Amounts vary.
Number Awarded: Varies.
Deadline: Contact the Foundation for details. Written proposals requested. Board meets on a quarterly basis.

Edna McConnell Clark Foundation

250 Park Avenue
New York, NY 10177-0026
212-551-9100
http://fdncenter.org/grantmaker/emclark/index.html
Disability Served: all

Purpose: The Foundation seeks to improve conditions and opportunities for people who live in poor and disadvantaged communities.
Eligibility: Nonprofit organizations are eligible to apply.
Financial Details: Amounts vary. In 1998 more than $25 million in grants was given. Grants ranged from $25,000 to $250,000.
Number Awarded: Varies.
Deadline: Proposals are accepted throughout the year.

Edyth Bush Charitable Foundation

199 East Welbourne Avenue
PO Box 1967
Winter Park, FL 32789
407-647-4322
http://fdncenter.org/grantmaker/bush/index.html
Disability Served: all

Purpose: The Foundation provides grants to support projects that help underprivileged and needy people.
Eligibility: Nonprofit organizations operating in Orange, Seminole, Osceola, and Lake County, Florida, may be eligible.
Financial Details: Amounts vary but grants average between $5,000 and $50,000.
Number Awarded: Varies.
Deadline: Contact the Foundation for details.

EL Wiegand Foundation

165 West Liberty Street
Reno, NV 89501
702-333-0320
Disability Served: all

Purpose: Provides grants for charitable purposes.
Eligibility: Educational institutions and health organizations are eligible to apply.
Financial Details: Amounts vary, depending on program need.
Number Awarded: Varies.
Deadline: Varies.

Elizabeth Firth Wade Endowment Fund

114 East De La Guerra Street, Suite 3
Santa Barbara, CA 93101
805-963-8822
Disability Served: all

Purpose: The Foundation provides grants for charitable purposes in the areas of human services, arts and culture, youth projects, and education.
Eligibility: Nonprofit organizations may apply.
Financial Details: Amounts vary and depend on need.
Number Awarded: Varies.
Deadline: Contact the Foundation for details.

Emma B. Howe Memorial Foundation

A200 Foshay Tower
Minneapolis, MN 55402
612-339-7343
Disability Served: all

Purpose: The Foundation provides grants to fund projects concerned with the economically disadvantaged, children, persons with disabilities who need rehabilitation, and victims of discrimination.
Eligibility: Charitable organizations devoted to helping those listed above are eligible to apply.
Financial Details: Amounts vary.
Number Awarded: Varies.
Deadline: Contact the Foundation for details.

Equifax Foundation

1600 Peachtree Street NW
Atlanta, GA 30309
404-885-8000
Disability Served: all

Purpose: Provides grants in the areas of health and welfare, arts and culture, civic and community services, and education.
Eligibility: Charitable organizations in areas where Equifax operates are eligible.
Financial Details: Amounts vary.
Number Awarded: Varies each year.
Deadline: Contact the Foundation for further information.

Eugene and Agnes E Meyer Foundation

1400 Sixteenth Street, NW, Suite 360
Washington, DC 20036
202-483-8294
Disability Served: all

Purpose: Provides grants to help finance projects having to do with learning disabilities, blindness, mental health, and vocational training.
Eligibility: Nonprofit organizations in the metropolitan area of Washington, DC, are eligible.
Financial Details: Amounts vary.
Number Awarded: Varies.
Deadline: Contact the Foundation for information.

Exxon Education Foundation

5959 Las Colinas Boulevard
Irving, TX 75039-2298
972-444-1104
http://www.exxon.com/exxoncorp/world/working_with_others.htm
Disability Served: all

Purpose: The Foundation provides funds to help support programs dedicated to improving the quality of education in the United States.
Eligibility: Charitable organizations and schools working on educational projects are eligible to apply.
Financial Details: Amounts vary and depend on project need. In 1998, more than $19 million was given.
Number Awarded: Varies each year.
Deadline: Contact the Foundation for details.

Field Foundation of Illinois, Inc.

200 South Wacker Drive, Suite 2080
Chicago, IL 60606
312-831-0910
Disability Served: all

Purpose: The Foundation offers grants in the areas of education, arts and culture, community affairs, welfare, and health issues in the Chicago metropolitan area.
Eligibility: Nonprofit organizations involved in the areas mentioned above may apply.
Financial Details: Amounts vary and depend on project need.
Number Awarded: Varies.
Deadline: Contact the Foundation for information.

Florence C. and Harry L. English Memorial

PO Box 4418
Atlanta, GA 30302
404-588-8246
Disability Served: all

Purpose: Provides grants to help programs for the speech impaired, mentally disabled, and physically disabled in the Atlanta area.
Eligibility: Charitable organizations in Atlanta are eligible to apply.
Financial Details: Amounts vary.
Number Awarded: Varies.
Deadline: Contact the Foundation for details.

Florence Nelson Foundation

120 Montgomery Street, Suite 2425
San Francisco, CA 94104
Disability Served: physically disabled

Purpose: The Foundation provides grants in the areas of education, arts and culture, health concerns, and civic projects.
Eligibility: Charitable organizations serving Santa Clara County are eligible.
Financial Details: Awards are determined by financial need.
Number Awarded: Varies.
Deadline: Write for details.

Florence V. Burden Foundation

630 Fifth Avenue, Suite 2900
New York, NY 10111
212-332-1150
Disability Served: all

Purpose: This private foundation provides grants in a variety of areas, including education, environment, family care giving, and employment and volunteer opportunities for the elderly.
Eligibility: Charitable organizations and schools are eligible to apply.
Financial Details: Amounts vary and depend on program need.
Number Awarded: Varies.
Deadline: Contact the Foundation for details.

Foundation for Seacoast Health

PO Box 4606
Portsmouth, NH 03801
603-433-4001
http://www.nh.ultranet.com/~ffsh/
Disability Served: all

Purpose: The Foundation provides grants to support programs in the Portsmouth, New Hampshire, area.
Eligibility: Charitable organizations serving the Portsmouth area are eligible.
Financial Details: Amounts vary.
Number Awarded: Varies each year.

Frank Adam Foundation

7701 Forsyth, Suite 1200
St Louis, MO 63105
Disability Served: all

Purpose: The Foundation provides grants to help fund projects in the areas of medicine and health services, child welfare, and more.
Eligibility: Nonprofit organizations and medical facilities are eligible. Other restrictions may apply, so contact the Foundation for details.
Financial Details: Amounts vary according to project need.
Number Awarded: Varies each year.
Deadline: Contact the Foundation for details.

Fred Gellert Family Foundation

One Embarcadero Center, Suite 2480
San Francisco, CA 94111
415-433-6174
Disability Served: all

Purpose: Provides funding in the areas of the arts, education, environment and population, health, and youth and family services. The purpose is to advance positive forces for social change to ensure quality of life for future generations.

Eligibility: Funding is limited to San Francisco, San Mateo, and Marin counties in California. Grants are available to nonprofit organizations only (no funds are given to individuals).
Financial Details: Amounts vary.

Gallo Foundation

PO Box 1130
Modesto, CA 95353
209-341-3599
Disability Served: all

Purpose: The Foundation supports projects for the physically disabled, the mentally disabled, child welfare programs, and the Special Olympics.
Eligibility: Nonprofit organizations dedicated to the areas mentioned above are eligible.
Financial Details: Amounts vary.
Number Awarded: Varies.
Deadline: Contact the Foundation for further details.

Gates Foundation

3200 Cherry Creek South Drive, #630
Denver, CO 80209
303-722-1881
Disability Served: all

Purpose: The Foundation provides grants for the purpose of improving the quality of life in Colorado with an emphasis on the Denver metropolitan area.
Eligibility: Charitable organizations dedicated to the health, well-being, and education of Coloradoans are eligible to apply.
Financial Details: Amounts vary.
Number Awarded: Varies each year.
Deadline: Contact the Foundation for details.

Gebbie Foundation

308 Hotel Jamestown Building
PO Box 1277
Jamestown, NY 14702-1277
716-487-1062
http://www.gebbie.org/
Disability Served: all

Purpose: Provides grants for charitable purposes in the areas of human services, community development, the arts, and children and education.
Eligibility: Nonprofit organizations in Chautauqua County and in western New York are eligible to apply.
Financial Details: Amounts vary.
Number Awarded: Varies each year.
Deadline: August 1, December 1, and April 1.

General Electric Fund

3135 Easton Turnpike
Fairfield, CT 06431
203-373-3216
http://www.ge.com/fund
Disability Served: all

Purpose: The Fund provides grants to fund programs in higher education, arts and culture, public policy, and global health.
Eligibility: Charitable organizations are eligible to apply.
Financial Details: Amounts vary. In 1996 more than $28 million in grants was awarded.
Number Awarded: Varies each year.
Deadline: Proposals are accepted throughout the year.

Giant Food Foundation, Inc.

PO Box 1804
Washington, DC 20013
Disability Served: all

Purpose: The Foundation provides grants in the areas of mental health, recreation, community programs, art, and education.
Eligibility: Charitable organizations in the greater Washington, DC, area may apply.
Financial Details: Amounts vary depending on project need.
Number Awarded: Varies each year.
Deadline: Varies.

Gladys Brooks Foundation

226 Seventh Street, Suite 101
Garden City, NY 11530
516-746-6103
Disability Served: all

Purpose: The Foundation provides grants to hospitals, clinics, educational institutions, and libraries.
Eligibility: Nonprofit organizations are eligible.
Financial Details: Amounts vary and depend on program need.

Number Awarded: Varies.
Deadline: Contact the Foundation for details.

Grover Hermann Foundation

Attn: Paul K. Rhoads
7200 Sears Tower
Chicago, IL 60606
312-876-1000
Disability Served: all

Purpose: The Foundation's primary areas of interest are education, public policy, community affairs, health care, and religious groups.
Eligibility: Charitable organizations with a focus on the areas listed above may apply.
Financial Details: Amounts vary.
Number Awarded: Varies.
Deadline: Varies.

Hall Family Foundation

PO Box 419580
Kansas City, MO 64141
816-274-8516
Disability Served: all

Purpose: The Foundation provides grants to help improve the quality of life for citizens of the Kansas City area.
Eligibility: Charitable organizations in the Kansas City area are eligible.
Financial Details: Amounts vary and depend on project need.
Number Awarded: Varies.
Deadline: Contact the Foundation for details.

Harry and Grace Steele Foundation

441 Old Newport Boulevard, Suite 301
Newport Beach, CA 92663
Disability Served: all

Purpose: The Foundation provides grants for charitable purposes.
Eligibility: Nonprofit organizations serving Southern California may apply.
Financial Details: Amounts vary.
Number Awarded: Varies.
Deadline: Contact the Foundation for further details.

Hartford Foundation for Public Giving

85 Gillett Street
Hartford, CT 06105
860-548-1888
http://www.hartnet.org/~hfpg1/
Disability Served: all

Purpose: This community foundation provides grants in the areas of education, recreation, and housing, particularly for those with developmental disabilities and hearing disabilities.
Eligibility: Nonprofit organizations serving the Hartford area are eligible to apply.
Financial Details: Amounts vary, but the Foundation normally does not make grants in excess of $75,000 to a new organization or in excess of $400,000 to an established organization.
Number Awarded: Varies.
Deadline: Applications may be submitted throughout the year.

Hawley Foundation

1530 Financial Center
666 Walnut
Des Moines, IA 50309
515-280-7071
Disability Served: all

Purpose: Provides grants to support projects in Des Moines.
Eligibility: Des Moines area organizations may apply. Areas of giving change each year, so contact the Foundation for details.
Financial Details: Amounts vary.

Herbert F. Parker Foundation

First Interstate Bank of Denver
Terminal Annex, Box 5825
Denver, CO 80217
303-293-2211
Disability Served: developmentally disabled

Purpose: The Foundation provides grants to help finance cancer research, recreational programs for youth, and the care of mentally disabled youth.
Eligibility: Nonprofit organizations are eligible to apply.
Financial Details: Amounts vary and depend on program need.
Number Awarded: Varies.

Deadline: Varies. Contact the Foundation for details.

Herbst Foundation

Three Embarcadero Center, 21st Floor
San Francisco, CA 94111
415-951-7508
Disability Served: all

Purpose: The Foundation provides funds for building projects and facilities in San Francisco County.
Eligibility: Nonprofit organizations involved in education and children's projects serving San Francisco County may apply.
Financial Details: Amounts vary and depend on project need.
Number Awarded: Varies each year.
Deadline: Applications are accepted throughout the year.

Heublein Foundation, Inc.

PO Box 388
Hartford, CT 06034
860-702-4000
Disability Served: all

Purpose: Provides grants for charitable projects in areas where Heublein employees reside or where a Heublein facility exists.
Eligibility: Nonprofit organizations in these areas with a focus on civic, health, or social issues may apply.
Financial Details: Amounts vary.
Number Awarded: Varies.
Deadline: Varies.

Hill Foundation

First Interstate Bank of Denver
Terminal Annex, Box 5825
Denver, CO 80217
Disability Served: all

Purpose: Provides grants to help finance projects in higher education, culture, or health and human services.
Eligibility: Charitable and university organizations are eligible to apply.
Financial Details: Amounts vary.
Number Awarded: Varies each year.

Houston Endowment

600 Travis Street, Suite 6400
Houston, TX 77002
713-238-8100
http://www.hou-endow.org
Disability Served: all

Purpose: The Endowment makes grants to Houston-area nonprofit organizations that serve people with disabilities.

Howard Heinz Endowment

30 CNG Tower
625 Liberty Avenue
Pittsburgh, PA 15222
412-281-5777
http://www.heinz.org
Disability Served: all

Purpose: Provides grants in the areas of arts and culture, education, economic opportunity, health and human services, and the environment.
Eligibility: Nonprofit organizations serving southwestern Pennsylvania may apply.
Financial Details: Amounts vary and depend on need.
Number Awarded: Varies.
Deadline: The Committee meets twice per year. Call for dates.

Hugh J. Andersen Foundation

PO Box 204
Bayport, MN 55003
612-439-1557, 888-439-9508
Disability Served: all

Purpose: Provides grants for the purpose of improving the community.
Eligibility: Charitable organizations in the St Croix Valley-Washington County in Minnesota and Pierce, Polk, and St Croix Counties in Wisconsin are eligible to apply.
Financial Details: Amounts vary. Request an amount on the application.
Number Awarded: Varies.
Deadline: November 15, March 15, June 15, and September 15.

Humboldt Area Foundation

PO Box 99
Bayside, CA 95524
707-442-2993
http://hafoundation.org
Disability Served: all

Purpose: This community foundation provides grants to improve the quality of life for residents of the counties of Humboldt, Del Norte, Siskiyou and Trinity.
Eligibility: Charitable organizations serving the North Coast area may apply.
Financial Details: Amounts vary and depend on need.
Number Awarded: Varies.
Deadline: February 1, May 1, August 1, and November 1.

Invacare Foundation

One Invacare Way
Elyria, OH 44036-2125
216-329-6000
http://www.invacare.com
Disability Served: all

Purpose: Provides grants intended to improve the lives of people with disabilities.
Eligibility: Charitable organizations are eligible to apply. Contact the Foundation for additional eligibility requirements.
Financial Details: Amounts vary. Applicants specify an amount on the application.
Number Awarded: Varies each year.
Deadline: The Application Review Committee meets during the first week of January, March, May, July, September, and November. Applications must be received no later than three weeks prior to a scheduled meeting.

ITT Hartford Insurance Group

Hartford Plaza
Hartford, CT 06115
860-547-4972
http://www.thehartford.com
Disability Served: all

Purpose: The Group supports projects in education and health, as well as United Way organizations.
Eligibility: Nonprofit groups servicing the Hartford area may apply.
Financial Details: Amounts vary.
Number Awarded: Varies.
Deadline: Contact the Group for information.

J. B. and Emily Van Nuys Charities

1800 Avenue of the Stars, Suite 435
Los Angeles, CA 90067
Disability Served: physically disabled

Purpose: Provides grants to help finance programs for the physically disabled.
Eligibility: Charitable organizations and Independent Living Programs are eligible.
Financial Details: Amounts vary.
Number Awarded: Varies.
Deadline: Contact the Charities for details.

James S. Copley Foundation

PO Box 1530
La Jolla, CA 92038
858-454-0411
Disability Served: all

Purpose: The Foundation provides support for community and civic services in the immediate circulation areas of Copley newspapers. Areas of interest include education, the arts, health and human services, youth development, and urban affairs.
Eligibility: Nonprofit organizations serving the Copley newspapers' immediate circulation areas may apply.
Financial Details: Amounts vary and depend on need and available funds.
Number Awarded: Varies each year.
Deadline: January 2 for spring meeting of trustees..

Jefferson Lee Ford III Memorial Foundation

9600 Collins Avenue
PO Box 546487
Bal Harbour, FL 33154
305-868-2630
Disability Served: all

Purpose: Provides grants for charitable purposes.
Eligibility: Nonprofit organizations concerned with the welfare of disabled children and persons with hearing and communicative impairments are eligible.
Financial Details: Amounts vary.

Number Awarded: Varies.
Deadline: Contact the Foundation for information.

Jessie Ball duPont Fund

225 Water Street, Suite 1200
Jacksonville, FL 32202-5176
http://www.dupontfund.org/index.html
Disability Served: all

Purpose: This grantmaking foundation limits its grantmaking to 327 eligible organizations to which Mrs. duPont personally contributed during the five calendars from 1960 through 1964.

Johnson Controls Foundation

PO Box 591, M.S. X-46
Milwaukee, WI 53201-0591
414-228-2296, 800-333-2222
Disability Served: all

Purpose: Provides grants for charitable purposes.
Eligibility: Charitable organizations are eligible to apply.
Financial Details: Amounts vary.
Number Awarded: Varies each year.
Deadline: Contact the Foundation for details.

Joseph Drown Foundation

1999 Avenue of the Stars, #1930
Los Angeles, CA 90067
310-277-4488
Disability Served: all

Purpose: Provides funds to help improve the quality of life for residents of California.
Eligibility: Charitable organizations serving California may apply.
Financial Details: Amounts vary.
Number Awarded: Varies.
Deadline: Varies.

Joseph P. Kennedy, Jr Foundation

1325 G Street, NW, Suite 500
Washington, DC 20005
202-393-1250
http://www.familyvillage.wisc.edu/jpkf
Disability Served: developmentally disabled

Purpose: The Foundation provides grants to programs focused on mental retardation, including public awareness projects, research programs, and prevention programs.
Eligibility: Nonprofit organizations focused on mental retardation may apply.
Financial Details: Amounts vary.
Number Awarded: Varies.
Deadline: Contact the Foundation for details.

Kenneth T. and Eileen L. Norris Foundation

11 Golden Shore, Suite 450
Long Beach, CA 90802
562-435-8444
http://www.norrisfoundation.org
Disability Served: all

Purpose: The Foundation offers grants in the areas of medicine and education.
Eligibility: Nonprofit organizations serving the Southern California area are eligible.
Financial Details: Amounts vary but average $5,000.
Number Awarded: Varies.
Deadline: Contact the Foundation for information.

Kinney-Lindstrom Foundation, Inc.

PO Box 520
Mason City, IA 50401
515-896-3888
Disability Served: all

Purpose: Provides grants for charitable purposes, primarily in the areas of arts and culture, programs for the physically disabled, and the Special Olympics.
Eligibility: Nonprofit organizations in Iowa may apply.
Financial Details: Amounts vary.
Number Awarded: Varies.
Deadline: Contact the Foundation for information.

Kiplinger Foundation, Inc.

1729 H Street, NW
Washington, DC 20006
202-887-6559
Disability Served: all

Purpose: Provides grants to fund programs in education, cultural projects, social welfare, and community activities.
Eligibility: Nonprofit organizations in the Greater Washington, DC, area are eligible to apply.
Financial Details: Amounts vary and depend on project need.
Number Awarded: Varies.
Deadline: Varies. Contact the Foundation for information.

Kresge Foundation

3215 West Big Beaver Road
Troy, MI 48007
248-643-9630
Disability Served: all

Purpose: The Foundation offers challenge grants for capital projects, such as building renovation, construction, and major equipment purchase.
Eligibility: Nonprofit organizations are eligible.
Financial Details: Amounts vary and depend on the project.
Number Awarded: Varies.
Deadline: Varies.

L. J. Skaggs and Mary C. Skaggs Foundation

1221 Broadway, 21st Floor
Oakland, CA 94612
510-451-3300
Disability Served: all

Purpose: The Foundation offers funds in the areas of performing arts, social concerns, historical projects, and special projects.
Eligibility: Charitable organizations focused on the areas mentioned above may apply.
Financial Details: Amounts vary.
Number Awarded: Varies.
Deadline: Varies.

Levi Strauss Foundation

1155 Battery Street, LS7N
San Francisco, CA 94111
415-501-6579
http://www.levistrauss.com
Disability Served: all

Purpose: The Foundation provides funds in the areas of AIDS, economic empowerment, youth empowerment, and social justice.
Eligibility: Charitable organizations involved in AIDS projects that serve areas where Levi Strauss & Company has facilities are eligible to apply.
Financial Details: Awards vary and depend on project need.
Number Awarded: Varies.
Deadline: See Web site for current priorities and application information..

Lila Wallace-Reader's Digest Fund

2 Park Avenue, 23rd Floor
New York, NY 10016
212-251-9800
http://www.wallacefunds.org
Disability Served: all

Purpose: The Fund provides grants in the areas of arts and culture, adult literacy, and urban parks.
Eligibility: Nonprofit organizations are eligible.
Financial Details: Awards vary, but in general the Fund does not make grants of less than $100,000.
Number Awarded: Varies.
Deadline: Letters of inquiry are accepted throughout the year, but the Fund rarely makes grants to unsolicited projects.

Liz Claiborne Foundation

1441 Broadway
New York, NY 10018
212-221-1927
http://www.lizclaiborne.com/foundate.html
Disability Served: all

Purpose: The Foundation supports projects in the areas of social welfare, education, health, culture, or the environment.
Eligibility: Charitable organizations involved in the areas listed above are eligible.
Financial Details: Award amounts vary.
Number Awarded: Varies.
Deadline: Contact the Foundation for further details.

Longwood Foundation, Inc.

100 West 10th Street, Suite 1109
Wilmington, DE 19801
302-654-2477
Disability Served: all

Purpose: The Foundation offers grants to support projects for the mentally and physically disabled in Delaware.
Eligibility: Nonprofit organizations dedicated to helping the mentally and physically disabled in Delaware are eligible.
Financial Details: Amounts vary.
Number Awarded: Varies.
Deadline: Varies.

Louis R. Lurie Foundation

555 California Street, Suite 5100
San Francisco, CA 94104
415-392-2470
Disability Served: all

Purpose: The Foundation provides grants in the areas of health, art, community services, and education.
Eligibility: Nonprofit organizations are eligible to apply.
Financial Details: Amounts vary according to program need.

Luke B. Hancock Foundation

360 Bryant Street
Palo Alto, CA 94301
650-321-5536
http://fdncenter.org/grantmaker/hancock/index.html
Disability Served: all

Purpose: The Foundation provides funds in a number of different areas, including vocational training for at-risk youth, emergency and transitional funding, education, and more.
Eligibility: Charitable organizations serving the South Bay of the San Francisco Bay area may apply.
Financial Details: Amounts vary and depend on need.
Number Awarded: Varies.
Deadline: Applications are reviewed in December and January. Contact the Foundation for additional details.

Lynde and Harry Bradley Foundation, Inc.

PO Box 92848
Milwaukee, WI 53202
414-291-9915
http://www.townhall.com/bradley/
Disability Served: all

Purpose: The Foundation offers grants in the areas of education, culture, and community services.
Eligibility: Charitable organizations and universities in Wisconsin are eligible to apply.
Financial Details: Amounts vary.

Mary A. Crocker Trust

Attn: Barbaree Jernigan
233 Post Street, 2nd Floor
San Francisco, CA 94108
415-982-0138
Disability Served: all

Purpose: The Trust provides funds in the areas of education, environment, and community services.
Eligibility: Charitable organizations in the San Francisco Bay area may apply.
Financial Details: Amounts vary but grants usually range from $10,000 to $25,000. Continuing support is not awarded.
Number Awarded: Varies. In 1996, forty-five grants were awarded.
Deadline: Applications are reviewed on a quarterly basis. Contact the Trust for details.

Mary Reynolds Babcock Foundation, Inc.

102 Reynolda Village
Winston-Salem, NC 27106
336-748-9222
http://www.mrbf.org
Disability Served: all

Purpose: The Foundation provides grants to support community projects.
Eligibility: Nonprofit organizations serving communities in the Southeast are eligible to apply.
Financial Details: Amounts vary but often range from $10,000 to $50,000.
Number Awarded: Varies each year.
Deadline: Contact the Foundation for information.

MCA Foundation

100 Universal City Plaza
Universal City, CA 91608
818-777-1208
Disability Served: all

Purpose: The Foundation offers grants in the areas of education, youth programs, arts and culture, and health and welfare.
Eligibility: Nonprofit organizations serving New York or California may apply.
Financial Details: Amounts vary.
Number Awarded: Varies.
Deadline: Varies.

McKesson Foundation, Inc.

One Post Street
San Francisco, CA 94104
415-983-8673
Disability Served: all

Purpose: The Foundation provides funds in the areas of food and shelter for families in crisis as well as education for junior high school aged students.
Eligibility: Nonprofit organizations involved in the areas mentioned above may apply.
Financial Details: Varies depending on need but grants range from $2,500 to $15,000. In 1996 a total of $2.1 million was awarded.
Number Awarded: Varies.
Deadline: Applications are accepted throughout the year.

McKnight Foundation

121 South Eighth Street
600 TCF Tower
Minneapolis, MN 55402
612-333-4220
Disability Served: all

Purpose: The Foundation provides grants in a number of areas, including social services, arts, housing, family services, the disadvantaged, rural development, child development, child welfare, women, youth, AIDS, community funds, environment, homeless, and international development.
Eligibility: Charitable organizations in Minnesota may apply.
Financial Details: Amounts vary.
Number Awarded: Varies.
Deadline: March 1, June 1, September 1, and December 1.

Meadows Foundation

Grants Administration Department
3003 Swiss Avenue
Dallas, TX 75204-6090
214-826-9431, 800-826-9431
http://www.mfi.org/
Disability Served: all

Purpose: The Foundation provides grants in the areas of arts and culture, civic and public affairs, education, and health and human services.
Eligibility: Nonprofit organizations serving the people of Texas are eligible.
Financial Details: Grants Grant amounts vary. No limits.
Number Awarded: Varies.
Deadline: None.

Metzger-Price Fund, Inc.

230 Park Avenue
New York, NY 10169
212-867-9500
Disability Served: all

Purpose: Provides funds for the purpose of helping organizations in New York City care for the needy, elderly, and infirm.
Eligibility: Nonprofit organizations in the New York metropolitan area are eligible.
Financial Details: Amounts vary.
Number Awarded: Varies.
Deadline: Contact the Fund for details.

Mildred Andrews Fund

1220 Huntington Building
Cleveland, OH 44115
Disability Served: all

Purpose: Provides grants to support charitable projects in the Cleveland area.
Eligibility: Nonprofit organizations serving the Cleveland area are eligible to apply.
Financial Details: Amounts vary.
Number Awarded: Varies each year.
Deadline: Write for information.

Montgomery Street Foundation

235 Montgomery Street, #1107
San Francisco, CA 94104
415-398-0600
Disability Served: all

Purpose: The Foundation provides grants in the areas of special education, health and human services, rehabilitation facilities, and mental health organizations and projects.
Eligibility: Nonprofit organizations involved in the areas mentioned above are eligible.
Financial Details: Amounts vary according to project need.
Number Awarded: Varies each year.
Deadline: Write for information.

Morris Stulsaft Foundation

100 Bush Street, Suite 825
San Francisco, CA 94104
415-986-7117
Disability Served: all

Purpose: The Foundation offers grants to support projects for children and youth, specifically in the areas of education, health, arts, recreation, and social services.
Eligibility: Charitable organizations serving the youth of the San Francisco Bay area are eligible.
Financial Details: Amounts vary but grants generally range from $3,000 to $40,000.
Number Awarded: Varies.
Deadline: Applications are accepted throughout the year and are reviewed six times per year.

Ordean Foundation

424 West Superior Street
Duluth, MN 55802
218-726-4785
Disability Served: all

Purpose: The Foundation provides grants for projects in a number of areas, including rehabilitation for the mentally ill, youth programs, and aid for the economically disadvantaged.
Eligibility: Nonprofit organizations servicing the Duluth and St. Louis County areas are eligible.
Financial Details: Amounts vary.
Number Awarded: Varies.
Deadline: Contact the Foundation for information.

Pacific Telesis Foundation

130 Kearney Street, Room 3351
San Francisco, CA 94105
415-394-3693
Disability Served: all

Purpose: Provides grants in the areas of education, United Way organizations, community services, and arts and culture.
Eligibility: Charitable organizations focused on the areas mentioned above may apply.
Financial Details: Amounts vary and depend on project need.
Number Awarded: Varies.
Deadline: Contact the Foundation for information.

Parker Foundation

4365 Executive Drive, Suite 1600
San Diego, CA 92121-2189
619-677-1431
Disability Served: all

Purpose: The Foundation provides grants for charitable purposes in San Diego County.
Eligibility: Nonprofit organizations serving San Diego County may apply.
Financial Details: Amounts vary.
Number Awarded: Varies.
Deadline: Varies. Contact the Foundation for information.

Pasadena Foundation

16 North Marengo Avenue, Suite 300
Pasadena, CA 91101
626-796-2097
http://www.PasadenaFoundation.org
Disability Served: all

Purpose: Provides funds to help improve the quality of life in Pasadena.
Eligibility: Nonprofit organizations serving the communities of Pasadena, Altadena, and Sierra Madre are eligible.
Financial Details: Awards vary.
Number Awarded: Varies.
Deadline: Contact the Foundation for information.

Peter Berkey Foundation
1260 Coast Village Circle
Santa Barbara, CA 93108
Disability Served: all

Purpose: Provides funds for charitable purposes.
Eligibility: Nonprofit organizations dedicated to helping the physically disabled or the Special Olympics may apply.
Financial Details: Amounts vary.
Number Awarded: Varies.
Deadline: Contact the Foundation for details.

Philadelphia Foundation
1234 Market Street, Suite 1900
Philadelphia, PA 19107
215-563-6417
http://www.phlfound.org/
Disability Served: all

Purpose: This community foundation provides grants in the areas of education, culture, health, housing and economic development, children and families, community affairs, and social services.
Eligibility: Nonprofit organizations serving the counties of Bucks, Chester, Delaware, Montgomery, and Philadelphia are eligible.
Financial Details: Amounts vary. In 1996 more than $140 million in grants was paid, with grant sizes ranging from $2,000 to $20,000.
Number Awarded: Varies each year. In 1996 more than 500 organizations received awards.
Deadline: Applications are due June 2 and November 3.

Prudential Foundation
751 Broad Street, 15th Floor
Newark, NJ 07102
973-802-7354
http://www.prudential.com/community/corporate/cmczz1004.html
Disability Served: all

Purpose: Provides grants for charitable projects in the areas of children's issues, community development, education, health and human services, business and civic affairs, and arts and culture.
Eligibility: Nonprofit organizations may apply. Priority is given to organizations in New Jersey and in cities where Prudential has a significant presence.
Financial Details: Awards vary widely. In 1995, a total of $18.3 million was awarded.
Number Awarded: Varies.
Deadline: Contact the Foundation for details.

Public Welfare Foundation, Inc.
2600 Virginia Avenue, NW, Suite 505
Washington, DC 20037
202-965-1800
Disability Served: all

Purpose: The Foundation supports programs that help the economically disadvantaged in any number of fields.
Eligibility: Nonprofit organizations that work in the areas of criminal justice, environment, health, population, disadvantaged youth, or disadvantaged elderly may apply.
Financial Details: Amounts vary.
Number Awarded: Varies.
Deadline: Contact the Foundation for details.

R. C. Baker Foundation
PO Box 6150
Orange, CA 92613
Disability Served: all

Purpose: Provides grants for charitable causes. Historically, aid has been given to educational institutions, scientific facilities, religious organizations, and youth programs.
Eligibility: Nonprofit organizations may apply.
Financial Details: Amounts vary and depend on need.
Number Awarded: Varies.
Deadline: Contact the Foundation for information.

Ralph M Parsons Foundation
1055 Wilshire Boulevard, Suite 1701
Los Angeles, CA 90017
213-482-3185
Disability Served: all

Purpose: The Foundation supports projects in the areas of education, social issues, health, and civic and community affairs.
Eligibility: Charitable organizations may apply.
Financial Details: Amounts vary.

Number Awarded: Varies.
Deadline: Varies. Write or call for information.

Rasmuson Foundation

National Bank of Alaska
PO Box 100600
Anchorage, AK 99510
907-267-5706
Disability Served: all

Purpose: The Foundation offers grants for recreation programs and projects designed to increase the quality of life of the mentally and physically disabled in Alaska.
Eligibility: Charitable organizations in Alaska are eligible.
Financial Details: Amounts vary and depend on program need.
Number Awarded: Varies.
Deadline: Contact the Foundation for details.

Retirement Research Foundation

8765 West Higgins Road, Suite 401
Chicago, IL 60631
773-714-8080
http://fdncenter.org/grantmaker/rrf/index.html
Disability Served: elderly

Purpose: This private foundation provides grants to support projects for the elderly.
Eligibility: Charitable organizations dedicated to improving the lives of the aged are eligible.
Financial Details: Amounts vary according to need.

Robert Sterling Clark Foundation

135 East 64th Street
New York, NY 10021
212-288-8900
http://fdncenter.org/grantmaker/rsclark/index.html
Disability Served: all

Purpose: Principal funding areas of this private foundation include arts and culture, government accountability, and family planning.
Eligibility: Nonprofit organizations involved in the areas listed above are eligible.
Financial Details: Amounts vary.
Number Awarded: Varies.
Deadline: Proposals are accepted throughout the year.

Roy and Christine Sturgis Charitable Trust

PO Box 92
Malvern, AR 72104
501-332-3899
Disability Served: all

Purpose: The Trust provides funds to support programs in the areas of medicine and health services, child welfare, and programs for the visually impaired and the physically disabled.
Eligibility: Nonprofit organizations serving Arkansas are eligible.
Financial Details: Amounts vary according to project need.
Number Awarded: Varies each year.
Deadline: Contact the Trust for details.

S. H. Cowell Foundation

260 California, Suite 501
San Francisco, CA 94111
415-397-0285
Disability Served: all

Purpose: The Foundation supports projects that focus on the underlying causes of poverty and social problems. Areas of interest include child care, family planning, disabled assistance, job training, education, and prevention of drug and alcohol problems.
Eligibility: Nonprofit organizations involved in the areas listed above may apply.
Financial Details: Amounts vary and depend on project need. Grants range from $15,000 to $700,000.
Number Awarded: Varies.
Deadline: Contact the Foundation for information.

San Diego Community Foundation

1420 Kettner Boulevard, Suite 500
San Diego, CA 92101
619-235-2300
http://www.sdcf.org/
Disability Served: all

Purpose: The Foundation funds projects designed to benefit the residents of the San Diego region. Areas of interest include health and human services, arts and culture, the environment, urban affairs, and education.
Eligibility: Nonprofit organizations involved in the areas described above may apply.

Financial Details: Amounts vary and depend on project need. In fiscal year 1995-1996 more than $12 million in grants was awarded.
Number Awarded: Varies.
Deadline: Contact the Foundation for dates.

San Francisco Foundation

225 Bush Street, Suite 500
San Francisco, CA 94104
415-733-8500
Disability Served: all

Purpose: Provides grants to support projects that benefit the residents of the San Francisco Bay area.
Eligibility: Nonprofit organizations serving the San Francisco Bay area are eligible to apply.
Financial Details: Amounts vary.
Number Awarded: Varies.
Deadline: Contact the Foundation for details.

Sarkeys Foundation

116 South Peters, Suite 219
Norman, OK 73069
405-364-3703
Disability Served: all

Purpose: To improve the quality of life in Oklahoma and the Southwest. Areas of interest include arts and culture, social service, health concerns, and education.
Eligibility: Nonprofit organizations in Oklahoma are eligible to apply.
Financial Details: Amounts vary.
Number Awarded: Varies.
Deadline: Contact the Foundation for information and application guidelines.

Sears-Roebuck Foundation

3333 Beverly Road
Hoffman Estates, IL 60179
847-286-7112
http://www.sears.com
Disability Served: all

Purpose: The Foundation provides grants in the areas of volunteerism, women, families, and cultural diversity.
Eligibility: Nonprofit organizations are eligible.
Financial Details: Awards vary.
Number Awarded: Varies.
Deadline: Applications are accepted throughout the year.

Sidney Stern Memorial Trust

PO Box 893
Pacific Palisades, CA 90272
Disability Served: all

Purpose: Provides grants in the areas of community affairs, youth services, arts and culture, health and science, education, and programs for the mentally and physically disabled.
Eligibility: Nonprofit organizations serving California may apply.
Financial Details: Amounts vary.
Number Awarded: Varies.
Deadline: Write for more information.

Square D Foundation

1415 South Roselle Road
Palatine, IL 60067
847-397-2600
Disability Served: all

Purpose: The Foundation provides funds in a number of areas, including education, civic and community affairs, health services, and arts and culture.
Eligibility: Nonprofit organizations may apply.
Financial Details: Amounts vary. Funds may be used for operating support or capital development.
Number Awarded: Varies.
Deadline: Varies.

Stockham Valves & Fitting, Inc.

4000 North Tenth Avenue
PO Box 10326
Birmingham, AL 35202
205-592-6361
Disability Served: all

Purpose: The William H. and Kate Stockham Foundation provides grants to support projects that will benefit the lives of the employees of Stockham Valves & Fitting, Inc.
Eligibility: Charitable organizations with proposals for projects designed to benefit the employees of Stockham Valves & Fitting, Inc. are eligible to apply.

Financial Details: Amounts vary.
Number Awarded: Varies.
Deadline: Varies.

Surdna Foundation, Inc.

330 Madison Avenue, 30th Floor
New York, NY 10017-5001
212-730-0030
http://fdncenter.org/grantmaker/rrf/index.html
Disability Served: all

Purpose: This private foundation provides funds in the areas of the environment, community revitalization, the arts, organizational capacity building grants, and effective citizenry.
Eligibility: Nonprofit organizations involved in the areas listed above are eligible.
Financial Details: Amounts vary depending on the area of interest.
Number Awarded: Varies.
Deadline: Letters of inquiry are accepted throughout the year. Contact the Foundation for further details.

The Seattle Foundation

425 Pike Street, Suite 510
Seattle, WA 98101
206-622-2294
Disability Served: all

Purpose: Provides grants for charitable purposes.
Eligibility: Nonprofit organizations in the Seattle metropolitan area are eligible to apply.
Financial Details: Amounts vary. In 1996, $4.5 million in grants was awarded.
Number Awarded: Varies each year.
Deadline: Contact the Foundation for details.

Tull Charitable Foundation

50 Hurt Plaza, Suite 1245
Atlanta, GA 30303
404-659-7079
Disability Served: all

Purpose: The Foundation provides funds to support major projects, including endowments and building projects.
Eligibility: Nonprofit organizations in Georgia may apply.
Financial Details: Amounts vary. Funds may not be used for operating support.
Number Awarded: Varies.
Deadline: Contact the Foundation for details.

UNUM Charitable Foundation

2211 Congress Street
Portland, ME 04122
207-770-2211
Disability Served: all

Purpose: The Foundation provides grants in the areas of aging, the disabled, economic development, the arts, AIDS, education, and family services.
Eligibility: Nonprofit organizations serving the Portland, Maine, area are eligible.
Financial Details: Amounts vary.
Number Awarded: Varies.
Deadline: None.

Van Ameringen Foundation, Inc.

509 Madison Avenue
New York, NY 10022-5501
212-758-6221
Disability Served: mental health

Purpose: The Foundation provides grants in the areas of mental health and social welfare.
Eligibility: Nonprofit organizations serving the urban Northeast from Boston to Washington, DC, may apply.
Financial Details: Amounts vary.
Number Awarded: Varies.
Deadline: Six weeks prior to board meetings, which take place in March, June, and November. Call for more details.

W. P. and H. B. White Foundation

540 Frontage Road, Suite 332
Northfield, IL 60093
847-446-1441
Disability Served: all

Purpose: The Foundation gives to organizations in the Chicago metropolitan area.
Eligibility: Nonprofit groups in Chicago involved with the visually impaired, youth, and those with mental illnesses are eligible.
Financial Details: Amounts vary.
Number Awarded: Varies.
Deadline: Write for details.

Walt Disney Company Foundation
500 South Buena Vista Street
Burbank, CA 91521
818-265-6500
Disability Served: all

Purpose: Provides grants to support projects in the areas of cerebral palsy and disabilities, including physical, mental, and visual disabilities.
Eligibility: Charitable organizations are eligible to apply. Organizations in areas where Walt Disney Company has branches are given priority.
Financial Details: Amounts vary.
Number Awarded: Varies each year.
Deadline: Varies. Contact the Foundation for details.

Weyerhaeuser Company Foundation
33663 Weyerhaeuser Way South
Tacoma, WA 98477
253-924-3159
Disability Served: all

Purpose: Provides grants for charitable purposes.
Eligibility: Nonprofit organizations are eligible to apply. Organizations in areas where Weyerhaeuser employees reside are given priority.
Financial Details: Amounts vary.

William G. Selby and Marie Selby Foundation
1800 Second Street, Suite 750
Sarasota, FL 34236
941-957-0442
Disability Served: all

Purpose: The Foundation supports capital projects in education, health and human services, and arts and culture.
Eligibility: Nonprofit organizations in Sarasota and neighboring communities are eligible.
Financial Details: Amounts vary.
Number Awarded: Varies.
Deadline: Call for details.

William Randolph Hearst Foundation
888 Seventh Avenue, 45th Floor
New York, NY 10106
212-586-5404
http://fdncenter.org/grantmaker/hearst/index.html
Disability Served: all

Purpose: Provides grants in the areas of education, health, social service, and culture.
Eligibility: Nonprofit organizations are eligible to apply.
Financial Details: Awards vary.
Number Awarded: Varies.
Deadline: Letters of inquiry are accepted throughout the year.

William Stamps Farish Fund
1100 Louisiana, Suite 1250
Houston, TX 77002
713-686-7373
Disability Served: all

Purpose: Provides grants for charitable purposes.
Eligibility: Nonprofit organizations in Texas are eligible to apply.
Financial Details: Amounts vary.
Number Awarded: Varies.
Deadline: Contact the Fund for details.

Winthrop Rockefeller Foundation
308 East Eighth Street
Little Rock, AR 72202
501-376-6854
Disability Served: all

Purpose: Provides grants for the improvement of the quality of life in Arkansas.
Eligibility: Nonprofit organizations dedicated to making changes and improvements in education, economic development, or civic affairs are eligible to apply.
Financial Details: Grant amounts vary. Applicants should specify an amount on the application.
Number Awarded: Varies from year to year.
Deadline: Varies. Contact the Foundation for information.

Publications

ABC's of Funding
Pin Dot Products
6001 Gross Point Road
Niles, IL 60648-4027
800-451-3553
Disability Served: all

This book provides background information on advocacy, business operations, and client services and their relation to assistive technology funding.

Accent Guide: 151 Tax Deductions You Can Take
Accent Books & Products
PO Box 700
Bloomington, IL 61702
309-378-2961, 800-787-8444
Disability Served: all

This guide gives information on how to deduct for medical expenses on federal income tax returns.

Acquisition Barriers: Assistive Technology and Iowans with Disabilities
Institute for Social and Economic Development
1901 Broadway, Suite 313
Iowa City, IA 52240
Disability Served: all

This publication is geared toward Iowa residents with disabilities and provides information on the funding sources available.

Aging: The Burden Study on Foundation Grantmaking Trends
The Foundation Center
79 Fifth Avenue, Department ZE
New York, NY 10003
212-620-4230, 800-424-9836
http://fdncenter.org
Disability Served: all

This publication explores the history of giving for projects focusing on the elderly.

AIDS Funding
The Foundation Center
79 Fifth Avenue, Department ZE
New York, NY 10003
212-620-4230, 800-424-9836
http://fdncenter.org
Disability Served: all

This publication provides information on foundations, public charities, and corporate giving programs.

America's Nonprofit Sector
The Foundation Center
79 Fifth Avenue, Department ZE
New York, NY 10003
212-620-4230, 800-424-9836
http://fdncenter.org
Disability Served: all

This publication provides background information on the nonprofit industry.

America's Voluntary Spirit
The Foundation Center
79 Fifth Avenue, Department ZE
New York, NY 10003
212-620-4230, 800-424-9836
http://fdncenter.org
Disability Served: all

This publication provides background information on volunteerism in the United States.

Analysis of Workers' Compensation Laws
US Chamber of Commerce
1615 H Street, NW
Washington, DC 20062
202-659-6000
Disability Served: all

This manual is published annually and discusses changes and effects of workers' compensation laws.

Annotated Bibliography on Funding for Technology (An)

REC on the Evaluation of Assistive Technology
National Rehabilitation Hospital
102 Irving Street, NW
Washington, DC 20010-2949
202-877-1932
Disability Served: all

This annotated bibliography provides resources and publications on funding for assistive technology.

Assistive Financing for Assistive Devices

Electronic Industries Foundation
919 18th Street, NW, Suite 900
Washington, DC 20006
202-955-5810
Disability Served: all

This guide discusses funding sources for assistive technology primarily in regard to loan guarantees.

Assistive Technology: A Funding Workbook

RESNA Press
1700 Moore Street, Suite 1540
Arlington, VA 22209-1903
703-524-6686
Disability Served: all

This workbook is designed to assist the reader in locating and developing funding sources for assistive technology. The workbook discusses public policy and outlines federal laws.

"Bakers Dozen of Excuses for Denying Funding"

United Cerebral Palsy Association
1522 K Street, NW, Suite 1112
Washington, DC 20005
800-872-5827
Disability Served: all

This article from *The Networker* discusses common excuses given by Medicaid, special education organizations, vocational rehabilitation organizations, and private insurance companies for denying funding requests for assistive technology.

Best Practices of Effective Nonprofit Organizations: A Practitioner's Guide

The Foundation Center
79 Fifth Avenue, Department ZE
New York, NY 10003
212-620-4230, 800-424-9836
http://fdncenter.org
Disability Served: all

This publication provides useful information for nonprofit organizations.

Buck Starts Here....Strategies for Legislative Advocacy and the Funding of Assistive Technology (The)

KATS Network Coordinating Center
427 Versailles Road
Frankfort, KY 40601
502-564-4665, 800-327-5287
Disability Served: all

This publication discusses funding sources for assistive technology in Kentucky.

Careers for Dreamers and Doers: A Guide to Management Careers in the Nonprofit Sector

The Foundation Center
79 Fifth Avenue, Department ZE
New York, NY 10003
212-620-4230, 800-424-9836
http://fdncenter.org
Disability Served: all

This guide is geared toward persons who are interested in working in the nonprofit industry.

Catalog of Federal Domestic Assistance

Government Printing Office
Superintendent of Documents
Washington, DC 20402
800-827-1000
http://www.gpo.gov
Disability Served: all

This publication is produced annually and discusses funding source availability.

Chronicle Guide to Grants
The Chronicle Guide to Grants
1255 23rd Street, NW
Washington, DC 20037
202-726-6200, 800-287-6072
Disability Served: all

This Guide provides a comprehensive listing of grants. It is available on CD-ROM.

Community Health Funding Report
CD Publications
8204 Fenton Street
Silver Spring, MD 20910
301-588-6380, 800-666-6380
Disability Served: all

CD Publications publishes newsletters announcing funding sources.

Comsearch: Broad Topics
The Foundation Center
79 Fifth Avenue, Department ZE
New York, NY 10003
212-620-4230, 800-424-9836
http://fdncenter.org
Disability Served: all

This publication contains samples of actual grants in a wide variety of fields.

Corporate Foundation Profiles
The Foundation Center
79 Fifth Avenue, Department ZE
New York, NY 10003
212-620-4230, 800-424-9836
http://fdncenter.org
Disability Served: all

This publication provides profiles of foundations and the grants they offer.

Creative Funding for Augmentative Communication Services
RESNA Press
1700 Moore Street, Suite 1540
Arlington, VA 22209-1903
703-524-6686
Disability Served: communication

This report gives strategies for locating and/or creating funding sources for the purchase of augmentative communication devices.

Crime and Justice
The Foundation Center
79 Fifth Avenue, Department ZE
New York, NY 10003
212-620-4230, 800-424-9836
http://fdncenter.org
Disability Served: all

This publication discusses funding for programs in law enforcement, crime prevention, juvenile justice, correctional facilities, rehabilitation, and victim assistance.

Directory of Funding Resources for Assistive Technology in Minnesota
STAR Program
300 Centennial Building
658 Cedar Street
St Paul, MN 55155
612-296-2771
Disability Served: all

This guide lists statewide resources that offer either funding or assistive technology loans in Minnesota.

Directory of Grants for Organizations Serving People with Disabilities, 8th Edition
Research Grant Guides
PO Box 1214
Loxahatchee, FL 33470
Disability Served: all

This directory provides information on more than 1,000 foundations, corporations, government agencies, and associations that offer grants to help persons with disabilities.

Directory of Japanese Giving
The Foundation Center
79 Fifth Avenue, Department ZE
New York, NY 10003
212-620-4230, 800-424-9836
http://fdncenter.org
Disability Served: all

This directory provides information and a listing of major Japanese foundations.

Directory of Missouri Grantmakers
The Foundation Center
79 Fifth Avenue, Department ZE
New York, NY 10003
212-620-4230, 800-424-9836
http://fdncenter.org
Disability Served: all

This is a directory of grantmaking foundations in the state of Missouri.

Directory of New and Emerging Foundations
The Foundation Center
79 Fifth Avenue, Department ZE
New York, NY 10003
212-620-4230, 800-424-9836
http://fdncenter.org
Disability Served: all

This publication provides a listing of more than 3,000 new and incorporated foundations in the United States.

Disability Funding News
CD Publications
8204 Fenton Street
Silver Spring, MD 20910
301-588-6380, 800-666-6380
Disability Served: all

This biweekly newsletter provides information on federal grants, foundations, and legal news.

Dollars for College—The Quick Guide to Financial Aid for Students with Disabilities
Ferguson Publishing Company
200 West Jackson Boulevard, Suite 700
Chicago, IL 60606
312-692-1000, 800-306-9941
http://www.fergpubco.com
Disability Served: all

Economics for Nonprofit Managers
The Foundation Center
79 Fifth Avenue, Department ZE
New York, NY 10003
212-620-4230, 800-424-9836
http://fdncenter.org
Disability Served: all

This guide is designed to assist managers of nonprofit organizations in economics and finances.

Establishing Nonprofit Foundations to Pay for Assistive Technology
RESNA Press
1700 Moore Street, Suite 1540
Arlington, VA 22209-1903
703-524-6686
Disability Served: all

This report discusses the possibilities of using foundations as an alternative funding source for the purchase of assistive technology.

Federal Educational and Scholarship Funding Guide
Grayco Publishing
PO Box 1291
West Warwick, RI 02893
401-821-2750
Disability Served: all

This guide provides in-depth profiles of foundations and agencies that provide grants for a wide variety of educational purposes.

Federal Funding to Fight AIDS
Government Information Services
4301 North Fairfax Drive, Suite 875
Arlington, VA 22203
703-528-1000, 800-225-5750
Disability Served: all

This guide provides a list of federal grants, loans, and programs available for funding the fight against AIDS.

Federal Grants & Contracts Weekly
Capitol Publications, Inc.
1101 King Street, #444
Alexandria, VA 22314-2053
703-683-4100, 800-655-5597
Disability Served: all

This weekly publication provides information on new grant opportunities, profiles of foundations and programs, advice on writing grants, and more. The publication focuses on the fields of research, training, and services.

Final Report of the National Task Force on Third Party Payment for Rehabilitation Equipment

Electronic Industries Foundation
919 18th Street, NW, Suite 900
Washington, DC 20006
202-955-5810
Disability Served: all

This book provides information on reimbursement and third party payment for rehabilitation equipment.

Financial Aid for Students with Disabilities

HEATH Resource Center
One Dupont Circle, NW
Washington, DC 20036-1193
800-544-3284, 800-333-INFO
Disability Served: all

This publication discusses funding sources, including funding for assistive technology while in college.

Financial Aid for the Disabled and Their Families 1996-1998

Reference Service Press
5000 Windplay Drive, Suite 4
El Dorado Hills, CA 95762
916-939-9620
http://www.rspfunding.com
Disability Served: all

This book provides comprehensive information on financial aid sources for the disabled, including scholarships, grants, and loans.

Finding the Common Denominator: A Supported Employment Guide to Long-Term Funding Supports and Services for People with Disabilities

Virginia Commonwealth University
Technical Assistance Center
1314 West Main Street
Box 2011
Richmond, VA 23284-2011
804-828-1222
Disability Served: all

This publication provides information on funding sources and services for people with disabilities.

Foundation Center's User-Friendly Guide

The Foundation Center
79 Fifth Avenue, Department ZE
New York, NY 10003
212-620-4230, 800-424-9836
http://fndcenter.org
Disability Served: all

This affordable publication is geared toward those new to grant-seeking and answers common questions regarding fund-raising.

Foundation Directory

The Foundation Center
79 Fifth Avenue, Department ZE
New York, NY 10003
212-620-4230, 800-424-9836
http://fndcenter.org
Disability Served: all

This directory outlines corporate, independent, and community foundations that award grants.

Foundation Fundamentals

The Foundation Center
79 Fifth Avenue, Department ZE
New York, NY 10003
212-620-4230, 800-424-9836
http://fndcenter.org
Disability Served: all

This guide provides general information about foundations and how to write grants.

Foundation Grants to Individuals

The Foundation Center
79 Fifth Avenue, Department ZE
New York, NY 10003
212-620-4230, 800-424-9836
http://fdncenter.org
Disability Served: all

This publication provides information on more than 1,200 corporate and independent foundations that award grants to individuals.

Foundation 1000

The Foundation Center
79 Fifth Avenue, Department ZE
New York, NY 10003
212-620-4230, 800-424-9836
http://fdncenter.org

Disability Served: all

This publication offers in-depth profiles of 1,000 foundations in the United States.

Funding and Assistive Technology: A STAR Program Workshop

STAR Program
300 Centennial Building
658 Cedar Street
St Paul, MN 55155
612-296-2771
Disability Served: all

This workbook is designed to be used as part of an assistive technology funding workshop.

Funding Assistive Technology Devices: A Resource Manual for Oregon

Oregon Technology Access Project
1871 NE Stephens
Roseburg, OR 97470
541-440-4791
Disability Served: all

This report provides information on funding sources for assistive technology in Oregon.

Funding for Augmentative Communication Aids

Pegijohn
6432 Fifth Avenue South
Richfield, MN 55423
Disability Served: communication

This report outlines funding sources and how to locate them for the purchase of augmentative communication devices.

Funding for Persons with Visual Impairments 1997

Reference Service Press
5000 Windplay Drive, Suite 4
El Dorado Hills, CA 95762
916-939-9620
http://www.rspfunding.com
Disability Served: vision

This book provides comprehensive information on financial aid sources for people with visual impairments, including scholarships, fellowships, grants, and loans. A large print edition as well as a disk version are available.

Funding Guide for the Purchase of Assistive Technology Devices and Services (A)

Nebraska Assistive Technology Project, Nebraska Department of Education
301 Centennial Mall South
PO Box 94987
Lincoln, NE 68509-0734
402-471-0734, 800-742-7594
Disability Served: all

This publication offers information about funding sources for the purchase of assistive technology, including where to look for funding and how to secure it.

Funding of Assistive Technology in Connecticut: A Guide for Consumers and their Advocates

Connecticut Rehabilitation Engineering Center, Institute for Human Resource Development
78 Eastern Boulevard
Glastonbury, CT 06033
Disability Served: all

This manual explains how and where to obtain funding for assistive technology in Connecticut.

Funding Resource Manual for Assistive Technology

Illinois Assistive Technology Project
411 East Adams
Springfield, IL 62701
217-522-7985, 800-852-5110
Disability Served: all

This publication provides detailed information on more than fifty public and alternative funding sources in Illinois.

Grants for Schools: How to Find and Win Funds for K12 Programs

Capitol Publications, Inc.
1101 King Street, #444
Alexandria, VA 22314-2053
703-683-4100, 800-655-5597
Disability Served: all

This publication discusses the availability of grants for K through twelve schools.

Guide to Federal Funding for Child Care and Early Childhood Development

Government Information Services
4301 North Fairfax Drive, Suite 875
Arlington, VA 22203
703-528-1000, 800-225-5750
Disability Served: all

This guide lists federal loans and grants available for child care and early childhood development programs.

Guide to Federal Funding for Hospitals and Health Centers

Government Information Services
4301 North Fairfax Drive, Suite 875
Arlington, VA 22203
703-528-1000, 800-225-5750
Disability Served: all

This guide provides information on federal grants and loans available for hospitals, medical centers, and other health facilities.

Guide to Federal Funding for Volunteer Programs & Community Service

Government Information Services
4301 North Fairfax Drive, Suite 875
Arlington, VA 22203
703-528-1000, 800-225-5750
Disability Served: all

This publication provides information on federal grants and loans available for child care and early childhood development programs.

Guide to Funding for International and Foreign Programs

The Foundation Center
79 Fifth Avenue, Department ZE
New York, NY 10003
212-620-4230, 800-424-9836
http://fdncenter.org
Disability Served: all

This is a directory of grants focused on international and foreign programs.

Guide to Funding Resources for Assistive Technology in Delaware

University of Delaware/AI duPont Institute
1600 Rockland Road
PO Box 269
Wilmington, DE 19899
302-651-6790
Disability Served: all

This publication explains how and where to obtain funding for assistive technology in Delaware.

Guide to Funding Resources for Assistive Technology in South Carolina (A)

Center for Rehabilitation Technology Services
1410-C Boston Avenue
West Columbia, SC 29171-0015
803-822-5362
Disability Served: all

This guide offers information on available funding resources and how to pursue funding for assistive technology in South Carolina.

Guide to Greater Washington, DC Grantmakers

The Foundation Center
79 Fifth Avenue, Department ZE
New York, NY 10003
212-620-4230, 800-424-9836
http://fdncenter.org
Disability Served: all

This is a directory of grantmaking foundations in the Washington, DC, area.

Guide to U.S. Foundations, Their Trustees, Officers, and Donors

The Foundation Center
79 Fifth Avenue, Department ZE
New York, NY 10003
212-620-4230, 800-424-9836
http://fdncenter.org
Disability Served: all

The Guide provides profiles on foundations across the nation.

Guidelines for Seeking Funding for Communication Aids
Trace Center, University of Wisconsin
1500 Highland Drive
Madison, WI 53705
608-262-6966
http://www.trace.wisc.edu
Disability Served: communication

This publication assists in organizing strategies for obtaining funding for communication devices.

Handbook on Private Foundations
The Foundation Center
79 Fifth Avenue, Department ZE
New York, NY 10003
212-620-4230, 800-424-9836
http://fdncenter.org
Disability Served: all

This directory provides information on private foundations.

Health Care and Finances: A Guide for Adult Children and Their Parents
American Council of Life Insurance and Health Insurance Association of America
1001 Pennsylvania Avenue, NW
Washington, DC 20004
202-624-2000
Disability Served: all

This report provides information regarding financial planning for health care needs.

Health Care Financing: A Guide for Families
National Maternal and Child
Health Resource Center
College of Law Building
The University of Iowa
Iowa City, IA 52242
319-335-9067
Disability Served: all

This book provides practical information regarding financing health care and assistive devices. The book also has a listing of resource agencies and organizations.

Hispanics and the Nonprofit Sector
The Foundation Center
79 Fifth Avenue, Department ZE
New York, NY 10003
212-620-4230, 800-424-9836
http://fndcenter.org
Disability Served: all

This publication explores giving to Hispanic organizations and programs.

How To Obtain Funding for Augmentative Communication Devices
Prentke Romich Company
1022 Heyl Road
Wooster, OH 44691
800-642-8255
Disability Served: communication

This publication outlines medical-based funding sources for purchasing augmentative communication devices.

How to Prepare a Complete Funding Justification for Medicaid Funding for AAC Devices & Services
United Cerebral Palsy Association
1522 K Street, NW, Suite 1112
Washington, DC 20005
800-872-5827
Disability Served: communication

This pamphlet describes how to receive funding for communication devices through Medicaid. The manual is also available on disk.

Human/Civil Rights Grants
The Foundation Center
79 Fifth Avenue, Department ZE
New York, NY 10003
212-620-4230, 800-424-9836
http://fdncenter.org
Disability Served: all

This is a directory of grants that are given for human and civil rights purposes.

IMPACT

Santa Fe Development Council
PO Box 749
Gainesville, FL 32602
352-338-2194
Disability Served: all

This biannual newsletter discusses fund-raising issues and provides profiles on foundations.

International Encyclopedia of Foundations

The Foundation Center
79 Fifth Avenue, Department ZE
New York, NY 10003
212-620-4230, 800-424-9836
http://fdncenter.org
Disability Served: all

This publication provides profiles of foundations located outside the United States. More than thirty-one countries are covered.

International Grant Guides

The Foundation Center
79 Fifth Avenue, Department ZE
New York, NY 10003
212-620-4230, 800-424-9836
http://fdncenter.org
Disability Served: all

This is a guide for those seeking international funding.

International Grantmaking: A Report on US Foundation Trends

The Foundation Center
79 Fifth Avenue, Department ZE
New York, NY 10003
212-620-4230, 800-424-9836
http://fdncenter.org
Disability Served: all

This publication provides information on international grants.

Japanese Corporate Connection: A Guide for Fundraisers

The Foundation Center
79 Fifth Avenue, Department ZE
New York, NY 10003
212-620-4230, 800-424-9836
http://fdncenter.org
Disability Served: all

This guide provides strategies for organizations seeking grants from Japanese foundations and corporations.

Many Faces of Funding

Phonic Ear, Inc.
3880 Cypress Drive
Petaluma, CA 94954-7600
800-227-0735
Disability Served: communication

This monthly publication discusses funding programs and sources, including federal, private, insurance, and educational sources. The publication is geared toward attaining communication devices.

Mental Health News Alert

CD Publications
8204 Fenton Street
Silver Spring, MD 20910
301-588-6380, 800-666-6380
Disability Served: all

CD Publications publishes newsletters announcing funding sources.

National Data Book of Foundations

The Foundation Center
79 Fifth Avenue, Department ZE
New York, NY 10003
212-620-4230, 800-424-9836
http://fdncenter.org
Disability Served: all

This book provides a comprehensive listing of more than 32,000 foundations in the United States.

National Directory of Corporate Giving

The Foundation Center
79 Fifth Avenue, Department ZE
New York, NY 10003
212-620-4230, 800-424-9836
http://fdncenter.org
Disability Served: all

The Directory provides profiles of corporations that provide funding through corporate giving programs.

National Directory of Grantmaking Public Charities
The Foundation Center
79 Fifth Avenue, Department ZE
New York, NY 10003
212-620-4230, 800-424-9836
http://fdncenter.org
Disability Served: all

This comprehensive directory provides information on public charities that provide grants.

National Guide to Funding for Children, Youth and Families
The Foundation Center
79 Fifth Avenue, Department ZE
New York, NY 10003
212-620-4230, 800-424-9836
http://fdncenter.org
Disability Served: all

This guide lists foundations and corporate giving programs that have a history of awarding funds to projects focused on children, youth, and families. The publication also lists sample grants.

National Guide to Funding for Community Development
The Foundation Center
79 Fifth Avenue, Department ZE
New York, NY 10003
212-620-4230, 800-424-9836
http://fdncenter.org
Disability Served: all

This is a directory of grants available in the community development arena.

National Guide to Funding for Elementary & Secondary Education
The Foundation Center
79 Fifth Avenue, Department ZE
New York, NY 10003
212-620-4230, 800-424-9836
http://fdncenter.org
Disability Served: all

This publication lists more than 1,400 foundations and corporate giving programs that award grants to projects supporting elementary and secondary education.

National Guide to Funding for Information Technology
The Foundation Center
79 Fifth Avenue, Department ZE
New York, NY 10003
212-620-4230, 800-424-9836
http://fdncenter.org
Disability Served: all

This is a directory of grants available in the information technology area.

National Guide to Funding for Libraries and Information Services
The Foundation Center
79 Fifth Avenue, Department ZE
New York, NY 10003
212-620-4230, 800-424-9836
http://fdncenter.org
Disability Served: all

This guide provides a listing of foundations and corporate giving programs that award grants to libraries.

National Guide to Funding for the Environment and Animal Welfare
The Foundation Center
79 Fifth Avenue, Department ZE
New York, NY 10003
212-620-4230, 800-424-9836
http://fdncenter.org
Disability Served: all

This is a directory of grants available for environmental and animal rights causes.

National Guide to Funding for Women and Girls
The Foundation Center
79 Fifth Avenue, Department ZE
New York, NY 10003
212-620-4230, 800-424-9836
http://fdncenter.org
Disability Served: all

This publication lists foundations and corporate giving programs that provide grants to projects supporting women and girls.

National Guide to Funding in Aging

The Foundation Center
79 Fifth Avenue, Department ZE
New York, NY 10003
212-620-4230, 800-424-9836
http://fdncenter.org
Disability Served: elderly

This publication offers information on foundations, organizations, and federal and state programs that provide funding for projects dedicated to the elderly.

National Guide to Funding in Arts and Culture

The Foundation Center
79 Fifth Avenue, Department ZE
New York, NY 10003
212-620-4230, 800-424-9836
http://fdncenter.org
Disability Served: all

This guide provides a listing of foundations and corporate giving programs that have a history of awarding grants for programs in the arts.

National Guide to Funding in Health

The Foundation Center
79 Fifth Avenue, Department ZE
New York, NY 10003
212-620-4230, 800-424-9836
http://fdncenter.org
Disability Served: all

This publication provides a listing of more than 2,500 foundations and corporate giving programs that have a record of awarding funds to research centers, hospitals, universities, and other medical projects.

National Guide to Funding in Higher Education

The Foundation Center
79 Fifth Avenue, Department ZE
New York, NY 10003
212-620-4230, 800-424-9836
http://fdncenter.org
Disability Served: all

This guide lists more than 3,000 foundations and corporate giving programs that have a history of awarding grants to universities, colleges, graduate programs, and research facilities.

National Guide to Funding in Substance Abuse

The Foundation Center
79 Fifth Avenue, Department ZE
New York, NY 10003
212-620-4230, 800-424-9836
http://fdncenter.org
Disability Served: chemical dependency

This publication provides information on funding sources for drug and alcohol abuse programs.

National Guide to Funding Religion

The Foundation Center
79 Fifth Avenue, Department ZE
New York, NY 10003
212-620-4230, 800-424-9836
http://fdncenter.org
Disability Served: all

This directory lists foundations and corporate giving programs that award grants to churches and religious programs.

Negotiating the Funding Maze

Family Child Learning Center
90 West Overdale Drive
Tallmadge, OH 44278
330-633-2055
Disability Served: communication

This publication offers strategies for obtaining funding for augmentative communication devices.

New York State Foundations

The Foundation Center
79 Fifth Avenue, Department ZE
New York, NY 10003
212-620-4230, 800-424-9836
http://fdncenter.org
Disability Served: all

This is a directory of foundations in the New York State area.

Nineteen Ninety-One Guide to Health Insurance for People with Medicare (1991)

Government Printing Office
Superintendent of Documents
Washington, DC 20402
800-827-1000
http://www.gpo.gov
Disability Served: all

This guide provides basic information regarding Medicare coverage and gives advice on acquiring supplemental health insurance.

Nonprofit Organization Operating Manual (A)

The Foundation Center
79 Fifth Avenue, Department ZE
New York, NY 10003
212-620-4230, 800-424-9836
http://fdncenter.org
Disability Served: all

This guide is designed for managers of nonprofit organizations.

On Line: Financing Strategies for Educational Technology

National School Boards Association
1680 Duke Street
Alexandria, VA 22314
703-838-6722
Disability Served: all

This publication discusses strategies for obtaining funding for educational technology.

PAM Repeater

PAM Assistance Center
601 West Maple Street
Lansing, MI 48906
517-371-5897
Disability Served: all

This publication describes issues pertinent to persons with disabilities and their families, including funding sources for purchasing assistive devices in Michigan.

Payment for Assistive Devices by the Veterans Administration

Electronic Industries Foundation
919 18th Street, NW, Suite 900
Washington, DC 20006
202-955-5810
Disability Served: all

This publication provides information on how to obtain funding for assistive devices from the Veterans Administration.

PRI Index: 500 Foundation Charitable Loans and Investments (The)

The Foundation Center
79 Fifth Avenue, Department ZE
New York, NY 10003
212-620-4230, 800-424-9836
http://fdncenter.org
Disability Served: all

This directory lists foundations that offer charitable loans and investments.

Profiles of Funding Sources

ASHA Speech-Language-Hearing Association
10801 Rockville Pike
Rockville, MD 20852
301-897-8682
Disability Served: all

This publication lists federal, private, and corporate funding sources.

Raise More Money for Your Nonprofit Organization

The Foundation Center
79 Fifth Avenue, Department ZE
New York, NY 10003
212-620-4230, 800-424-9836
http://fdncenter.org
Disability Served: all

This guide provides useful information regarding fund-raising for nonprofit organizations.

Resource Manual (The)

Carroll Center for the Blind
Computer Access for the Blind in
Education and Employment
770 Centre Street
Newton, MA 02158

617-969-6200
http://carroll.org
Disability Served: vision

This book provides a comprehensive look at funding sources and how to secure funding.

Resource Manual for Funding Assistive Technology Devices (A)

Coalition for Assistive Technology in Oregon
PO Box 431
Wincester, OR 97495
503-440-4791
Disability Served: all

This manual discusses funding sources and how to go about locating funding for the purchase of assistive technology.

Source Book Profiles

The Foundation Center
79 Fifth Avenue, Department ZE
New York, NY 10003
212-620-4230, 800-424-9836
http://fdncenter.org
Disability Served: all

This book provides in-depth profiles of major foundations in the United States.

Student Guide

US Department of Education
400 Maryland Avenue, SW
Washington, DC 20202
202-732-1134
Disability Served: all

The Guide provides a listing of student aid programs administered by the US Department of Education.

Subsidy Programs for Assistive Devices

Electronic Industries Foundation
919 18th Street, NW, Suite 900
Washington, DC 20006
202-955-5810
Disability Served: all

This publication provides information on various subsidy programs and how they function.

Substance Abuse Funding News

CD Publications
8204 Fenton Street
Silver Spring, MD 20910
301-588-6380, 800-666-6380
Disability Served: all

This newsletter announces new funding sources for chemical dependency programs.

Twenty-First Century Nonprofit (The 21st)

The Foundation Center
79 Fifth Avenue, Department ZE
New York, NY 10003
212-620-4230, 800-424-9836
http://fdncenter.org
Disability Served: all

This publication discusses trends in the nonprofit industry.

Who Gets Grants: Foundation Grants to Nonprofit Organizations

The Foundation Center
79 Fifth Avenue, Department ZE
New York, NY 10003
212-620-4230, 800-424-9836
http://fdncenter.org
Disability Served: all

This publication provides information on nonprofit organizations that have received grants.

Research

The following organizations and foundations provide funds to research facilities and university organizations for research that is often scientific or medical in nature.

Allen P. and Josephine B. Green Foundation

222 South Jefferson Street
PO Box 523
Mexico, MO 65265
573-581-5568

Disability Served: all

Purpose: Provides grants for issues that will benefit mankind.
Eligibility: Organizations in Missouri are eligible to apply.
Financial Details: Varies.
Number Awarded: Varies.
Deadlines: April 1 and October 1.

American Hearing Research Foundation

55 East Washington Street, Suite 2022
Chicago, IL 60602-2103
312-726-9670
Disability Served: hearing

Purpose: Provides grants for the purpose of research to help hearing impaired people.
Eligibility: Organizations dedicated to helping the hearing impaired are eligible to apply.
Financial Details: Grants are for $15,000.

Arc (The)

500 East Border Street, Suite 300
Arlington, TX 76010
817-261-6003, 800-433-5255
http://www.thearc.org/welcome.html
Disability Served: developmentally disabled

Purpose: Provides research grants for the study of the prevention of mental retardation.
Eligibility: Grants must be used to research the prevention of mental retardation.
Financial Details: Award amounts vary.
Number Awarded: Varies each year.
Deadline: Check with The Arc for dates.

Bireley Foundation

144 North Brand Boulevard
Glendale, CA 91203
Disability Served: all

Purpose: Provides grants for the purpose of medical research.
Eligibility: Organizations involved in the research of adolescent medicine may apply.
Financial Details: Amounts vary.
Number Awarded: Varies.
Deadline: Contact the Foundation for information.

Burroughs Wellcome Fund

4709 Creekstone Drive, Suite 100
Durham, NC 27703
919-991-5100
http://www.bwfund.org/index.html
Disability Served: all

Purpose: Provides funds to support biomedical research.
Eligibility: Research institutions or facilities involved in biomedical research are eligible to apply. Individual researchers must be nominated by their institution.
Financial Details: Amounts vary. In 1996 a total of $27.2 million was awarded.
Number Awarded: Varies. In 1996 more than 150 institutions and 300 individuals received funds.
Deadline: Contact the Fund for details.

Christopher Reeve Paralysis Foundation

500 Morris Avenue
Springfield, NJ 07081
973-379-2690, 800-225-0292
http://www.paralysis.org
Disability Served: physically disabled

Purpose: This nonprofit organization supports research to find a cure for paralysis caused by spinal cord injury and other central nervous system disorders.
Eligibility: Individuals researching the cure for paralysis caused by spinal cord injury or other central nervous system disorders are eligible to apply.
Financial Details: $50,000 one-year grants are offered.
Number Awarded: Varies.
Deadline: Proposals are reviewed twice yearly. Contact the CRPF for dates.

Cystic Fibrosis Foundation

6931 Arlington Road
Bethesda, MD 20814
301-951-4422, 800-FIGHT-CF
http://www.cff.org/research.htm
Disability Served: all

Purpose: Provides grants for research related to cystic fibrosis.
Eligibility: Qualified individuals dedicated to researching cystic fibrosis are eligible to apply.

Financial Details: Amounts vary widely.
Number Awarded: The Foundation sponsors a number of different awards and grants. Contact the Foundation for additional information.
Deadline: Deadlines vary.

E. Matilda Ziegler Foundation for the Blind

c/o Swisher International Group
20 Thorndal Circle, 2nd Floor
Darien, CT 06820
203-356-9000
Disability Served: vision

Purpose: Provides grants for the research of blindness.
Eligibility: Programs dedicated to the research of the causes, cures, and prevention of blindness are eligible to apply.
Financial Details: Amounts vary.
Number Awarded: Varies each year.
Deadline: Proposals are considered during the Foundation's annual meeting, which occurs during the fourth quarter. Contact the Foundation for details.

Fortis Foundation

One World Trade Center, Suite 5001
New York, NY 10048
212-859-7000
Disability Served: all

Purpose: The Foundation provides grants for medical research.
Eligibility: Research institutions and universities involved in medical research are eligible.
Financial Details: Amounts vary but often range from $500 to $5,000.

Hermundslie Foundation

3672 North Harrison Road
Tucson, AZ 85749
Disability Served: vision

Purpose: Provides grants for the purpose of eye research.
Eligibility: Individuals dedicated to researching the cause and cure of eye diseases and conditions are eligible to apply.
Financial Details: Amounts vary.
Number Awarded: Varies.
Deadline: Contact the Foundation for details.

Jane Coffin Childs Memorial Fund for Medical Research

Shawmut Bank
777 Main Street, MSN 242
Hartford, CT 06115
800-742-9688
Disability Served: all

Purpose: The Fund supports medical research projects.
Eligibility: Research facilities and organizations involved with medical research may apply for grants.
Financial Details: Amounts vary.
Number Awarded: Varies.
Deadline: Contact the Fund for details.

Lowe Foundation

Colorado Judicial Center
Two East 14th Avenue
Denver, CO 80203
303-837-3785
Disability Served: developmentally disabled

Purpose: The Foundation provides grants for education, research, and training in the area of mental retardation.
Eligibility: Nonprofit organizations that provide research and education in mental retardation are eligible to apply.
Financial Details: Amounts vary.
Number Awarded: Varies.
Deadline: Varies. Contact the Foundation for dates.

May Mitchell Royal Foundation

Comerica Bank
201 McDonald Street
Midland, MI 48640
517-839-2256
Disability Served: vision

Purpose: Provides funds for the purpose of eye research.
Eligibility: Research facilities or organizations studying the cause, cure, and prevention of eye disease may apply.
Financial Details: Amounts vary.
Number Awarded: Varies.
Deadline: Contact the Foundation for details.

Multiple Sclerosis Foundation, Inc.

6350 North Andrews Avenue
Ft Lauderdale, FL 33309
954-776-6805, 800-441-7055
http://www.msfacts.org
Disability Served: multiple sclerosis

Purpose: Provides grants to universities for the research of the cause, cure, prevention, and treatment of multiple sclerosis.
Eligibility: Applicants must be affiliated with an accredited university.
Financial Details: Award amounts vary.
Number Awarded: Varies each year.
Deadline: Check with the Foundation for deadline dates.

National Ataxia Foundation

15500 Wayzata Boulevard, #750
Wayzata, MN 55391
612-473-9289
http://www.ataxia.org
Disability Served: physically disabled

Purpose: Provides grants for the research of ataxia.
Eligibility: Qualified individuals researching ataxia are eligible to apply.
Financial Details: Research grants range from $3,000 to $15,000.
Number Awarded: Two to six research grants are awarded each year.
Deadline: June 30.

National Hemophilia Foundation

110 Greene Street, Suite 303
New York, NY 10012
212-219-8180, 800-424-2634
http://www.hemophilia.org
Disability Served: all

Purpose: Provides scholarships and grants for the purpose of researching hemophilia.
Eligibility: Funds are limited to research scientists and hemophilia chapters, organizations, and treatment centers.
Financial Details: Grant amounts vary. The scholarship is for $2,000.
Number Awarded: One scholarship and ten to fifteen grants are awarded each year.
Deadline: Contact the Foundation for specific dates.

National Parkinson Foundation

1501 NW 9th Avenue, Bob Hope Road
Miami, FL 33136
800-327-4545
http://www.parkinson.org/grants.htm
Disability Served: physically disabled

Purpose: Provides grants for the research of Parkinson's disease.
Eligibility: Research facilities studying the causes, cures, and prevention of Parkinson's Disease are eligible.
Financial Details: Awards vary.
Number Awarded: Varies.
Deadline: Contact the Foundation for further details.

National Society to Prevent Blindness

500 East Remington Road
Schaumburg, IL 60173
847-843-2020
Disability Served: vision

Purpose: Provides Burroughs Welcome Fellowships to fund research activities in the field of blindness prevention.
Eligibility: Persons who hold the M.D. degree and who have completed a residency in ophthalmology are eligible.
Financial Details: Amounts vary.
Number Awarded: Varies.
Deadline: Contact the Society for information.

Phil N. Allen Charitable Trust

Bank of America
PO Box 5848
Palo Alto, CA 94306
650-324-4433
Disability Served: multiple sclerosis

Purpose: The Trust offers grants for multiple sclerosis research.
Eligibility: Research facilities focusing on the causes, cures, and prevention of multiple sclerosis may apply.
Financial Details: Amounts vary.
Number Awarded: Varies.
Deadline: Contact the Trust for information.

Retinitis Pigmentosa Foundation

1401 West Mount Royal Avenue, 4th Floor
Baltimore, MD 21217-4245

410-225-9400, 800-683-5555
Disability Served: vision

Purpose: The Foundation offers funding for medical research.
Eligibility: Research facilities dedicated to finding the causes, cures, and prevention of Retinitis Pigmentosa may apply.
Financial Details: Amounts vary.
Number Awarded: Varies.
Deadline: Contact the Foundation for details.

W. M. Keck Foundation

555 South Flower Street, Suite 3230
Los Angeles, CA 90071
213-680-3833
http://www.wmkeck.org/
Disability Served: all

Purpose: The Foundation supports scientific, engineering, and medical research programs at accredited universities and colleges.
Eligibility: Accredited four-year colleges and universities are eligible to apply.
Financial Details: Varies.
Number Awarded: Varies each year.
Deadline: Phase I inquiries are due May 15 for the December grant cycle, and November 15 for the June grant cycle.

Technology

These companies and organizations provide funding to help persons with disabilities purchase assistive technology and necessary equipment.

American Council of the Blind of Indiana

Attn: Director, Indiana School for the Blind
7725 North College Avenue
Indianapolis, IN 46240
317-638-7552
Disability Served: vision

Purpose: The Council helps Indiana residents who are blind through the Hank Hofstetter Grant Program.
Eligibility: Indiana residents who are blind are eligible to apply.
Financial Details: Amounts vary. Write for further information.
Number Awarded: Varies.
Deadline: Varies.

Artists' Fellowship, Inc.

47 Fifth Avenue
New York, NY 10003
Disability Served: all

Purpose: Provides financial aid to artists.
Eligibility: Professional painters, graphic artists, or sculptors living in the U.S. and in financial distress because of serious illness, disability, or age are eligible to apply for a one-time grant. Funds are not intended to pay college tuition or other costs.
Financial Details: Varies.
Number Awarded: Varies.
Deadline: Contact the fellowship for information.

Blue Ridge Independent Living Center

1502-D Williamson Road NE
Roanoke, VA 24012
540-342-1231
Disability Served: all

Purpose: To assist people with disabilities to be independent and to provide grants for purchasing assistive technology.
Eligibility: Funds are limited to individuals residing in the fifth planning district of Virginia and surrounding areas.
Financial Details: Amounts vary.
Number Awarded: Number varies.
Deadline: Contact the Center for additional information.

Chrysler Motors Organization

Physically Challenged Assistance Program
PO Box 3124
Bloomfield Hills, MI 48302
800-255-9877
Disability Served: physically disabled

Purpose: Provides cash reimbursements for the purpose of adapting Chrysler vehicles for persons with disabilities.
Eligibility: Physically disabled individuals who purchase Chrysler vehicles and need to have

them converted or adapted are eligible.
Financial Details: Reimbursements are for up to $1,000 on full-size vans and up to $750 on other vehicles.
Number Awarded: Varies.
Deadline: No deadline applies.

Department of Veterans Affairs—Vocational Rehabilitation

Federal Building, 125 South State Street
PO Box 11500
Salt Lake City, UT 84147
801-524-5450, ext. 1
Disability Served: all

Purpose: Provides funds for the purchase of necessary equipment or supplies in relation to an occupational goal.
Eligibility: Veterans with a disability rating are eligible to apply.
Financial Details: Amounts vary and depend on need.
Number Awarded: Varies.
Deadline: Varies. Contact the agency for details.

Easter Seal Rehabilitation Center of Mobile

2419 Gordon Smith Drive
Mobile, AL 36617
334-478-8582
Disability Served: all

Purpose: Provides funds for the purchase of necessary equipment.
Eligibility: Residents in the seven counties in southwestern Alabama serviced by the Easter Seal Rehabilitation Center of Mobile who are unable to purchase costly equipment are eligible to apply.
Financial Details: Amounts vary.
Number Awarded: Varies each year.
Deadline: Varies.

Fireman's Fund Foundation

777 San Marin Drive
Novato, CA 94998
415-899-2757
Disability Served: all

Purpose: Provides grants to persons with disabilities for whatever purposes they deem necessary.
Eligibility: Disabled residents of Marin and Sonoma Counties may apply.
Financial Details: Amounts vary.
Number Awarded: Varies.
Deadline: Contact the Foundation for information.

Nevada Rehabilitation Division

Department of Human Resources
305 East King Street, Room 502
Carson City, NV 89710
702-687-4440
Disability Served: all

Purpose: This state agency offers low-interest loans for the purpose of financing assistive technology purchases.
Eligibility: Nevada residents with disabilities are eligible.
Financial Details: Amounts vary according to need.

Telesensory Systems

Mitari/Canon Financing Program, Paul Lewis
455 North Bernardo Avenue
Mountain View, CA 94039-7455
650-616-8700
http://www.telesensory.com/bpd/optacon.htm
Disability Served: vision

Purpose: Provides low interest financing for the purpose of purchasing the Optacon II, a reading device for the visually impaired.
Eligibility: Blind individuals who need financial assistance to purchase the Optacon II may apply.
Financial Details: Contact the company for details regarding the loan.
Number Awarded: Varies.
Deadline: Does not apply.

Tucson Community Foundation

6842 East Tanque Verde
Tucson, AZ 85715
520-722-1707
Disability Served: all

Purpose: The Foundation provides grants to help those with disabilities purchase equipment.
Eligibility: Tucson residents with disabilities are eligible to apply.
Financial Details: Amounts vary.
Number Awarded: Varies.
Deadline: Contact the Foundation for details.

Organizations & Associations

Alliance for Technology Access Organizations

The Alliance for Technology Access is a network of community-based resource centers that provide information and support services to children and adults with disabilities, particularly in regard to assistive technology.

ALASKA

Alaska Services for Enabling Technology
PO Box 6485
207 Moller Drive
Sitka, AK 99835
907-747-7615
Disability Served: all

ALABAMA

Birmingham Alliance for Technology Access Center
Birmingham Independent Living Center
206 13th Street South
Birmingham, AL 35233
205-251-2223, 205-251-0605
Disability Served: all

Technology Assistance for Special Consumers
915 Monroe Street
PO Box 443
Huntsville, AL 35804
205-532-5996
http://tasc.ataccess.org
Disability Served: all

ARKANSAS

Technology Resource Center
c/o Arkansas Easter Seal Society
3920 Woodland Heights Road
Little Rock, AR 72212
501-227-3600
Disability Served: all

ARIZONA

Technology Access Center of Tucson
PO Box 13178
4710 East 29th Street
Tucson, AZ 85732-3178
520-745-5588, ext. 412
Disability Served: all

CALIFORNIA

Alliance for Technology Access
2175 East Francisco Boulevard, Suite L
San Rafael, CA 94901
415-455-4575, 800-455-7970
http://www.ATAccess.org
Disability Served: all

Center for Accessible Technology
2547 8th Street, #12A
Berkeley, CA 94710
510-841-3224
http://www.el.net/CAT
Disability Served: all

Computer Access Center
6234 87th Street
Los Angeles, CA 90045
310-388-1597
http://www.cac.org
Disability Served: all

SACC Assistive Technology Center
Simi Valley Hospital, North Campus
PO Box 1325
Simi Valley, CA 93062
805-582-1881
Disability Served: all

Sacramento Center for Assistive Technology
701 Howe Avenue, Suite E-5
Sacramento, CA 95825
916-927-7228
http://www.quiknet.com/~scat
Disability Served: all

Special Technology Center
590 Castro Street
Mountain View, CA 94041
650-961-6789
Disability Served: all

Team of Advocates for Special Kids
100 West Cerritos Avenue
Anaheim, CA 92805
714-533-8275
Disability Served: all

FLORIDA

Center for Independence, Technology & Education
215 East New Hampshire Street
Orlando, FL 32804
407-898-2483
Disability Served: all

GEORGIA

Tech-Able, Inc.
1112A Brett Drive
Conyers, GA 30094
770-922-6768
Disability Served: all

HAWAII

Aloha Special Technology Access Center
710 Green Street
Honolulu, HI 96813
808-523-5547
http://www.aloha.net/~stachi
Disability Served: all

IDAHO

United Cerebral Palsy of Idaho, Inc.
5530 West Emerald
Boise, ID 83706
208-377-8070
Disability Served: all

ILLINOIS

Northern Illinois Center for Adaptive Technology
3615 Louisiana Road
Rockford, IL 61108-6195
815-229-2163
Disability Served: all

Technical Aids & Assistance for the Disabled Center
1950 West Roosevelt Road
Chicago, IL 60608
312-421-3373, 800-346-2939
http://homepage.interaccess.com/~taad
Disability Served: all

INDIANA

Assistive Technology Training and Information Center
Attn: A Resource Center on Independent Living
PO Box 2441
Vincennes, IN 47591
812-886-0575
Disability Served: all

KANSAS

OCCK, Inc.—Technology Resource Solutions for People
1710 West Schilling Road
Salina, KS 67402-1160
785-827-9383
Disability Served: all

KENTUCKY

AbleTech Assistive Technology Resource Center
36 West Fifth Street
Covington, KY 41011
606-491-8700
Disability Served: all

ATA Eastern Technical Assistance Office
1531 Dawn Drive
Louisville, KY 40216
502-449-0645
Disability Served: all

Bluegrass Technology Center
169 North Limestone Street
Lexington, KY 40507
606-255-9951, 800-209-7767
http://www.kde.state.ky.us
Disability Served: all

Enabling Technologies of Kentuckiana (enTECH)
301 York Street
Louisville, KY 40203
502-574-1637, 800-890-1840
Disability Served: all

Western Kentucky Assistive Technology Consortium
PO Box 266
Murray, KY 42071
502-759-4233
http://www.kde.state.ky.us/assistive/Assistive_Technology.html
Disability Served: all

MASSACHUSETTS

Massachusetts Special Technology Access Center
12 Mudge Way 1-6
Bedford, MA 01730
617-275-2446
Disability Served: all

MARYLAND

Learning Independence Through Computers, Inc. (LInc.)
1001 Eastern Avenue, 3rd Floor
Baltimore, MD 21202
410-659-5462
http://www.linc.org
Disability Served: all

MICHIGAN

Assistive Technology Resource Center
Riley Center, 9601 Vine
Allen Park, MI 48101
313-928-0841, 313-928-0408
Disability Served: all

Living and Learning Resource Centre
600 West Maple Street
Lansing, MI 48906
517-487-0883, 800-833-1996
Disability Served: all

Michigan's Assistive Technology Resource
PIAM, 1023 South US 27
St Johns, MI 48879-2423
517-224-0333, 800-274-7426
Disability Served: all

MINNESOTA

Minnesota STAR Program
300 Centennial Building
658 Cedar Street
St Paul, MN 55155
612-296-2771, 800-657-3862 (MN)
http://www.state.mn.us/
Disability Served: all

PACER Computer Resource Center
4826 Chicago Avenue South
Minneapolis, MN 55417
617-827-2966, 800-53PACER (MN)
http://www.pacer.org/crc/crc.htm
Disability Served: all

MISSOURI

Adaptive Computing Technology Center
University of Missouri at Columbia
4816 Santana Circle
Columbia, MO 65211
573-882-2000
http://crprcep7.drake.edu
Disability Served: all

Technology Access Center
12110 Clayton Road
St Louis, MO 63131
314-989-8404
http://stlouis.missouri.org/501c/mostltac
Disability Served: all

MONTANA

Parents Let's Unite for Kids
526 North 32nd Street
Billings, MT 59101
406-255-0540, 800-222-7585
http://www.pluk.org
Disability Served: all

NORTH CAROLINA

Carolina Computer Access Center
Metro School
700 East Second Street
Charlotte, NC 28202
704-342-3004
http://ccac.ataccess.org
Disability Served: all

NORTH DAKOTA

Pathfinder Parent Training and Information Center
ATA Computer Resource Center
1600 2nd Avenue SW, Suite 19
Minot, ND 58701
701-837-7500, 800-245-5840
http://www.ndcd.org
Disability Served: all

NEW HAMPSHIRE

New Hampshire Assistive Technology Center—NHATECH
5 Right Way Path
Laconia, NH 03246
603-528-3060
Disability Served: all

NEW JERSEY

Center for Enabling Technology
622 Route 10 West, Suite 22B
Whippany, NJ 07981
973-428-1455
Disability Served: all

Computer Center for People with disAbilities
c/o Family Resource Associates, Inc.
35 Haddon Avenue
Shrewsbury, NJ 07702
908-747-5310
Disability Served: all

NEW YORK

Center for Assistive Technology
University of Buffalo
515 Kimball Tower
Buffalo, NY 14214-3079
716-829-3141, 800-628-2281
http://wings.buffalo.edu/go?cat
Disability Served: all

Resource Center for Independent Living
401-409 Columbia Street, Box 210
Utica, NY 13503-0210
315-797-4642
http://rcil.com
Disability Served: all

OHIO

Technology Resource Center
301 Valley Street
Dayton, OH 45404
937-222-5222
Disability Served: all

RHODE ISLAND

TechACCESS of Rhode Island
110 Jefferson Boulevard, Suite I
Warwick, RI 02888-3854
401-463-0202, 800-916-TECH
http://techaccess-ri.org
Disability Served: all

TENNESSEE

East Tennessee Technology Access Center
3525 Emory Road, NW
Powell, TN 37849
423-947-2191
http://www.korrnet.org/ettac
Disability Served: all

Technology Access Center of Middle Tennessee
2222 Metro Center Boulevard, Suite 126
Nashville, TN 37221
615-248-6733, 800-368-4651
Disability Served: all

West Tennessee Special Technology Access Resource Center
PO Box 3683
60 Lynoak Cove
Jackson, TN 38305
901-668-3888, 800-464-5619
http://www.starcenter.tn.org
Disability Served: all

UTAH

Computer Center for Citizens with Disabilities
c/o Utah Center for Assistive Technology
2056 South 1100 East
Salt Lake City, UT 84106
801-485-9152
Disability Served: all

VIRGINIA

Tidewater Center for Technology Access
960 Windsor Oaks Boulevard
Virginia Beach, VA 23462
757-474-8650
http://tcta.ataccess.org
Disability Served: all

VIRGIN ISLANDS

Virgin Islands Resource Center for the Disabled, Inc.
PO Box 1825
St Thomas, VI 00803
809-777-ABLE
Disability Served: all

WASHINGTON

Washington Technology Access Center
8511 15th Avenue NE
Seattle, WA 98115-3199
206-526-1240
Disability Served: all

WISCONSIN

Communication Aids and Systems Clinic
1500 Highland Avenue, Room 315
Madison, WI 53705-2274
608-263-2522
http://trace.wisc.edu
Disability Served: all

WEST VIRGINIA

Eastern Panhandle Technology Access Center, Inc.
PO Box 987
300 South Lawrence Street
Charleston, WV 25414
304-725-6473
Disability Served: all

Project G.L.U.E
c/o Children's Therapy Clinic
2345 Chesterfield Avenue
Charleston, WV 25304
304-342-6501
Disability Served: all

Americans with Disabilities Act Organizations

These organizations provide information on the Americans with Disabilities Act, including compliance assistance, explanation of regulations, referral services, and more.

ADA Technical Assistance Program
Southeast Disability and
Business Technical Center
1776 Peachtree Street, Suite 310N
Atlanta, GA 30309
404-888-0022
Disability Served: all

This state agency provides information regarding the Americans with Disabilities Act and provides assistance to help businesses and organizations reach ADA compliance.

Architectural and Transportation Barriers Compliance Board
1111 18th Street, NW, Suite 501
Washington, DC 20036
800-USA-ABLE
Disability Served: all

The Board provides information on ADA Accessibility Guidelines and technical assistance on architectural, transportation, and communications accessibility issues.

Federal Communications Commission
445 Twelfth Street Southwest
Washington, DC 20554
888-2255-5322
TTY: 888-835-5322
http://www.fcc.gov
Disability Served: all

The FCC addresses ADA regulations and issues in telecommunications.

Foundation on Employment and Disability
3820 Del Amo Boulevard, #201
Torrance, CA 90503
Disability Served: all

The Foundation provides ADA information through publications, presentations, toll-free hotlines, and more.

Internal Revenue Service
Office of the Chief Counsel
PO Box 7604
Ben Franklin Station
Washington, DC 20044
202-566-3292
Disability Served: all

The IRS offers technical assistance on ADA tax code provisions.

National Conference on Building Codes and Standards
505 Huntmar Park Drive, Suite 210
Herndon, VA 22070
703-437-0100
Disability Served: all

This organization advocates for ADA standards and policy changes.

National Institute on Disability & Rehabilitation Research

OSERS/ED
330 C Street, SW, Room 3060
Switzer Building
Washington, DC 20202-8133
202-205-8134
Disability Served: all

NIDRR provides leadership and support for programs of disability and rehabilitation research and administers the Technology Related Assistance for Individuals with Disabilities Act and ADA technical assistance centers.

United States Access Board

1331 F Street, NW, Suite 1000
Washington, DC 20004-1111
202-272-5434, 800-USA-ABLE
http://www.access-board.gov
Disability Served: physically disabled

The Board provides information on ADA and the Architectural Barriers Act for designers, building owners, and government agencies.

United States Department of Justice, ADA Information Line

PO Box 66738
Washington, DC 20035-6738
800-514-0301 (Voice)
TTY: 800-514-0383
http://www.usdoj.gov/crt/ada/adahom1.htm
Disability Served: all

The Department of Justice answers questions about the Americans with Disabilities Act (ADA) and provides free publications by mail and fax through the ADA Information Line.

United States Small Business Administration

Office of Advocacy, Office of Economic Research
409 Third Street SW, 5th Floor
Washington, DC 20416
202-205-6530
http://sba.gov/advo
Disability Served: all

This office provides information and assistance on ADA regulations that affect small businesses.

Education Organizations

These organizations provide educational assistance, information, programs, and materials for persons with disabilities.

ACT, Inc.

PO Box 4028
Iowa City, IA 52243
319-337-1332
http://www.act.org
Disability Served: all

This organization develops educational programs, exams, and services for students and educational institutions. The most frequently used program is the ACT Assessment. Students with documented disabilities may be eligible for testing accommodations.

Addiction Intervention with the Disabled Resource Center

Kent State University
Sociology Department
Kent, OH 44242
330-672-2121
http://www.kent.edu
Disability Served: chemical dependency

The Center provides publications and resources on substance abuse and chemical dependency for persons with reading difficulties and other impairments.

Alliance for Parental Involvement in Education

PO Box 59
East Chatham, NY 12060-0059
518-392-6900
Disability Served: all

This nonprofit organization advocates for an increase in parental involvement in education.

American College Testing Program

PO Box 168
2201 North Dodge Street
Iowa City, IA 52243
319-337-1332
Disability Served: all

This organization develops educational programs, exams, and services for students and educational institutions.

American Council for the Blind

1155 15th Street, NW, Suite 1004
Washington, DC 20005
202-467-5081
http://www.acb.org
Disability Served: vision

This national membership organization is dedicated to promoting the independence and well being of blind and visually impaired people. Services include a monthly magazine, a hotline, student scholarships, and information and retrieval.

American School Health Association

PO Box 708
Kent, OH 44240
330-678-1601
http://www.ashaweb.org
Disability Served: all

This organization disseminates information on school health to parents and professionals.

Assistive Technology/Special Schools Program

200 Kolmus Drive
Costa Mesa, CA 92626
714-966-4140
http://sped.ocoe.k12.ca.us
Disability Served: all

This program provides assistive technology services for students with disabilities in Orange County. Students are trained in the use of computer systems and assistive technology.

Association for Individually Guided Education

Hutchinson United School District #3008
PO Box 1908
Hutchinson, KS 67504
316-655-4881
Disability Served: all

This association focuses on the individual educational needs of students and adults.

Augmentative and Alternative Communication Assessment Program

Los Angeles Unified School District
c/o Widney High School
2302 South Gramercy Place
Los Angeles, CA 90018
213-732-1976
Disability Served: all

This program provides evaluations, equipment fitting, and training for individuals aged three to twenty-one years.

Child and Family Outreach Programs

Eastern Washington University, MS-56
705 West First
Spokane, WA 99201
509-623-4229
Disability Served: all

This organization provides services to children from birth to age 3 through its Early Head Start program. It also provides training and technical assistance on children with disabilities to child care providers.

Clearinghouse Depository for Handicapped Students

502 Jay Street, Room 390
Sacramento, CA 95814
916-445-5103
Disability Served: all

This organization is a clearinghouse of educational materials and equipment for special education.

College Board

ATP Services for Handicapped Students
PO Box 6671
Princeton, NJ 08541-6671
609-771-7300
http://www.collegeboard.org
Disability Served: all

The Board offers special test-taking arrangements for persons with disabilities.

Distance Education and Training Council

1601 18th Street, NW
Washington, DC 20009-2529

202-234-5100
http://www.detc.org
Disability Served: all

The Council provides information on correspondence and distance education.

Educational Referral Service
2222 Eastlake Avenue East
Seattle, WA 98102
206-323-1838
Disability Served: all

This organization assesses the learning needs of children and helps plan educational programs.

Federal Student Aid Information Center
US Department of Education
Office of Postsecondary Education
PO Box 84
Washington, DC 20044
800-433-3243
http://www.ed.gov/prog_info/SFA/StudentGuide
Disability Served: all

The Center provides information on financial aid to fund a college education.

Florida Department of Education/Bureau of Education for Exceptional Students
Florida Education Center
325 West Gaines Street, Suite 614
Tallahassee, FL 32399-0400
850-488-1570
http://www.firn.edu.doe.commhome/#mhom
Disability Served: all

The Department of Education strives to improve the educational services for students with special needs.

Foundation on Employment and Disability (The)
3820 Del Amo Boulevard, Suite 201
Torrance, CA 90503
310-214-3430
Disability Served: all

The Foundation sponsors programs to encourage students with disabilities to enter technical fields and works with employers to promote greater hiring of minorities. TFED also provides information on education and careers in the sciences.

Gifted Child Society
190 Rock Road
Glen Rock, NJ 07452-1736
201-444-6530
http://www.gifted.org
Disability Served: all

The Society offers training programs for educators of special needs children.

Handicapper Educational Services
Wayne State University
583 Student Center Building
Detroit, MI 48202
313-577-1851
Disability Served: all

This group provides advocacy services for college students with disabilities.

Institute on Disability/UAP
University of New Hampshire
7 Leavitt Lane, Suite 101
Durham, NH 03824
603-862-4320
http://iod.unh.edu
Disability Served: all

The Institute advocates for improved services and programs for the disabled.

Microcomputer Resource Lab
Los Angeles Unified School District
15530 Hesby Street
Encino, CA 91436
818-997-2330, ext. 186
Disability Served: all

The Lab provides technology assessments for students with disabilities in the Los Angeles Unified School District. The Lab also offers computer training for special education teachers.

Multisensory Learning Associates
1 Katherine Road
Rehoboth, MA 02769
508-252-6482

Disability Served: developmentally disabled, physically disabled

This organization provides services and training programs to parents and teachers in reading, writing, spelling, and phonological awareness (administrators). It also gives consultations, presentations, and workshops anywhere in the world. An extensive catalog of teaching materials is available.

National Center for Research in Vocational Education/Office of Student Service

University of Illinois Site
345 Education Boulevard
1310 South Sixth
Champaign, IL 61820
217-333-0807
Disability Served: all

The Center provides programs and services and conducts research on vocational education and the transition from school to work.

National Council on Rehabilitation Education

Utah State University
Department of Special Education
Logan, UT 84322
801-797-3241
Disability Served: all

The Council represents educators, researchers, and others and promotes the education of persons with disabilities. The Council also provides vocational rehabilitation services and develops standards for rehabilitation personnel.

National Technical Institute for the Deaf

Rochester Institute for the Deaf
Division of Public Affairs
52 Lomb Memorial Drive
Rochester, NY 14623-5604
716-475-6400
http://www.isc.rit.edu/~418www/
Disability Served: hearing

NTID provides postsecondary education to students with hearing impairments.

New Jersey Institute of Technology

Pre-College Program
323 Martin Luther King Boulevard
Newark, NJ 07102
201-596-3574
Disability Served: all

With support from the National Science Foundation, a training program has been established to help teachers learn how to promote interest in science and mathematics among students with disabilities.

Porter County Special Education Cooperative

750 Ransom Road
Valparaiso, IN 46383
219-464-9607
Disability Served: communication

This organization provides evaluations for students in the area of speech and language, including augmentative communication.

Special Education Technology—British Columbia (SET-BC)

105-1750 West 75th Avenue
Vancouver, BC V6P 6G2 Canada
604-261-9450
Disability Served: all

This program provides assistive technology services to school districts, including consultation, evaluation of student needs, and program planning.

TASH: The Association for Persons with Severe Handicaps

11201 Greenwood Avenue North
Seattle, WA 98133
206-443-9592
Disability Served: all

TASH is a membership organization of educators, parents, administrators, and other educational professionals. TASH provides numerous publications, materials, and resources.

United States Department of Education

Division of Student Services
1250 Maryland Avenue, SW, Suite 600
Washington, DC 20202
Disability Served: all

TRIO Programs (Talent Search, Educational Opportunity Centers, and Special Services for Disadvantaged Students) operate to aid students with disabilities. Contact local schools for details on programs in your area.

Government Bodies

These nonprofit government agencies provide free programs to help people with disabilities find employment, pursue an education, receive legal representation and social services, and gain greater independence in their communities.

FEDERAL

Social Security Library

US Social Security Administration
PO Box 17330
Baltimore, MD 21235
301-965-6113
Disability Served: all

U.S. Administration on Aging

330 Independence Avenue, SW
Washington, DC 20201
202-619-0724
http://www.aoa.dhhs.gov/
Disability Served: all

U.S. Administration on Developmental Disabilities

U.S. Department of Health and Human Services
200 Independence Avenue, SW
Washington, DC 20201
202-690-6590
Disability Served: developmentally disabled

U.S. Center for Mental Health Services

U.S. Department of Health and Human Services,
5600 Fishers Lane
Rockville, MD 20857
301-443-0001
http://www.samhsa.gov/cmhs/cmhs.htm
Disability Served: mental health

U.S. Department of Education

600 Independence Avenue, SW
Washington, DC 20202-0498
800-USA-LEARN
//www.ed.gov/
Disability Served: all

U.S. Department of Health and Human Services

200 Independence Avenue, SW
Washington, DC 20201
202-619-0257
http://www.hhs.gov/
Disability Served: all

U.S. Health Care Financing Administration

U.S. Department of Health and Human Services
200 Independence Avenue, SW
Washington, DC 20201
202-690-5974
http://www.hcfa.gov/
Disability Served: all

U.S. National Council on Disability

1331 F Street, NW, Suite 1050
Washington, DC 20004-1107
202-272-2004
Disability Served: all

U.S. National Institutes of Health

U.S. Department of Health and Human Services
Building One
One Center Drive
Bethesda, MD 20892-0148
301-496-2433
http://www.nih.gov/
Disability Served: all

U.S. President's Committee on Employment of People with Disabilities
U.S. Department of Labor
1331 F Street, NW
Washington, DC 20004-1107
202-376-6200
Disability Served: all

U.S. Social Security Administration
Office of the Commissioner, Altmeyer Building
6401 Security Boulevard
Baltimore, MD 21235
410-965-3120
http://www.ssa.gov/
Disability Served: all

U.S. Special Education and Rehabilitative Services
U.S. Department of Education
330 C Street, SW
Washington, DC 20202-2500
202-205-5465
http://www.ed.gov/offices/osers/
Disability Served: all

U.S. Veterans Benefits Administration
U.S. Department of Veterans Affairs
810 Vermont Avenue, NW
Washington, DC 20420
202-273-7004
http://www.va.gov/dvavba.htm
Disability Served: all

U.S. Veterans Health Administration
U.S. Department of Veterans Affairs
810 Vermont Avenue, NW
Washington, DC 20420
202-273-6280
http://www.va.gov/dvavh.htm
Disability Served: all

U.S. Workers Compensation Programs
U.S. Department of Labor, FPB
200 Constitution Avenue, NW
Washington, DC 20210
202-219-7503
http://www.dol.gov/dol.esa/public/owcp_org.htm
Disability Served: all

STATE

ALABAMA

Alabama Commission on Aging
PO Box 301851
Montgomery, AL 36130-1851
334-242-5743
Disability Served: all

Alabama Department of Education
PO Box 302101
Montgomery, AL 36130-2101
334-242-9950
Disability Served: all

Alabama Department of Mental Health and Mental Retardation
PO Box 301410
Montgomery, AL 36130-1410
334-242-3107
Disability Served: mental health

Alabama Department of Public Health
PO Box 303017
Montgomery, AL 36130-3017
334-613-5300
http://www.alapubhealth.org/
Disability Served: all

Alabama Department of Rehabilitation Services
PO Box 301801
Montgomery, AL 36130-1801
334-281-8780, 800-441-7607
Disability Served: all

Alabama Division of Worker's Compensation
649 Monroe Street
Montgomery, AL 36131
334-242-2868
Disability Served: all

Alabama Institute for the Deaf and Blind
205 East South Street
Talladega, AL 35160
205-761-3201
Disability Served: hearing, vision

ALASKA

Alaska Department of Education
801 West 10th Street, Suite 200
Juneau, AK 99801
907-465-2800
http://www.educ.state.ak.us/
Disability Served: all

Alaska Department of Health and Social Services
350 Main Street, Room 204
PO Box 11061
Juneau, AK 99811-0601
907-465-3030
Disability Served: all

Alaska Division of Mental Health and Developmental Disabilities
350 Main Street, Room 214
PO Box 110620
Juneau, AK 99811-0620
907-465-3370
Disability Served: developmentally disabled, mental health

Alaska Division of Senior Services
PO Box 110209
Juneau, AK 99811-0209
907-465-3250
Disability Served: all

Alaska Division of Vocational Rehabilitation
801 West 10th Street, Suite A
Juneau, AK 99801-1894
907-465-2814
http://www.educ.state.ak.us/VocRehab/
Disability Served: all

Alaska Division of Worker's Compensation
PO Box 25512
Juneau, AK 99802-5512
907-465-2790
Disability Served: all

Social Security Disability Determination Service—Alaska
701 East Tudor, Suite 250
Anchorage, AK 99503-7498
907-562-0460
Disability Served: all

ARIZONA

Arizona Council for the Hearing Impaired
1400 West Washington, Room 126
Phoenix, AZ 85007
602-542-3323
http://www.state.az.us/achi
Disability Served: hearing

Arizona Department of Health Services
1740 West Adams
Phoenix, AZ 85007
602-542-1024
http://www.hs.state.az.us/
Disability Served: all

Arizona Division of Aging and Community Services
PO Box 6123
Phoenix, AZ 85005
602-542-6572
Disability Served: all

Arizona Division of Behavioral Health Services
2122 East Highland
Phoenix, AZ 85016
602-381-8999
http://www.hs.state.az.us/bhs
Disability Served: mental health

Arizona Division of Developmental Disabilities
PO Box 6123
Phoenix, AZ 85005
602-542-6853
Disability Served: developmentally disabled

Arizona Division of Employment and Rehabilitation Services
PO Box 6123
Phoenix, AZ 85005
602-542-4910
Disability Served: all

Arizona Education Services Department
1535 West Jefferson
Phoenix, AZ 85007
602-542-6417
http://www.ade.state.az.us/
Disability Served: all

Social Security Disability Determination Service—Arizona (Tucson)
PO Box 40060
Tucson, AZ 85717-0060
520-881-7330
http://www.ssa.gov/
Disability Served: all

ARKANSAS

Arkansas Department of Education
#4 Capitol Mall
Little Rock, AR 72201
501-682-4475
http://arkedu.k12.ar.us/
Disability Served: all

Arkansas Department of Health
4815 West Markham
Little Rock, AR 72205
501-661-2000
http://health.state.ar.us/
Disability Served: all

Arkansas Division of Aging and Adult Services
1417 Donaghey Plaza South
Little Rock, AR 72201
501-682-8150
Disability Served: all

Arkansas Division of Developmental Disabilities Services
Fifth Floor, Donaghey Plaza North
Little Rock, AR 72201
501-682-8665
Disability Served: developmentally disabled

Arkansas Division of Mental Health Services
4313 West Markham
Little Rock, AR 72205
501-682-9000
Disability Served: mental health

Arkansas Division of Services for the Blind
522 Main Street, Suite 100
PO Box 3237
Little Rock, AR 72203
501-682-5463, 800-960-9270
Disability Served: vision

Arkansas Rehabilitation Services
1616 Brookwood Drive
Little Rock, AR 72202
501-296-1600
http://www.state.ar.us/ars/ars2.html
Disability Served: all

Arkansas Worker's Compensation Commission
Fourth & Spring Streets
Little Rock, AR 72203-0950
501-682-3930, 800-622-4472
http://www.awcc.state.ar.us/
Disability Served: all

CALIFORNIA

California Department of Aging
1600 K Street
Sacramento, CA 95814
916-322-3887
http://www.aging.state.ca.us/
Disability Served: all

California Department of Education
721 Capitol Mall
PO Box 944272
Sacramento, CA 94244-2720
http://goldmine.cde.ca.gov/
Disability Served: all

California Department of Health Services
714 P Street, Room 1253
Sacramento, CA 95814
916-657-1425
Disability Served: all

California Department of Mental Health
1600 Ninth Street, Room 151
Sacramento, CA 95814
916-654-2309
http://www.dmh.cahwnet.gov/
Disability Served: mental health

California Department of Rehabilitation
PO Box 944222
Sacramento, CA 94244-2220
916-445-8638
http://www.rehab.cahwnet.gov/
Disability Served: all

California Division of Worker's Compensation
PO Box 420603
San Francisco, CA 94142
415-975-0700
Disability Served: all

Social Security Administration Region IX—San Francisco
75 Hawthorne Street
San Francisco, CA 94105
415-744-4896
http://www.ssa.gov/
Disability Served: all

Social Security Disability Determination Service—California (Fresno North)
PO Box 1072
Fresno, CA 93714-1072
209-297-3506
http://www.ssa.gov/
Disability Served: all

Social Security Disability Determination Service—California (Los Angeles East)
PO Box 3819, Terminal Annex
Los Angeles, CA 90051-3819
213-736-7900
http://www.ssa.gov/
Disability Served: all

Social Security Disability Determination Service—California (Los Angeles North)
PO Box 60999, Terminal Annex
Los Angeles, CA 90060-0999
213-736-7000
http://www.ssa.gov/
Disability Served: all

Social Security Disability Determination Service—California (Los Angeles South)
PO Box 3819, Terminal Annex
Los Angeles, CA 90051-3819
213-736-4086
http://www.ssa.gov/
Disability Served: all

Social Security Disability Determination Service—California (Los Angeles West)
PO Box 60999, Terminal Annex
Los Angeles, CA 90060-0999
213-736-7500
http://www.ssa.gov/
Disability Served: all

Social Security Disability Determination Service—California (Oakland East)
PO Box 24225
Oakland, CA 94623
510-286-1823
http://www.ssa.gov/
Disability Served: all

Social Security Disability Determination Service—California (Oakland West)
PO Box 24225
Oakland, CA 94623
510-286-1534
http://www.ssa.gov/
Disability Served: all

Social Security Disability Determination Service—California (Roseville)
PO Box 619020
Roseville, CA 95661
916-744-4111
http://www.ssa.gov/
Disability Served: all

Social Security Disability Determination Service—California (Sacramento)
PO Box 997120
Sacramento, CA 95899-7120
916-322-3973
http://www.ssa.gov/
Disability Served: all

Social Security Disability Determination Service—California (San Diego East)
PO Box 85326
San Diego, CA 92186-2058
619-467-2018
http://www.ssa.gov/
Disability Served: all

Social Security Disability Determination Service—California (San Diego West)
PO Box 85326
San Diego, CA 92186-5326
619-467-2010
http://www.ssa.gov/
Disability Served: all

COLORADO

Colorado Department of Education
201 East Colfax Avenue
Denver, CO 80203
303-866-6600
http://www.cde.state.co.us/
Disability Served: all

Colorado Department of Public Health and Environment
4300 Cherry Creek Drive South
Denver, CO 80246-1530
303-692-2000
Disability Served: all

Colorado Developmental Disabilities Services
3824 West Princeton Circle
Denver, CO 80236
303-866-7450
Disability Served: developmentally disabled

Colorado Division of Aging and Adult Services
110 16th Street, Suite 200
Denver, CO 80202
Disability Served: all

Colorado Division of Vocational Rehabilitation
110 16th Street, Second Floor
Denver, CO 80202
303-620-4132
Disability Served: all

Colorado Division of Worker's Compensation
1515 Arapahoe Street
Denver, CO 80202
303-575-8700
Disability Served: all

Colorado Mental Health Services
3824 West Princeton Circle
Denver, CO 80236
303-866-7400
Disability Served: mental health

Social Security Administration Region VIII—Denver

1961 Stout Street
Denver, CO 80294-3538
303-844-4441
http://www.ssa.gov/
Disability Served: all

Social Security Disability Determination Service—Colorado

10065 East Harvard Avenue, Suite 207
Denver, CO 80231-5941
http://www.ssa.gov/
Disability Served: all

CONNECTICUT

Connecticut Board of Education and Services for the Blind

170 Ridge Road
Wethersfield, CT 06109
860-566-5800, 860-278-6920
Disability Served: vision

Connecticut Deaf and Hearing Impaired Commission

1245 Farmington Avenue
West Hartford, CT 06107
860-566-7414
Disability Served: hearing

Connecticut Department of Education

PO Box 2219
Hartford, CT 06145
860-566-5677
http://www.state.ct.us/sde
Disability Served: all

Connecticut Department of Mental Health and Addiction Services

410 Capitol Avenue, Fourth Floor
Hartford, CT 06134
860-418-7000
Disability Served: mental health

Connecticut Department of Mental Retardation

460 Capitol Avenue
Hartford, CT 06106
860-418-6000
http://www.state.ct.us/dmr/
Disability Served: mental health

Connecticut Department of Public Health

410 Capitol Avenue
PO Box 340308
Hartford, CT 06134-0308
860-509-8000
http://www.state.ct.us/dph/
Disability Served: all

Connecticut Division of Elderly Services

25 Sigourney Street
Hartford, CT 06106
860-424-5025
Disability Served: all

Connecticut Governor's Committee on Employment of People with Disabilities

200 Folly Brook Boulevard
Wethersfield, CT 06109
860-566-8061
Disability Served: all

Connecticut Worker's Compensation Commission

21 Oak Street
Hartford, CT 06106
860-493-1500
Disability Served: all

Social Security Disability Determination Service—Connecticut

PO Box 2363
Hartford, CT 06101-8585
860-298-2136
http://www.ssa.gov/
Disability Served: all

DISTRICT OF COLUMBIA

District of Columbia Board of Education

415 12th Street, NW
Washington, DC 20004

202-724-8724
Disability Served: all

District of Columbia Department of Health
800 Ninth Street, SW, Third Floor
Washington, DC 20024
202-645-5556
Disability Served: all

District of Columbia Mental Health Services Commission
2700 Martin Luther King, Jr. Avenue, SE, Building A, Room 105
Washington, DC 20032
202-373-7166
Disability Served: mental health

District of Columbia Mental Retardation and Developmental Disabilities Services
609 H Street, NE
Washington, DC 20002
202-673-7657
Disability Served: developmentally disabled, mental health

District of Columbia Office of Aging
441 Fourth Street, NW
Washington, DC 20001
202-724-5622
Disability Served: all

District of Columbia Rehabilitation Services
609 H Street, NE
Washington, DC 20002
202-727-2337
Disability Served: all

District of Columbia Workers' Compensation Office
1200 Upshur Street, NW
Washington, DC 20011
202-576-6265
Disability Served: all

Social Security Disability Determination Service—Washington, DC
717 14th Street
Washington, DC 20005
202-727-8622
http://www.ssa.gov/
Disability Served: all

DELAWARE

Delaware Department of Education
PO Box 1402
Federal & Lookerman Streets
Dover, DE 19903
302-739-4601
http://www.doe.state.de.us/
Disability Served: all

Delaware Developmental Disabilities Planning Council
821 Silver Lake Boulevard, Suite 108
Dover, DE 19904
302-739-3333
http://www.state.ct.us/ddc/
Disability Served: developmentally disabled

Delaware Division for the Visually Impaired
1901 North duPont Highway
Biggs Building
New Castle, DE 19720
302-577-3333
Disability Served: vision

Delaware Division of Mental Retardation
Jesse Cooper Building
Federal & Water Streets
Dover, DE 19901
Disability Served: all

Delaware Division of Public Health
Jesse Cooper Building
Federal & Water Streets
Dover, DE 19901
Disability Served: all

Delaware Division of Services for the Aging and Adults with Physical Disabilities
1901 North duPont Highway
Main Building, Second Floor Annex
New Castle, DE 19720
Disability Served: all

Delaware Division of Vocational Rehabilitation
4425 North Market Street
Wilmington, DE 19802
302-761-8349
Disability Served: all

Social Security Disability Determination Service—Delaware
PO Box 9969
Fox Valley Offices
4425 North Market Street, Third Floor
Wilmington, DE 19809-0969
302-761-8325
http://www.ssa.gov/
Disability Served: all

FLORIDA

Florida Agency for Health Care Administration
2727 Mahan Drive
Tallahassee, FL 32303
904-922-3809
Disability Served: all

Florida Department of Education
Turlington Building
325 West Gaines Street
Tallahassee, FL 32399-0400
850-488-1234
http://www.firn.edu/doe
Disability Served: all

Florida Department of Elder Affairs
4040 Esplanade Way
Tallahassee, FL 32399-7000
800-96-ELDER, 850-414-2000
http://www.state.fl.us/doea/
Disability Served: all

Florida Division of Workers Compensation
2012 Capitol Circle, SE
Hartman Building
Tallahassee, FL 32399-2152
904-488-2514
Disability Served: all

GEORGIA

Georgia Department of Education
2054 Twin Towers East
Atlanta, GA 30334
800-311-3627, 404-656-2446
http://www.doe.k12.ga.us/
Disability Served: all

Georgia Division of Aging Services
Two Peachtree Street, NW, Suite 18-403
Atlanta, GA 30303-3176
404-657-5258
Disability Served: all

Georgia Division of Mental Health, Mental Retardation, and Substance Abuse
Two Peachtree Street, NW
Atlanta, GA 30303
404-657-2260
Disability Served: mental health

Georgia Division of Public Health
Two Peachtree Street, NW
Atlanta, GA 30303-3186
404-657-2700
http://www.ph.dhr.state.ga.us/
Disability Served: all

Georgia Workers Compensation Board
270 Peachtree Street, NW
Atlanta, GA 30303-1299
404-656-2034
Disability Served: all

Social Security Administration Region IV—Atlanta
101 Marietta Tower, Suite 1804
Atlanta, GA 30323
404-331-2998

http://www.ssa.gov/
Disability Served: all

GUAM

Social Security Disability Determination Service—Guam
Central Avenue, Building 1313
Tiyan, Guam 96913
http://www.ssa.gov/
Disability Served: all

HAWAII

Hawaii Department of Education
PO Box 2360
Honolulu, HI 96804
808-586-3310
Disability Served: all

Hawaii Department of Health
PO Box 3378
Honolulu, HI 96801
808-586-4442
http://www.hawaii.gov/health/
Disability Served: all

Hawaii Developmental Disabilities Council
919 Ala Moana Boulevard, Room 113
Honolulu, HI 96814
808-586-8100
Disability Served: developmentally disabled

Hawaii Division of Adult Mental Health
1250 Punchbowl Street
Honolulu, HI 96813
808-586-4686
Disability Served: mental health

Hawaii Division of Vocational Rehabilitation and Blind Services
PO Box 339
Honolulu, HI 96809-0339
808-586-5366
Disability Served: all

Hawaii Persons with Disabilities Commission
919 Ala Moana Boulevard, Room 101
Honolulu, HI 96814
808-586-8121
Disability Served: all

Social Security Disability Determination Service—Hawaii
PO Box 2458
Honolulu, HI 96804-2458
808-944-8755
http://www.ssa.gov/
Disability Served: all

IDAHO

Idaho Commission for the Blind and Visually Impaired
PO Box 83720
Boise, ID 83720-0012
208-334-3220
Disability Served: vision

Idaho Commission on Aging
PO Box 83720
Boise, ID 83720-0007
208-334-3833
http://www.state.id.us/icoa/
Disability Served: all

Idaho Council for the Deaf and Hard of Hearing
1720 Westgate Drive
Boise, ID 83704
800-433-1323, 208-334-0879
Disability Served: hearing

Idaho Council on Developmental Disabilities
280 North 8th Street, Suite 208
PO Box 83720
Boise, ID 83720
208-334-2178
Disability Served: developmentally disabled

Idaho Deaf and Hard of Hearing Council
PO Box 83720
Boise, ID 83720-0036

208-334-5700
Disability Served: hearing

Idaho Department of Education
PO Box 83720
Boise, ID 83720-0027
208-332-6800
http:////www.sde.state.id.us/Dept/
Disability Served: all

Idaho Department of Health and Welfare
PO Box 83720
Boise, ID 83720-0036
208-334-5506
http://www.state.id.us/dhw/
Disability Served: all

Idaho Department of Vocational Rehabilitation
PO Box 83720
Boise, ID 83720-0096
208-334-3390
http://www.state.id.us/idvr/
Disability Served: all

Idaho Developmental Disabilities Council
280 North 8th Street
Boise, ID 83720
208-334-2178
Disability Served: developmentally disabled

Idaho Mental Health and Substance Abuse Bureau
PO Box 83720
Boise, ID 83720
208-334-5700
Disability Served: mental health

Social Security Disability Determination Service—Idaho
1505 McKinney
Boise, ID 83704
208-327-7333
Disability Served: all

ILLINOIS

Illinois Board of Education
100 North First Street
Springfield, IL 62777
217-782-2221
http://www.isbe.state.il.us/
Disability Served: all

Illinois Department of Aging
421 East Capitol Avenue #100
Springfield, IL 62701-1789
217-785-2870
http://www.state.il.us/aging/
Disability Served: all

Illinois Department of Public Health
535 West Jefferson Street
Springfield, IL 62761
217-782-4977
http://www.idph.state.il.us/
Disability Served: all

Illinois Developmental Disabilities Services
416 Stratton Building
Springfield, IL 62675
217-524-0453
Disability Served: developmentally disabled

Illinois Mental Health Services
100 South Grand Avenue
Springfield, IL 62762
217-782-7555
Disability Served: mental health

Illinois Rehabilitation Services
100 South Grand Avenue
Springfield, IL 62762
217-785-0234
Disability Served: all

Social Security Administration Region V—Chicago
PO Box 8280
Chicago, IL 60680
312-353-1733
http://www.ssa.gov/
Disability Served: all

Social Security Disability Determination Service—Illinois
100 North First Street
Springfield, IL 62702
217-782-8283
http://www.ssa.gov/
Disability Served: all

INDIANA

Indiana Department of Education
Room 229, State House
Indianapolis, IN 46204-2798
317-232-0808
http://www.doe.state.in.us/
Disability Served: all

Indiana Department of Health
Two North Meridian Street
Indianapolis, IN 46204
317-233-1325
http://www.state.in.us/doh/
Disability Served: all

Indiana Division of Disability, Aging, and Rehabilitative Services
PO Box 7083
Indianapolis, IN 46207-7083
317-232-1147
Disability Served: all

Indiana Division of Mental Health
PO Box 7083
Indianapolis, IN 46207-7083
317-233-3367
Disability Served: mental health

Indiana Worker's Compensation Board
402 West Washington Street, Room W-196
Indianapolis, IN 46204
800-824-COMP
http://www.state.in.us/wkcomp/
Disability Served: all

Social Security Disability Determination Service—Indiana
225 North New Jersey Street
Indianapolis, IN 46204
317-232-6466
http://www.ssa.gov/
Disability Served: all

IOWA

Iowa Department for the Blind
524 Fourth Street
Des Moines, IA 50309-2364
515-281-1334
http://www.state.ia.us/government/dfb/index.html
Disability Served: vision

Iowa Department of Education
Grimes State Office Building
Des Moines, IA 50319-0146
515-281-3436
http://www.state.ia.us/educate/depteduc/index.html
Disability Served: all

Iowa Department of Elder Affairs
Clemens Building, Third Floor
200 Tenth Street
Des Moines, IA 50309-3609
515-281-5188
Disability Served: all

Iowa Department of Public Health
321 East Twelfth Street
Lucas State Office Building
Des Moines, IA 50319
515-281-5605
http://www.idph.state.ia.us/
Disability Served: all

Iowa Division of Deaf Services
321 East Twelfth Street
Lucas State Office Building
Des Moines, IA 50319
515-281-7121
Disability Served: hearing

Iowa Division of Mental Health and Developmental Disabilities
Hoover State Office Building, Fifth Floor
Des Moines, IA 50319
Disability Served: developmentally disabled, mental health

Iowa Division of People with Disabilities
321 East Twelfth Street
Lucas State Office Building
Des Moines, IA 50319
515-281-5238
Disability Served: all

Iowa Division of Vocational Rehabilitation
Grimes State Office Building
Des Moines, IA 50319-0146
515-281-6731
Disability Served: all

KANSAS

Kansas Commission on Disabilities Concern
1430 SW Topeka Avenue
Topeka, KS 66612-1877
913-296-1722
Disability Served: all

Kansas Department of Education
120 SE Tenth Avenue
Topeka, KS 66612
913-296-3202
Disability Served: all

Kansas Department on Aging
Docking State Office Building
915 SW Harrison, Room 150-S
Topeka, KS 66612-1500
913-296-4986
Disability Served: all

Kansas Division of Health
900 SW Jackson, Suite 665
Topeka, KS 66612-1290
913-296-1086
Disability Served: all

Kansas Division of Rehabilitation Services
300 SW Oakley, First Floor
Biddle Building
Topeka, KS 66606
913-296-3911
Disability Served: all

Kansas Division of Workers Compensation
401 SW Topeka Boulevard
Topeka, KS 66603-3182
913-296-4000
Disability Served: all

KENTUCKY

Kentucky Commission for the Deaf and Hard of Hearing
632 Versailles Road
Frankfort, KY 40601
502-573-3594
Disability Served: hearing

Kentucky Department for the Blind
PO Box 757
Frankfort, KY 40602
502-564-4754
Disability Served: vision

Kentucky Department of Education
Capitol Plaza Tower
500 Mero Street
Frankfort, KY 40601
502-564-3141
Disability Served: all

Kentucky Department of Health Services
275 East Main Street
Frankfort, KY 40621
502-564-3970
Disability Served: all

Kentucky Department of Mental Health and Mental Retardation
275 East Main Street
Frankfort, KY 40621
502-564-4527
Disability Served: mental health

Kentucky Division of Aging Services
275 East Main Street
Frankfort, KY 40621
502-564-6930
Disability Served: all

Kentucky Vocational Rehabilitation Department
209 St. Clair Street
Frankfort, KY 40601
502-564-6742
Disability Served: all

Kentucky Workers Compensation Board
1047 US 127 South, Suite 4
Frankfort, KY 40601
502-564-5550
Disability Served: all

LOUISIANA

Louisiana Department of Education
PO Box 94064
Baton Rouge, LA 70804-9064
504-342-3602
http://www.doe.state.la.us/
Disability Served: all

Louisiana Department of Health and Hospitals
PO Box 629
Baton Rouge, LA 70821-0629
504-342-9503
http://204.58.127.20/dhh/
Disability Served: all

Louisiana Division of Citizens with Developmental Disabilities
PO Box 629
Baton Rouge, LA 70821-0629
504-342-0095
Disability Served: developmentally disabled

Louisiana Division of Mental Health
PO Box 629
Baton Rouge, LA 70821-0629
504-342-2540
Disability Served: mental health

Louisiana Office of Public Health Services
PO Box 3214
New Orleans, LA 70160
504-342-8092
Disability Served: all

Louisiana Office of Workers' Compensation
PO Box 94040
Baton Rouge, LA 70804-9094
504-342-7561
Disability Served: all

Louisiana Rehabilitative Services
PO Box 94371
Baton Rouge, LA 70804-9371
Disability Served: all

MAINE

Maine Bureau of Elder and Adult Services
Whitten Road
Augusta, ME 04333-0011
207-624-5335
Disability Served: all

Maine Bureau of Health
11 State House Station
35 Anthony Avenue
Augusta, ME 04333-0011
207-287-3201
Disability Served: all

Maine Department of Education
23 State House Station
Augusta, ME 04333-0023
207-287-5112
http://www.state.me.us/education/homepage.htm
Disability Served: all

Maine Department of Mental Health, Mental Retardation, and Substance Abuse Services
40 State House Station
Augusta, ME 04333
207-287-4223
Disability Served: mental health

Maine Workers Compensation Board
27 State House Station
Augusta, ME 04333
207-287-3751
Disability Served: all

MARYLAND

Maryland Blind Industries and Services
2901 Strickland Street
Baltimore, MD 21223-2796
410-233-4567
Disability Served: vision

Maryland Department of Education
200 West Baltimore Street
Baltimore, MD 21201
888-246-0016
http://www.msde.state.md.us/
Disability Served: all

Maryland Department of Health and Mental Hygiene
201 West Preston Street
Baltimore, MD 21201
410-767-6860
http://www.charm.net/~epi9/
Disability Served: all

Maryland Developmental Disabilities Council
300 West Lexington Street, Box 10
Baltimore, MD 21201
410-333-3688
Disability Served: developmentally disabled

Maryland Division of Vocational Rehabilitation
2301 Argonne Drive
Baltimore, MD 21218
410-554-9400
Disability Served: all

Maryland Office for Individuals with Disabilities
300 West Lexington Street, Box 10
Baltimore, MD 21201
http://www.mdtap.org/oid.html
Disability Served: all

Maryland Office on Aging
301 West Preston Street, Suite 1807
Baltimore, MD 21201
410-767-1100, 800-AGE-DIAL
Disability Served: all

Maryland Worker's Compensation Commission
61 North Liberty Street
Baltimore, MD 21201-3735
410-767-0900, 800-492-0479
http://www.charm.net/~wcc/
Disability Served: all

Social Security Disability Determination Service—Maryland
PO Box 6338
Timonium, MD 21094-6338
410-308-4500
http://www.ssa.gov/
Disability Served: all

MASSACHUSETTS

Massachusetts Commission for the Blind
88 Kingston Street
Boston, MA 02111-2227
617-727-5550
Disability Served: vision

Massachusetts Commission for the Deaf and Hard of Hearing
210 South Street, Fifth Floor
Boston, MA 02111
617-695-7500
Disability Served: hearing

Massachusetts Department of Education
350 Main Street
Malden, MA 02148
617-388-3300
http://info.doe.mass.edu/
Disability Served: all

Massachusetts Department of Elder Affairs
One Ashburton Place, Fifth Floor
Boston, MA 02108
617-727-7750
Disability Served: all

Massachusetts Department of Mental Health
25 Stanford Street
Boston, MA 02114
617-727-5600
Disability Served: mental health

Massachusetts Department of Mental Retardation Services
160 North Washington Street
Boston, MA 02114
617-727-5608
Disability Served: all

Massachusetts Department of Public Health
250 Washington Street
Boston, MA 02108-4619
617-624-6000
Disability Served: all

Massachusetts Developmental Disabilities Agency
174 Portland Street, Fifth Floor
Boston, MA 02114-1714
617-727-4178
Disability Served: developmentally disabled

Massachusetts Disabled Person Protection Commission
99 Bedford Street, Room 200
Boston, MA 02111
617-727-6465
Disability Served: all

Massachusetts Rehabilitation Commission
27-43 Wormwood Street
Boston, MA 02210
617-204-3600
Disability Served: all

Social Security Administration Region I—Boston
JFK Federal Building, Room 1900
Boston, MA 02203
617-565-2881
http://www.ssa.gov/
Disability Served: all

Social Security Disability Determination Service—Massachusetts (Boston)
110 Chauncy Street
Boston, MA 02111
617-654-7729
http://www.ssa.gov/
Disability Served: all

Social Security Disability Determination Service—Massachusetts (Worcester)
22 Front Street
PO Box 8009
Worcester, MA 01614-9981
508-752-5001
http://www.ssa.gov/
Disability Served: all

MICHIGAN

Michigan Department of Community Health
Lewis Cass Building, Sixth Floor
320 South Walnut Street
Lansing, MI 48913
517-335-3500
http://www.mdch.state.mi.us/
Disability Served: all

Michigan Department of Education
608 West Allegan Street
Hannal Building
Lansing, MI 48933
http://www.state.mi.us/mde/
Disability Served: all

Michigan Developmental Disabilities Council
Lewis Cass Building, Sixth Floor
320 South Walnut
Lansing, MI 48913
517-334-6769
Disability Served: developmentally disabled

Michigan Mental Health and Substance Abuse Services
Lewis Cass Building, Sixth Floor
320 South Walnut
Lansing, MI 48913
517-335-0196
Disability Served: mental health

Michigan Office of Services to the Aging
611 West Ottawa
PO Box 30676
Lansing, MI 48909-8176
517-373-8230
http://mass.iog.wayne.edu/
Disability Served: all

Social Security Disability Determination Service—Michigan (Detroit)
Michigan Plaza Building, Tenth Floor
1200 Sixth Street
Detroit, MI 48226
313-256-3108
http://www.ssa.gov/
Disability Served: all

Social Security Disability Determination Service—Michigan (Kalamazoo)
Commercial Building, Fifth Floor
151 South Rose Street
Kalamazoo, MI 49007-4715
616-337-3550
http://www.ssa.gov/
Disability Served: all

Social Security Disability Determination Service—Michigan (Lansing)
608 West Allegan Street, Third Floor
Lansing, MI 48933
517-373-6636
http://www.ssa.gov/
Disability Served: all

Social Security Disability Determination Service—Michigan (Traverse City)
315 East Front Street
Traverse City, MI 49684
616-929-5550
http://www.ssa.gov/
Disability Served: all

MINNESOTA

Minnesota Aging Initiative Project
444 Lafayette Road
St. Paul, MN 55155
612-297-3209
Disability Served: all

Minnesota Council on Disability
121 East Seventh Place, Suite 107
St. Paul, MN 55101
612-296-6785
http://www.disability.state.mn.us
Disability Served: all

Minnesota Department of Children, Families, and Learning
Capitol Square Building
550 Cedar Street
St. Paul, MN 55101
612-296-2358
http://children.state.mn.us/
Disability Served: all

Minnesota Department of Health
PO Box 64975
St. Paul, MN 55164-0975
612-215-5800
Disability Served: all

Minnesota Division of Deaf and Hard of Hearing Services
444 Lafayette Road
St. Paul, MN 55155-3833
612-297-1299
Disability Served: hearing

Minnesota Division of Mental Health Services
444 Lafayette Road
St. Paul, MN 55155
612-297-3510
Disability Served: mental health

Minnesota Division of Workers Compensation
443 Lafayette Road
St. Paul, MN 55155
612-296-6490
Disability Served: all

Minnesota Office of Blind Services
2200 University Avenue West, Suite 240
St. Paul, MN 55114
612-642-0508
Disability Served: vision

Minnesota Rehabilitation Services Branch
390 North Robert Street
St. Paul, MN 55101
612-296-1822
Disability Served: all

Minnesota Vocational Rehabilitation Unit
443 Lafayette Road
St. Paul, MN 55155
612-297-3753
Disability Served: all

Social Security Disability Determination Service—Minnesota
Metro Square Building, Suite 300
Seventh and Robert Streets
St. Paul, MN 55101
612-296-5959
http://www.ssa.gov/
Disability Served: all

MISSISSIPPI

Mississippi Department of Education
PO Box 771
Jackson, MS 39205
601-359-3513
http://mdek12.state.ms.us/
Disability Served: all

Mississippi Department of Health
PO Box 1700
Jackson, MS 39215-1700
601-960-7634
http://www.msdh.state.ms.us/
Disability Served: all

Mississippi Department of Mental Health
1101 Robert E. Lee Building
Jackson, MS 39201
601-359-1288
Disability Served: mental health

Mississippi Department of Rehabilitation Services
PO Box 1698
Jackson, MS 39215-1698
601-853-5100
Disability Served: all

Mississippi Division of Aging and Adult Services
PO Box 352
Jackson, MS 39205-0352
601-359-4480
Disability Served: all

Mississippi Workers Compensation Commission
PO Box 5300
Jackson, MS 39296-5300
601-987-4200
Disability Served: all

MISSOURI

Missouri Department of Elementary and Secondary Education
PO Box 480
205 Jefferson Street
Jefferson City, MO 65102-0480
573-751-3469
http://services.dese.state.mo.us/
Disability Served: all

Missouri Department of Health
PO Box 570
920 Wildwood Drive
Jefferson City, MO 65102
573-751-6062

http://www.health.state.mo.us/
Disability Served: all

Missouri Department of Mental Health
1706 East Elm Street
PO Box 687
Jefferson City, MO 65102
573-751-3070
http://www.state.mo.us/dmh/modmh.htm
Disability Served: mental health

Missouri Division of Aging
PO Box 1337
Jefferson City, MO 65102
573-751-3082
Disability Served: all

Missouri Division of Mental Retardation and Developmental Disability
1706 East Elm Street
PO Box 687
Jefferson City, MO 65102
573-751-4054
Disability Served: developmentally disabled

Missouri Division of Services for the Deaf and Hard of Hearing
1706 East Elm Street
PO Box 687
Jefferson City, MO 65102
573-751-0768
Disability Served: hearing

Missouri Division of Vocational Rehabilitation
3024 West Truman Boulevard
Jefferson City, MO 65109
573-751-3251
Disability Served: all

Missouri Division of Workers Compensation
3315 West Truman Boulevard
Jefferson City, MO 65102-0504
573-751-4231
Disability Served: all

Missouri Rehabilitation Services for the Blind
PO Box 88
Jefferson City, MO 65103
573-751-4249
Disability Served: vision

Social Security Administration Region VII—Kansas City
601 East Twelfth Street, Room 436
Kansas City, MO 64106
816-426-6191
http://www.ssa.gov/
Disability Served: all

MONTANA

Montana Office of Addictive and Mental Disorders
PO Box 202951
Helena, MT 59620-2951
406-444-3964
Disability Served: mental health

Montana Office of Disability Services
PO Box 4210
Helena, MT 59604
406-444-2590
Disability Served: all

Montana Office of Public Instruction
PO Box 202501
Room 106, State Capitol
Helena, MT 59620-2501
406-444-7362
http://www.161.7.114.15/OPI/opi.html
Disability Served: all

Montana Public Health and Human Services Department
PO Box 4210
Helena, MT 59604
406-444-5622
http://www.dphhs.mt.gov/
Disability Served: all

Montana Workers Compensation Court
PO Box 537
Helena, MT 59624
406-444-7794
Disability Served: all

Social Security Disability Determination Service—Montana
2550 Prospect Avenue
Helena, MT 59601
http://www.ssa.gov/
Disability Served: all

NEBRASKA

Nebraska Aging Services
PO Box 95044
Lincoln, NE 68509
402-471-4617
Disability Served: all

Nebraska Department of Education
PO Box 94987
Lincoln, NE 68509-4987
402-471-3560
http://www.nde.state.ne.us/
Disability Served: all

Nebraska Department of Health and Human Services
PO Box 95044
Lincoln, NE 68509
402-471-9197
Disability Served: all

Nebraska Developmental Disability Services
PO Box 95044
Lincoln, NE 68509
402-479-5110
Disability Served: developmentally disabled

Nebraska Office of Mental Health and Substance Abuse
PO Box 95044
Lincoln, NE 68509
402-471-8417
Disability Served: mental health

Nebraska Rehabilitation Services
PO Box 94987
Lincoln, NE 68509-4987
402-471-3667
Disability Served: all

Nebraska Rehabilitation Services for the Visually Impaired
PO Box 95044
Lincoln, NE 68509
402-471-2891
Disability Served: vision

NEVADA

Nevada Department of Education
700 East Fifth Street
Carson City, NV 89701-5096
702-687-9200
http://nsn.scs.unr.edu/nvdow/
Disability Served: all

Nevada Division of Aging Services
340 North 11th Street, Suite 103
Las Vegas, NV 89101
702-486-3545
Disability Served: all

Nevada Division of Mental Hygiene and Mental Retardation
505 East King Street, Room 602
Carson City, NV 89701-4761
702-687-5943
Disability Served: mental health

Nevada Division of Rehabilitation
505 East King Street, Room 502
Carson City, NV 89701
702-687-4440
Disability Served: all

Nevada Governor's Committee on the Employment of People with Disabilities
4001 South Virginia Street
Reno, NV 89502
702-688-1111
Disability Served: all

Social Security Disability Determination Service—Nevada
1050 East William Street, Suite 300
Carson City, NV 89710
702-687-4430
http://www.ssa.gov/
Disability Served: all

NEW HAMPSHIRE

New Hampshire Bureau of Blind Services
78 Regional Drive
Concord, NH 03301
603-271-3815
Disability Served: vision

New Hampshire Bureau of Vocational Rehabilitation Services
78 Regional Drive
Concord, NH 03301
603-271-3814
Disability Served: all

New Hampshire Department of Education
101 Pleasant Street
Concord, NH 03301-3860
603-271-6646
http://www.state.nh.us/doe/education.html
Disability Served: all

New Hampshire Department of Health and Human Services
Six Hazen Drive
Concord, NH 03301
603-271-4331
http://www.state.nh.us/dhhs
Disability Served: all

New Hampshire Division of Behavioral Health
105 Pleasant Street
Concord, NH 03301
603-271-5007
Disability Served: mental health

New Hampshire Division of Elderly and Adult Services
115 Pleasant Street
Annex Building One
Concord, NH 03301-3843
603-271-4394
Disability Served: all

New Hampshire Governor's Commission on Disability
57 Regional Drive
Concord, NH 03301
603-271-2773
Disability Served: all

New Hampshire Workers Compensation Division
95 Pleasant Street
Concord, NH 03301
603-271-3176
Disability Served: all

Social Security Disability Determination Service—New Hampshire
PO Box 452
Concord, NH 03302-0452
603-271-3341
http://www.ssa.gov/
Disability Served: all

NEW JERSEY

New Jersey Commission for the Blind
153 Halsey Street
Newark, NJ 07102
973-648-2324
Disability Served: vision

New Jersey Deaf and Hard of Hearing Division
PO Box 074
Capitol Center
Trenton, NJ 08625-0074
609-984-7281
Disability Served: hearing

New Jersey Department of Education
PO Box 500
Trenton, NJ 08625-0500
609-292-4450

http://www.state.nj.us/education/
Disability Served: all

New Jersey Department of Health and Senior Services

John Fitch Plaza, CN360
Trenton, NJ 08625-0360
609-292-7837
http://www.state.nj.us/health/
Disability Served: all

New Jersey Developmental Disabilities Division

PO Box 726, Capitol Center
Trenton, NJ 08625-0726
609-292-7260
Disability Served: developmentally disabled

New Jersey Mental Health Services Division

PO Box 727, Capitol Center
Trenton, NJ 08625-0727
609-777-0702
Disability Served: mental health

New Jersey Office of Elder and Disabled Affairs

CN 712
Trenton, NJ 08625-0712
609-588-2611
Disability Served: all

New Jersey Rehabilitation and Disability Program

PO Box 052
Trenton, NJ 08625
609-984-6550
Disability Served: all

New Jersey Workers Compensation Division

PO Box 110
Trenton, NJ 08625-0110
609-2312414
Disability Served: all

Social Security Disability Determination Service—New Jersey (New Brunswick)

506 Jersey Avenue
New Brunswick, NJ 08901
732-418-8685
http://www.ssa.gov/
Disability Served: all

Social Security Disability Determination Service—New Jersey (Newark)

124 Halsey Street, Fourth Floor
Newark, NJ 07102
973-648-3572
http://www.ssa.gov/
Disability Served: all

NEW MEXICO

New Mexico Agency on Aging

LaVilla Riviera Building
228 East Palace Avenue
Santa Fe, NM 87501
505-827-7640
Disability Served: all

New Mexico Department of Education

Education Building
300 Don Gaspar
Santa Fe, NM 87501-2786
505-827-6516
http://sde.state.nm.us/
Disability Served: all

New Mexico Department of Health

1190 St. Francis Drive
PO Box 26110
Santa Fe, NM 87502-6110
505-827-2613
Disability Served: all

New Mexico Division of Behavioral Health Services

1190 St. Francis Drive
PO Box 26110
Santa Fe, NM 87502-6110
505-827-2601
Disability Served: mental health

New Mexico Division of Vocational Rehabilitation
Education Building
300 Don Gaspar
Santa Fe, NM 87501-2786
505-827-3511
Disability Served: all

New Mexico Workers Compensation Administration
PO Box 27198
Albuquerque, NM 87125
505-841-6074
http://www.state.nm.us/wca/
Disability Served: all

NEW YORK

New York Commission on Quality of Care for the Mentally Disabled
99 Washington Avenue, Suite 1002
Albany, NY 12210
518-473-4057
Disability Served: all

New York Department of Education
Education Building, Washington Avenue
Albany, NY 12234
518-474-5844
http://www.nysed.gov/
Disability Served: all

New York Department of Health
Corning Tower, Empire State Plaza
Albany, NY 12237-0001
518-474-2011
http://www.health.state.ny.us/
Disability Served: all

New York Mental Retardation and Developmental Disabilities Agency
44 Holland Avenue
Albany, NY 12229
518-473-1997
Disability Served: developmentally disabled

New York Office of Aging
Building Two, Empire State Plaza
Albany, NY 12223-1251
518-474-4425
http://www.aging.state.ny.us/nysofa/
Disability Served: all

New York Office of Mental Health
44 Holland Avenue
Albany, NY 12229
518-474-4403
http://www.omh.state.ny.us/
Disability Served: mental health

New York Vocational and Educational Services for Individuals with Disabilities
Room 1606, One Commerce Plaza
Albany, NY 12234
518-474-2714
Disability Served: all

New York Workers Compensation Board
180 Livingston Street
Brooklyn, NY 11248
718-802-6700
http://www.wcb.state.ny.us/
Disability Served: all

Social Security Administration Region II—New York
26 Federal Plaza, Room 40-102
New York, NY 10278
212-264-2500
http://www.ssa.gov/
Disability Served: all

Social Security Disability Determination Service—New York (Brooklyn)
300 Cadman Plaza West, 13th Floor
Brooklyn, NY 11201-2701
718-522-8013
http://www.ssa.gov/
Disability Served: all

Social Security Disability Determination Service—New York (Buffalo)
Ellicott Square Building, Room 650
295 Main Street
Buffalo, NY 14203-2412
716-847-3927
http://www.ssa.gov/
Disability Served: all

Social Security Disability Determination Service—New York (Endicott)

Building #16, Second Floor
Glendale Technology Park
Endicott, NY 13760
607-741-4188
http://www.ssa.gov/
Disability Served: all

Social Security Disability Determination Service—New York (Jamaica)

92-31 Union Hall Street, Sixth Floor
Jamaica, NY 11433-1127
718-262-4336
http://www.ssa.gov/
Disability Served: all

Social Security Disability Determination Service—New York (Manhattan)

22 Cortlandt Street, Fourth Floor
New York, NY 10007-3107
212-240-3516
http://www.ssa.gov/
Disability Served: all

NORTH CAROLINA

North Carolina Department of Public Instruction

301 North Wilmington Street
Raleigh, NC 27601-2825
919-715-1299
http://www.dpi.state.nc.us/
Disability Served: all

North Carolina Developmental Disability Council

PO Box 29526
Raleigh, NC 27626-0526
919-733-6566
Disability Served: developmentally disabled

North Carolina Division for the Deaf and Hard of Hearing

PO Box 29526
Raleigh, NC 27626-0526
919-733-5199
Disability Served: hearing

North Carolina Division of Aging

PO Box 29526
Raleigh, NC 27626-0526
919-733-3983
Disability Served: all

North Carolina Division of Mental Health, Developmental Disabilities, and Substance Abuse Services

PO Box 29526
Raleigh, NC 27626-0526
919-733-7011
Disability Served: mental health

North Carolina Division of Vocational Rehabilitation Services

PO Box 29526
Raleigh, NC 27626-0526
919-733-3364
Disability Served: all

North Carolina Health Director's Office

PO Box 27687
Raleigh, NC 27611
919-715-4125
Disability Served: all

North Carolina Services for the Blind

309 Ash Avenue
Raleigh, NC 27606
919-733-9822
Disability Served: vision

NORTH DAKOTA

North Dakota Department of Health

600 East Boulevard Avenue
Bismarck, ND 58505-0200
701-328-2372
http://www.ehs.health.state.nd.us/ndhd/
Disability Served: all

North Dakota Department of Public Instruction
600 East Boulevard Avenue
Bismarck, ND 58505-0440
701-328-4572
http://www.sendit.nodak.edu/dpi/
Disability Served: all

North Dakota Division of Aging Services
600 East Boulevard Avenue
Bismarck, ND 58505
701-328-2577
Disability Served: all

North Dakota Division of Disabilities Services
600 East Boulevard Avenue
Bismarck, ND 58505
701-328-2768
Disability Served: all

North Dakota Division of Mental Health and Substance Abuse
600 East Boulevard Avenue
Bismarck, ND 58505
701-328-2769
Disability Served: mental health

North Dakota Workers Compensation Bureau
500 East Front Avenue
Bismarck, ND 58504-5685
701-328-3800
Disability Served: all

Social Security Disability Determination Service—North Dakota
600 South Second Street, Suite 4
Bismarck, ND 58504-5603
http://www.ssa.gov/
Disability Served: all

OHIO

Ohio Bureau of Services for the Visually Impaired
400 East Campus View Boulevard
Columbus, OH 43235-4604
614-438-1255
Disability Served: vision

Ohio Department of Aging
50 West Broad Street, Ninth Floor
Columbus, OH 43215-5928
614-466-5500
Disability Served: all

Ohio Department of Education
66 South Front Street, Room 810
Columbus, OH 43215-4183
614-466-2329
http://www.ode.ohio.gov/
Disability Served: all

Ohio Department of Health
PO Box 118
Columbus, OH 43266-0588
614-466-2253
http://www.ohio.gov/doh/
Disability Served: all

Ohio Department of Mental Health
30 East Broad Street, Eighth Floor
Columbus, OH 43215
614-466-2337
http://www.mh.state.oh.us/
Disability Served: mental health

Ohio Department of Mental Retardation and Developmental Disabilities
30 East Broad Street, Room 1280
Columbus, OH 43266-0415
614-466-5214
http://www.ohio.gov/dmr/
Disability Served: developmentally disabled

Ohio Rehabilitation Services Commission
400 East Campus View Boulevard
Columbus, OH 43235-4604
614-438-1210
Disability Served: all

Ohio Workers Compensation Bureau
30 West Spring Street, 29th Floor
Columbus, OH 43266 0538
614-466-8751

http://www.bwc.state.oh.us/
Disability Served: all

Social Security Disability Determination Service—Ohio
400 East Campus View Boulevard
Columbus, OH 43235-4604
614-438-1501
http://www.ssa.gov/
Disability Served: all

OKLAHOMA

Oklahoma Department of Education
2500 North Lincoln Boulevard
Oklahoma City, OK 73105
405-521-3301
http://www.sde.state.ok.us/
Disability Served: all

Oklahoma Department of Health
1000 NE Tenth Street
Oklahoma City, OK 73117-1299
405-271-4200
http://www.health.state.ok.us/
Disability Served: all

Oklahoma Department of Mental Health
PO Box 53277
Oklahoma City, OK 73152-3277
405-522-3908
http://www.state.ok.us/~dmhsas/
Disability Served: mental health

Oklahoma Department of Rehabilitation Services
3535 NW 58th Street, Suite 500
Oklahoma City, OK 73112
405-951-3400
Disability Served: all

Oklahoma Division of Aging Services
PO Box 25352
Oklahoma City, OK 73125
405-521-2327
Disability Served: all

Oklahoma Division of Developmental Disabilities Services
PO Box 25352
Oklahoma City, OK 73125
405-521-6267
Disability Served: developmentally disabled

Oklahoma Office of Handicapped Concerns
2712 Villa Prom Shephard Mall
Oklahoma City, OK 73107-2423
405-521-3756
Disability Served: all

Social Security Disability Determination Service—Oklahoma
240 West Wilshire, Suite B6
Oklahoma City, OK 73116
405-840-7770
http://www.ssa.gov/
Disability Served: all

OREGON

Oregon Commission for the Blind
535 SE 12th Street
Portland, OR 97214
503-731-3221
http://www.cfb.state.or.us/
Disability Served: vision

Oregon Department of Education
255 Capitol Street NE
Salem, OR 97310-0203
503-373-3573
http://www.ode.state.or.us/
Disability Served: all

Oregon Division of Health
PO Box 14450
Portland, OR 97214-0450
503-731-4000
Disability Served: all

Oregon Division of Mental Health and Developmental Disabilities Services
2575 Bittern Street NE
Salem, OR 97310
503-945-9499
Disability Served: developmentally disabled, mental health

Oregon Division of Senior and Disabled Services
500 North Summer Street NE
Salem, OR 97310-1015
503-945-5811
Disability Served: all

Oregon Division of Vocational Rehabilitation
500 North Summer Street NE
Salem, OR 97310-1018
503-945-5880
Disability Served: all

Oregon Workers Compensation Division
350 Winter Street NE
Salem, OR 97310
503-945-7881
Disability Served: all

PENNSYLVANIA

Office of Vocational Rehabilitation
1700 Labor and Industry Building
Seventh and Forster Streets
Harrisburg, PA 17120
717-787-5244
http://www.dli.state.pa.us/ovr/index.htm
Disability Served: all

Pennsylvania Department of Aging
400 Market Street, Sixth Floor
Rachel Carson State Office Building
Harrisburg, PA 17107-2301
717-783-1550
Disability Served: all

Pennsylvania Department of Education
333 Market Street
Harrisburg, PA 17126-0333
717-787-5820
http://www.cas.psu.edu/pde.html
Disability Served: all

Pennsylvania Department of Health
PO Box 90
Harrisburg, PA 17108
717-787-6436
http://www.state.pa.us/PA_Exec/Health
Disability Served: all

Pennsylvania Division of Mental Health
Box 2675
Harrisburg, PA 17105
717-787-6443
Disability Served: mental health

Pennsylvania Division of Mental Retardation
Box 2675
Harrisburg, PA 17105
717-787-3700
Disability Served: developmentally disabled

Pennsylvania Workers Compensation Bureau
Labor and Industry Building
Harrisburg, PA 17120
717-787-5421
Disability Served: all

Social Security Administration Region III—Philadelphia
PO Box 8788
Philadelphia, PA 19107
215-597-0596
http://www.ssa.gov/
Disability Served: all

Social Security Disability Determination Service—Pennsylvania (Harrisburg)
1171 South Cameron, Room 104
Harrisburg, PA 17104
717-783-3620
http://www.ssa.gov/
Disability Served: all

Social Security Disability Determination Service—Pennsylvania (Wilkes-Barre)
264 Highland Park Boulevard
PO Box R
Wilkes-Barre, PA 18702
717-824-8971
http://www.ssa.gov/
Disability Served: all

PUERTO RICO

Social Security Disability Determination Service—Puerto Rico
Plaza Mercantile Building, 14th Floor
Stop 27 1/2, Ponce de Leon Avenue
Hato Rey, PR 00918
787-754-8925
http://www.ssa.gov/
Disability Served: all

RHODE ISLAND

Rhode Island Department of Elderly Affairs
160 Pine Street
Providence, RI 02903
401-277-2894
http://www.state.ri.us/stdept/sd23.htm
Disability Served: all

Rhode Island Department of Health
Three Capitol Hill
Providence, RI 02908-5097
401-277-2231
http://www.state.ri.us/stdept/sd29.htm
Disability Served: all

Rhode Island Department of Mental Health, Retardation, and Hospitals
600 New London Avenue
Cranston, RI 02920
401-464-3201
http://www.state.ri.us/stdept/sd45.htm
Disability Served: mental health

Rhode Island Division of Developmental Disabilities
600 New London Avenue
Cranston, RI 02920
401-464-3234
Disability Served: developmentally disabled

Rhode Island Office of Elementary and Secondary Education
Shepard Building
255 Westminster Street
Providence, RI 02903
401-277-4600
Disability Served: all

Rhode Island Workers Compensation Unit
610 Manton Avenue
Providence, RI 02909
401-457-1701
Disability Served: all

Social Security Disability Determination Service—Rhode Island
40 Fountain Street
Providence, RI 02903
401-222-3182
http://www.ssa.gov/
Disability Served: all

SOUTH CAROLINA

South Carolina Department of Disabilities and Special Needs
PO Box 4706
Columbia, SC 29240
803-737-6444
http://www.state.sc.us/ddsn/
Disability Served: all

South Carolina Department of Education
1429 Senate Street
Columbia, SC 29201
803-734-8815
http://www.state.sc.us/sde/
Disability Served: all

South Carolina Office of Health Services
2600 Bull Street
Columbia, SC 29201
803-737-3900
Disability Served: all

South Carolina Workers Compensation Commission
PO Box 1715
Columbia, SC 29202-1715
803-737-5744
Disability Served: all

SOUTH DAKOTA

Social Security Disability Determination Service—South Dakota
817 West Russell, Suite 101
Sioux Falls, SD 57104-1317
http://www.ssa.gov/
Disability Served: all

South Dakota Department of Health
600 East Capitol
Pierre, SD 57501-3185
605-773-3361
http://www.state.sd.us/state/executive/doh/
Disability Served: all

South Dakota Division of Rehabilitation Services
500 East Capitol
Pierre, SD 57501
605-773-6283
Disability Served: all

South Dakota Division of Services to the Blind and Visually Impaired
500 East Capitol
Pierre, SD 57501
605-773-3228
Disability Served: vision

South Dakota Office of Adult Services on Aging
700 Governors Drive
Pierre, SD 57501
605-773-3656
Disability Served: all

TENNESSEE

Tennessee Aging Commission
500 Deaderick Street, Ninth Floor
Nashville, TN 37243-0860
615-741-2056
Disability Served: all

Tennessee Department of Education
Sixth Floor, Andrew Johnson Tower
710 James Robertson Parkway
Nashville, TN 37243-0375
615-741-2731
http://www.state.tn.us/education/
Disability Served: all

Tennessee Division of Blind Services
400 Deaderick Street
Nashville, TN 37248-0001
615-313-4914
Disability Served: vision

Tennessee Division of Mental Health Services
Tenth Floor, Andrew Johnson Tower
710 James Robertson Parkway
Nashville, TN 37243-0675
615-532-6767
Disability Served: mental health

Tennessee Division of Mental Retardation Services
Andrew Johnson Tower
710 James Robertson Parkway
Nashville, TN 37243-0675
615-532-6530
Disability Served: developmentally disabled

Tennessee Hearing Impaired Council
400 Deaderick Street
Nashville, TN 37248-0001
615-313-4913
Disability Served: hearing

Tennessee Rehabilitative Services
400 Deaderick Street
Nashville, TN 37248-0001
615-313-4714
Disability Served: all

TEXAS

Social Security Administration Region VI—Dallas
1301 Young Street, Suite 130
Dallas, TX 75202-5433
214-767-4281
http://www.ssa.gov/
Disability Served: all

Texas Commission for the Blind
PO Box 12866
Austin, TX 78711-2866
512-451-8494
http://link.tsl.state.tx.us/.www/TCB.dir
Disability Served: vision

Texas Commission for the Deaf and Hard of Hearing
PO Box 12904
Austin, TX 78711-2904
512-451-8494
http://www.state.tx.us/agency/335.html
Disability Served: hearing

Texas Department of Aging
Box 12786
Austin, TX 78711
512-424-6840
http://link.tsl.state.tx.us/tx/TDOA
Disability Served: all

Texas Department of Health
1100 West 49th Street
Austin, TX 78756-3199
512-548-7375
http://www.tdh.state.tx.us/
Disability Served: all

Texas Department of Mental Health and Mental Retardation
PO Box 12668
Austin, TX 78711-2668
512-206-4588
http://www.mhmr.state.tx.us/
Disability Served: mental health

Texas Developmental Disabilities Planning Council
4900 North Lamar Street
Austin, TX 78751-2399
512-424-4080
Disability Served: developmentally disabled

Texas Division of Workers Compensation
PO Box 149104
Austin, TX 78714-9104
512-322-3486
Disability Served: all

Texas Education Agency
1701 North Congress Avenue
Austin, TX 78701-1494
512-463-9008
http://www.tea.state.tx.us/
Disability Served: all

Texas Rehabilitation Commission
4900 North Lamar Street
Austin, TX 78751-2399
512-424-4003
http://www.rehab.state.tx.us/frtgate.html
Disability Served: all

UTAH

Utah Department of Health
Box 142802
Salt Lake City, UT 84114-2802
801-538-6111
http://www.hlunix.hl.state.ut.us/
Disability Served: all

Utah Developmental Disabilities Council
555 East 300 South, Room 201
Salt Lake City, UT 84102
801-533-4128
Disability Served: developmentally disabled

Utah Division of Aging and Adult Services
PO Box 45500
Salt Lake City, UT 84145-0500
801-538-3910
Disability Served: all

Utah Division of Mental Health
PO Box 45500
Salt Lake City, UT 84145-0500
801-538-4270
Disability Served: mental health

Utah Division of Services for People with Disabilities
PO Box 45500
Salt Lake City, UT 84145-0500
801-538-4200
Disability Served: all

Utah Services for the Deaf and Hard of Hearing
5709 South 1500 West
Salt Lake City, UT 84123
801-263-4860
Disability Served: hearing

Utah Services for the Visually Handicapped
309 East 100 South
Salt Lake City, UT 84111
801-533-9393
Disability Served: vision

VERMONT

Social Security Disability Determination Service—Vermont
Two Pilgrim Park Road, Second Floor
Waterbury, VT 05676
802-241-2463
http://www.ssa.gov/
Disability Served: all

Vermont Department of Aging and Disability
103 South Main Street, State Complex
Waterbury, VT 05671-0201
802-241-2400
Disability Served: all

Vermont Department of Developmental and Mental Health Services
103 South Main Street
State Complex
Waterbury, VT 05671-1601
802-241-2610
Disability Served: mental health

Vermont Department of Education
State Office Building
120 State Street
Montpelier, VT 05620
802-828-3147
http://www.state.vt.us/educ/
Disability Served: all

Vermont Department of Social and Rehabilitation Services
103 South Main Street, State Complex
Waterbury, VT 05671-2401
802-241-2101
Disability Served: all

Vermont Workers Compensation and Minimum Wage Division
National Life Building, Drawer 20
Montpelier, VT 05620-3401
802-828-2286
Disability Served: all

VIRGIN ISLANDS

Social Security Disability Determination Service—Virgin Islands
Nisky Shopping Center, First Floor
St. Thomas, VI 00802
http://www.ssa.gov/
Disability Served: all

VIRGINIA

Social Security Disability Determination Service—Virginia (Fairfax)
11150 Main Street, Suite 200
Fairfax, VA 22030-5066
703-934-7405
http://www.ssa.gov/
Disability Served: all

Social Security Disability Determination Service—Virginia (Richmond)
8004 Franklin Farms Drive
PO Box K-300
Richmond, VA 23288-0300
804-662-7026
http://www.ssa.gov/
Disability Served: all

Social Security Disability Determination Service—Virginia (Roanoke)
111 Franklin Road, SE, Suite 250
Roanoke, VA 24011

540-857-7748
http://www.ssa.gov/
Disability Served: all

Social Security Disability Determination Service—Virginia (Virginia Beach)
PO Box 5090
Virginia Beach, VA 23471-0900
804-363-3800
http://www.ssa.gov/
Disability Served: all

Virginia Department for the Deaf and Hard of Hearing
1602 Rolling Hills Drive
Ratcliffe Building, Suite 203
Richmond, VA 63229
804-662-9502
Disability Served: hearing

Virginia Department for the Rights of Virginians with Disabilities
Ninth Street Office Building, Ninth Floor
Richmond, VA 23219
804-225-2042
Disability Served: all

Virginia Department for the Visually Handicapped
397 Azalea Avenue
Richmond, VA 23227
804-371-3145
Disability Served: vision

Virginia Department of Aging
1600 Forest Avenue, Suite 102
Richmond, VA 63229
804-662-9333
Disability Served: all

Virginia Department of Education
PO Box 2120
Richmond, VA 23216-2120
804-371-0576
Disability Served: all

Virginia Department of Health
PO Box 2448
Richmond, VA 23218
804-786-3561
Disability Served: all

Virginia Department of Mental Health, Retardation, and Substance Abuse Services
PO Box 1797
Richmond, VA 23218
804-786-3921
Disability Served: mental health

Virginia Department of Rehabilitative Services
8004 Franklin Farms Drive
PO Box K300
Richmond, VA 23288
804-662-7000
Disability Served: all

WASHINGTON

Social Security Administration Region X—Seattle
2201 Sixth Avenue
Seattle, WA 98121
206-615-2105
http://www.ssa.gov/
Disability Served: all

Social Security Disability Determination Service—Washington (Renton)
1119 SW Seventh Street
Renton, WA 98057-3025
206-277-7000, 800-843-4440
Disability Served: all

Social Security Disability Determination Service—Washington (Spokane)
1330 North Washington, #2080, MS/B32-13
Spokane, WA 99201-2314
509-533-2200, 800-572-5299
Disability Served: all

Social Security Disability Determination Service—Washington (Tumwater)
Airdustrial Park, Building L2
Tumwater, WA 98504
206-753-2990
Disability Served: all

Washington Aging and Adult Services
PO Box 45050
Olympia, WA 98504-5050
360-902-7797
Disability Served: all

Washington Department of Health
PO Box 47890
Olympia, WA 98504-7890
360-753-5871
http://www.doh.wa.gov/
Disability Served: all

Washington Department of Public Instruction
PO Box 47200
Olympia, WA 98504-7200
360-753-6738
http://www.ospi.wednet.edu/
Disability Served: all

Washington Health and Rehabilitative Services
PO Box 45060
Olympia, WA 98504-5060
360-902-7799
Disability Served: all

WEST VIRGINIA

Social Security Disability Determination Service—West Virginia (Charleston)
Mason Building, Second Floor
1206 Quarrier Street
Charleston, WV 25301
304-353-4200
http://www.ssa.gov/
Disability Served: all

Social Security Disability Determination Service—West Virginia (Clarksburg)
153 West Main Street, Suite 607
Clarksburg, WV 26301
304-624-0200
http://www.ssa.gov/
Disability Served: all

West Virginia Bureau of Public Health
Building Three, Room 518
State Capitol Complex
Charleston, WV 25305-0501
304-558-2971
Disability Served: all

West Virginia Commission on Aging
1900 Kanawha Boulevard
State Capitol Complex
Charleston, WV 25305
304-558-3317
Disability Served: all

West Virginia Department of Education
Building Six, Room 358
State Capitol Complex
Charleston, WV 25305-0330
304-558-2681
Disability Served: all

West Virginia Division of Developmental Disabilities
Building Six, Room 617
State Capitol Complex
Charleston, WV 25305
304-558-0627
Disability Served: developmentally disabled

West Virginia Division of Mental Health and Community Rehabilitative Services
Building Six, Room 617
State Capitol Complex
Charleston, WV 25305
304-558-0627
Disability Served: mental health

West Virginia Division of Rehabilitation Services
State Capitol Complex
PO Box 50890
Charleston, WV 25305-0890
304-766-4601
Disability Served: all

West Virginia Workers Compensation Division

PO Box 3151
4700 MacCorkle Avenue SE
Charleston, WV 25332
304-926-5048
Disability Served: all

WISCONSIN

Social Security Disability Determination Service—Wisconsin

722 Williamson Street
Madison, WI 53703
608-266-1981
http://www.ssa.gov/
Disability Served: all

Wisconsin Aging Bureau

PO Box 7851
Madison, WI 53707-7851
608-266-3840
Disability Served: all

Wisconsin Community Mental Health Bureau

PO Box 7851
Madison, WI 53707-7851
608-266-3249
Disability Served: mental health

Wisconsin Department of Public Instruction

PO Box 7841
Madison, WI 53707-7841
608-266-1771
http://badger.state.wi.us/agencies/dpi/
Disability Served: all

Wisconsin Developmental Disabilities Bureau

PO Box 7851
Madison, WI 53707-7851
608-266-9329
Disability Served: developmentally disabled

Wisconsin Division of Health

PO Box 309
Madison, WI 53707-0309
608-266-1511
Disability Served: all

Wisconsin Division of Vocational Rehabilitation

PO Box 7852
Madison, WI 53707-7852
608-266-2168
Disability Served: all

WYOMING

Social Security Disability Determination Service—Wyoming

1780 West Land Road, Suite 107
Cheyenne, WY 82001-3333
http://www.ssa.gov/
Disability Served: all

Wyoming Department of Education

Hathaway Building, Second Floor
2300 Capitol Avenue
Cheyenne, WY 82002-0050
307-777-7675
http://www.k12.wy.us/
Disability Served: all

Wyoming Division of Behavioral Health Community Programs

446 Hathaway Building
Cheyenne, WY 82002-0710
307-777-7094
Disability Served: mental health

Wyoming Division of Developmental Disabilities

117 Hathaway Building
Cheyenne, WY 82002
307-777-7821
Disability Served: developmentally disabled

Wyoming Division of Public Health

Hathaway Building, Fourth Floor
Cheyenne, WY 82002-0480
307-777-6186
Disability Served: all

Wyoming Division of Vocational Rehabilitation

Herschler Building
122 West 25th Street
Cheyenne, WY 82002
307-777-7389
Disability Served: all

Wyoming Division of Workers Safety and Compensation
Herschler Building
122 West 25th Street
Cheyenne, WY 82002-0070
307-777-7441
Disability Served: all

Wyoming Office of Aging
139 Hathaway Building
Cheyenne, WY 82002-0710
307-777-6780
Disability Served: all

Hospitals and Other Medical Organizations

These medical facilities serve persons with disabilities, injuries, chronic ilnesses, and debilitating conditions. Services vary, and some hospitals cater to specific illnesses or conditions.

Bloorview Children's Hospital
25 Buchan Court
Willowdale, ON M2J 4S9 Canada
416-494-2222
Disability Served: all

Children's Medical Services—Atlanta Clinic
2600 Skyland Drive, NE
Atlanta, GA 30319
404-679-4700
Disability Served: all

Children's National Medical Center
111 Michigan Avenue, NW
Washington, DC 20010
202-884-5000
Disability Served: all

Department of Medicine and Surgery Veterans Administration
810 Vermont Avenue, NW
Washington, DC 20420
202-223-2596
Disability Served: all

Gillette Children's Specialty Healthcare
200 East University Avenue
St Paul, MN 55101
612-291-2848, 800-578-4266
Disability Served: all

Medic Alert
2323 Colorado Avenue
Turlock, CA 95382
800-432-5378
http://www.medicalert.org
Disability Served: all

National Rehabilitation Hospital
102 Irving Street, NW
Washington, DC 20010-2949
202-877-1440
Disability Served: all

Poudre Valley Hospital
1024 Lemay Avenue
Ft Collins, CO 80524
970-495-7000
Disability Served: all

RehabCare Group
Lakeway Regional Hospital
726 McFarland
Morristown, TN 37814
615-586-2930
Disability Served: all

Shriners Hospital for Children—Spokane
PO Box 2472
Spokane, WA 99210-2472
509-455-7844
Disability Served: all

Shriners Hospitals for Children, Portland
3101 SW Sam Jackson Park Road
Portland, OR 97201
503-241-5090
http://www.shcc.org
Disability Served: orthopedic

Independent Living Centers

Independent Living Centers provide services to people with disabilities, including information and referral, independent living skills instruction, personal assistant services, advocacy, group and individual counseling, assistive technlogy resources,and socialization and recreation activities.

ALABAMA

Birmingham Independent Living Center
206 13th Street South
Birmingham, AL 35233
205-251-2223
Disability Served: all

Independent Living Center
5304 B Overlook Road
Mobile, AL 36618
334-460-0301
Disability Served: all

ARKANSAS

Delta Resource Center for Independent Living
400 Main, Suite 118
Pine Bluff, AR 71601
870-535-2222
Disability Served: all

Mainstream Living
1818 South University
Little Rock, AR 72204
501-280-0012
Disability Served: all

Our Way, Inc.
10434 West 36th Street
Little Rock, AR 72204
501-225-5030
Disability Served: physically disabled

Sources for Community Independent Living Services
212 Poplar
Fayetteville, AR 72703
501-442-5600
Disability Served: all

Spa Area Independent Living Services, Inc.
600 Main
Hot Springs, AR 71913
501-624-7710
Disability Served: all

Twin River Community Living Facility
201 Dodd Creek Road
Mountain Home, AR 72653
870-425-4515
Disability Served: all

ALASKA

Access Alaska, Inc.
3710 Woodland Drive, Suite 900
Anchorage, AK 99517
907-248-4777, 800-770-4488
http://www.alaska.net/~access
Disability Served: all

Hope Cottages, Inc.
540 West International Airport Road, #100
Anchorage, AK 99518
907-561-5335
Disability Served: all

Independent Living Center of the Kenai Peninsula, Kodiak, and the Aleutian Islands
PO Box 2474
Homer, AK 99603
907-235-7911
http://www.xyz.net/~ilc
Disability Served: all

Southeastern Alaska Independent Living, Inc.
PO Box 35097
2490 Industrial Boulevard
Juneau, AK 99803
907-789-9665
Disability Served: all

ARIZONA

Arizona Bridge to Independent Living
1229 East Washington Street
Phoenix, AZ 85034
602-256-2245, 800-280-2245
http://www.abil.org
Disability Served: all

Community Outreach Program for the Deaf
268 West Adams Street
Tucson, AZ 85705
520-792-1906
Disability Served: hearing

DIRECT Center for Independence
1023 North Tyndall Avenue
Tucson, AZ 85719
520-624-6452, 800-342-1853
http://www.azstarnet.com/~direct
Disability Served: all

New Horizons Independent Living Center, Inc.
8085 East Manly, Suite 1
Prescott Valley, AZ 86314
520-772-1266
http://www.northlink.com/~nhilc
Disability Served: all

Services Maximizing Independent Living
1495 South Fourth Avenue
Yuma, AZ 85366
520-329-6881
Disability Served: all

CALIFORNIA

Access Center of San Diego
1295 University Avenue, Suite 10
San Diego, CA 92103
619-293-3500
Disability Served: all

Adult Independence Development Center
1601 Civic Center Drive, #100
Santa Clara, CA 95050-4109
408-985-1243
Disability Served: all

Center for Independence of the Disabled
875 O'Neill Avenue
Belmont, CA 94002
415-595-0783
Disability Served: all

Center for Independent Living of Fresno
3475 West Shaw Avenue, #101
Fresno, CA 93711
209-276-6777
Disability Served: all

Central Coast Center for Independent Living
234 Capitol Street, Suites A-B
Salinas, CA 93901
831-757-2968
Disability Served: all

Central Coast Center for Independent Living (CCCIL)
1395 41st Avenue, #B
Capitola, CA 95010
408-462-8720
Disability Served: all

Community Rehabilitation Services
4716 Cesar Chavez Avenue
Los Angeles, CA 90022
213-266-0453
Disability Served: all

Community Resources for Independence
2999 Cleveland Avenue, Suite D
Santa Rosa, CA 95403
707-528-2745
Disability Served: all

Community Resources for Independent Living
439 A Street
Hayward, CA 94541
510-881-5743
Disability Served: all

Disabled Resources Center, Inc.
2750 East Spring Street, Suite 100
Long Beach, CA 90806
562-427-1000
Disability Served: all

FREED—Foundation of Resources for Equality and Employment for the Disabled
154 Hughes Road, Suite 1
Grass Valley, CA 95945
916-272-1732
http://www.freed.org
Disability Served: all

Humboldt Access Project, Inc.
812 6th Street
Eureka, CA 95501
707-445-8404
Disability Served: all

Independence Northwest, Inc.
14402 Haynes Street, Suite 103
Van Nuys, CA 91401
818-785-6934
Disability Served: all

Independent Living Center of Kern County
1927 Eye Street
Bakersfield, CA 93301-4409
805-325-1063
Disability Served: all

Independent Living Center of Southern California (Lancaster Office)
356-B East Avenue
Lancaster, CA 93535
805-945-6602
Disability Served: all

Independent Living Resource Center
423 West Victoria
Santa Barbara, CA 93101
805-963-0595
Disability Served: physically disabled

Independent Living Resource Center of Contra Costa County
3811 Alhambra Avenue
Martinez, CA 94553
510-229-9200
Disability Served: all

Independent Living Resource Center San Francisco
649 Mission Street, Third Floor
San Francisco, CA 94105
415-543-6222
Disability Served: all

Independent Living Services of Northern California
555 Rio Lindo Avenue
Chico, CA 95926-1847
530-893-8527
Disability Served: all

Marin Center for Independent Living
710 Fourth Street
San Rafael, CA 94901
415-459-6245
Disability Served: all

Modesto Independent Living Center
221 McHenry Avenue
Modesto, CA 95354
209-521-7260
http://www.drail.org
Disability Served: all

Mother Lode Independent Living Center
83 South Stewart, #305
Sonora, CA 95370
209-532-0963
Disability Served: all

Placer Independent Resource Services
11768 Atwood Road, Suite 29
Auburn, CA 95603
530-885-6100
Disability Served: all

Resources for Independent Living
1211 H Street, #B
Sacramento, CA 95814
916-446-3074
Disability Served: all

Rolling Start, Inc.
570 West 4th Street, #103
San Bernardino, CA 92401-2810
909-884-2129
Disability Served: all

San Gabriel Valley (Branch Office)
963 West Badillo Street
Covina, CA 91722
818-967-0995
Disability Served: all

San Joaquin Independent Living Center
4505 Precissi, Suite A
Stockton, CA 95207
209-477-8143
Disability Served: all

Service Center for Independent Living
109 South Spring Street
PO Box 1296
Claremont, CA 91711-1296
909-621-6722
Disability Served: all

Southeast Center for Independent Living
12458 Rives Avenue, #202
Downey, CA 90242
562-862-6531
Disability Served: all

Westside Center for Independent Living
12901 Venice Boulevard
Los Angeles, CA 90066
310-390-3611
http://www.wcil.org
Disability Served: all

COLORADO

Atlantis Community Inc.
PO Box 9598
Denver, CO 80209-3195
303-733-9324
Disability Served: all

Center for Independence
1600 Ute Avenue, Suite 100
Grand Junction, CO 81501
970-241-0315
Disability Served: all

Center for People with Disabilities
948 North Street, Suite 7
Boulder, CO 80304
303-442-8662
Disability Served: all

Center on Deafness
1900 Grant Street, Suite 1010
Denver, CO 80203
303-839-8022
Disability Served: hearing

Colorado Springs Independence Center
21 East Las Animas
Colorado Springs, CO 80903
719-471-8181
Disability Served: all

Connections for Independent Living
1024 Ninth Avenue, Suite E
Greeley, CO 80631
970-352-8682, 800-887-5828
Disability Served: all

Disability Center for Independent Living
777 Grant Street, #100
Denver, CO 80203
303-837-1020
Disability Served: all

Disabled Resource Services
424 Pine Street, Suite 101
Ft Collins, CO 80524
970-482-2700
http://www.fortnet.org/FCAUW
Disability Served: all

Goodwill Home Care Program
247 South Santa Fe Avenue
Pueblo, CO 81003
719-544-9336
Disability Served: all

Greeley Center for Independent Living
2780 28th Avenue
Greeley, CO 80631
970-339-2444
Disability Served: all

Sangre De Cristo Center for Independent Living
803 West Fourth Street
Pueblo, CO 81003-3207
719-546-1271
Disability Served: all

CONNECTICUT

Chapel Haven, Inc.
1040 Whalley Avenue
New Haven, CT 06515
203-397-1714
Disability Served: all

Disabilities Network of Eastern Connecticut
107 Route 32
North Franklin, CT 06254
860-823-1898
Disability Served: all

Disability Resource Center of Fairfield County
80 Ferry Boulevard
Stratford, CT 06497
203-378-6977
Disability Served: all

Independence Northwest, Inc.
1183 New Haven Road, Suite 200
Naugatuck, CT 06770
203-729-3299
Disability Served: all

Independence Unlimited, Inc.
2138 Silas Deane Highway, #2
Rocky Hill, CT 06067
860-257-3221
Disability Served: all

New Horizons, Inc.
37 Bliss Road
Unionville, CT 06085
203-675-4711
Disability Served: all

DELAWARE

Easter Seal Independent Living Center
24 Read's Way
New Castle, DE 19720-2405
302-324-4488
Disability Served: all

Independent Living, Inc.
1800 North Broom Street, Suite 210
Wilmington, DE 19802
302-429-6693
Disability Served: all

DISTRICT OF COLUMBIA

DC Center for Independent Living
1400 Florida Avenue, NE, Suite 3
Washington, DC 20002
202-388-0033
Disability Served: all

FLORIDA

Briarwood Center for Independent Living
1023 SE 4th Avenue, Suite 23
Gainesville, FL 32601
352-378-7474
Disability Served: all

Caring and Sharing Center for Independent Living, Inc.
1130 94th Avenue North
St Petersburg, FL 33702
813-577-0065
Disability Served: all

Center for Independent Living in Central Florida, Inc.
720 North Denning Drive
Winter Park, FL 32789
407-623-1070
Disability Served: all

Center for Independent Living of Jacksonville
5243 Beach Boulevard
Jacksonville, FL 32207
904-399-8484
Disability Served: all

Center for Independent Living of Northern Florida
572C Appleyard Drive
Tallahassee, FL 32304
850-575-9621
Disability Served: all

Center for Independent Living of Southwest Florida
3626 Evans Avenue
Ft Myers, FL 33901
941-277-1447
Disability Served: all

Independent Living Center of Broward
8857 West McNab Road
Tamarac, FL 33321
954-722-6400
Disability Served: all

Pinellas Center for the Visually Impaired, Inc.
6925 112th Circle North, Suite 103
Largo, FL 33773
813-544-4433
Disability Served: vision

Self-Reliance, Inc. Center for Independent Living
12310 North Nebraska Avenue, Suite F
Tampa, FL 33612
813-975-6560
Disability Served: all

SFADA, Inc.
1335 NW 14th Street, Suite 200
Miami, FL 33125
305-325-0901
Disability Served: all

Suncoast Center for Independent Living
1945 Northgate Boulevard
Sarasota, FL 34234
941-351-9545
Disability Served: all

GEORGIA

Disability Action Center of Georgia
246 Sycamore Street, #100
Decatur, GA 30030
404-687-8890
Disability Served: all

DisABILITY LINK
755 Commerce Drive, Suite 415
Decatur, GA 30030-2618
404-687-8890, 800-239-2507 (GA)
TTY: 404-687-9175
Disability Served: all

Living Independence For Everyone (LIFE), Inc.
17-21 East Travis Street
Savannah, GA 31406
912-920-2414
Disability Served: all

Roosevelt Warm Springs Institute for Rehabilitation
PO Box 1000
Warm Springs, GA 31830
706-655-5000
http://www.rooseveltrehab.org/
Disability Served: all

Southwest District Independent Living Program
PO Box 50753
Albany, GA 31703
912-446-0977
Disability Served: all

HAWAII

Big Island Center for Independent Living
1190 Waianuenue Avenue
Hilo, HI 96720
808-935-3777
Disability Served: all

Hawaii Center for Independent Living
414 Kuwili Street, Suite 102
Honolulu, HI 96817
808-522-5400
http://hcil.org
Disability Served: all

Kailua Kona Center for Independent Living—West Hawaii
PO Box 2197
Kealakekua, HI 96750
808-323-2221
Disability Served: all

Kauai Center for Independent Living
PO Box 3529
Lihue, HI 96766
808-245-4034
Disability Served: all

Maui Center for Independent Living
1464 Lower Main Street, Suite 105
Wailuku, HI 96793
808-242-4966
Disability Served: all

IDAHO

Access for Idaho
PO Box 4185
Pocatello, ID 83201
208-232-2747
Disability Served: all

Disability Action Center NW
124 East Third Street
Moscow, ID 83843
208-883-0523
Disability Served: all

Eastern Idaho Center for Independence
PO Box 86
Blackfoot, ID 83221
208-785-9648
Disability Served: all

Housing Southwest #2
1108 West Finch Drive
Nampa, ID 83651
208-467-7461
Disability Served: all

Idaho Commission for the Blind
341 West Washington Street
Boise, ID 83702
208-334-3220
http://www.icbvi.state.id.us
Disability Served: vision

LInc. (Branch Office)
1002 Shoshone Street East
Twin Falls, ID 83301
208-733-1712
Disability Served: all

Living Independence Network Corporation
708 West Franklin Street
Boise, ID 83702
208-336-3335
Disability Served: all

ILLINOIS

Access Living
310 South Peoria, Suite 201
Chicago, IL 60607
312-226-5900
Disability Served: all

Center for Comprehensive Services
PO Box 2825
Carbondale, IL 62902
618-529-3060
Disability Served: all

Central Illinois Center for Independent Living
614 West Glen
Peoria, IL 61614
309-682-3500
Disability Served: all

Dupage Center for Independent Living
739 Roosevelt Road
Building 8, Suite 109
Glen Ellyn, IL 60137
TTY: 630-469-2300
Disability Served: all

Fox River Valley Center for Independent Living
730 West Chicago Street
Elgin, IL 60123
847-695-5818
Disability Served: all

Illinois-Iowa Independent Living Center
PO Box 6156
Rock Island, IL 61204-6156
319-324-1460
Disability Served: all

IMPACT, Inc.
2735 East Broadway
Alton, IL 62002
618-462-1411
Disability Served: all

Independent Living Centers
120 East A Street
Belleville, IL 62220-1401
618-235-9988
Disability Served: all

Lake County Center for Independent Living
706 East Hawley
Mundelein, IL 60060
847-949-4440
Disability Served: all

Living Independence for Everyone (IL)
1328 East Empire Street
Bloomington, IL 61701
309-663-5433, 888-543-3245
Disability Served: all

Northwestern Illinois Center for Independent Living
229 First Avenue, Suite 2
Rock Falls, IL 61071
815-625-7860
TTY: 815-625-6863
http://www.incil.org/nicil.html
Disability Served: all

Opportunities for Access
3300 West Broadway, Suite 5
Mt Vernon, IL 62864
618-244-9212, 800-938-7400
Disability Served: all

Options Center for Independent Living
61 Meadowview Center
Kankakee, IL 60901
815-936-0100
Disability Served: all

PACE, Inc.
1317 East Florida Avenue, Suite 27
Urbana, IL 61801
217-344-5433
TTY: 217-344-5024
Disability Served: all

Progress Center for Independent Living
7521 Madison Street
Forest Park, IL 60130
708-209-1500
Disability Served: all

Southern Illinois Center for Independent Living
PO Box 627
100 North Glenview Drive
Carbondale, IL 62903
618-457-3318
Disability Served: all

Springfield Center for Independent Living
426 West Jefferson
Springfield, IL 62702
217-523-2587
http://www.angelfire.com/sc/drnsc/drn
Disability Served: all

Will Grundy Center for Independent Living
2415 #A West Jefferson Street
Joliet, IL 60435
815-729-0162
Disability Served: all

INDIANA

Damar Homes, Inc.
PO Box 41
Camby, IN 46113
317-856-5201
Disability Served: all

Everybody Counts, Inc.
9111 Broadway
Merrillville, IN 46410
219-769-5055, 888-769-3636
Disability Served: all

Indianapolis Resource Center for Independent Living
8383 Craig Street, Suite 130
Indianapolis, IN 46250
317-596-6440
Disability Served: all

League for the Blind & Disabled, Inc.
5800 Fairfield Avenue, Suite 210
Ft Wayne, IN 46807
219-745-5491
http://www.ft-wayne.in.us/health/lbd/lbd.html
Disability Served: all

IOWA

Central Iowa Center for Independent Living
1024 Walnut Street
Des Moines, IA 50309-3424
515-243-1742, 888-503-2287
http://www.raccoon.com/~cicil/
Disability Served: all

Evert Conner Rights & Resources Center for Independent Living
20 East Market Street
Iowa City, IA 52240
319-338-3870
Disability Served: all

Hope Haven, Inc.
1800 19th Street
Rock Valley, IA 51247
712-476-2737
http://www.hopehealth.org
Disability Served: all

League of Human Dignity, Inc.
1417-1/2 West Broadway
Council Bluffs, IA 51501
712-323-6863, 800-843-5774
Disability Served: all

KANSAS

Coalition for Independence
4631 Orville, #102
Kansas City, KS 66102
913-287-0999
Disability Served: all

Cowley County Developmental Services
PO Box 133
Arkansas City, KS 67005
316-442-3575, 316-221-6140
Disability Served: developmentally disabled

Independence, Inc.
2001 Haskell Avenue
Lawrence, KS 66046
785-841-0333
http://lawrence.ks.us/~indepinc
Disability Served: all

Independent Living Resource Center (KS)
3330 West Douglas, Suite 101
Wichita, KS 67203-5415
316-942-6300
Disability Served: all

Kansas Rehabilitation Center for the Blind
2516 West Sixth Street
Topeka, KS 66606
785-296-3311
Disability Served: vision

LINK, Inc.
2401 East 13th Street
Hays, KS 67601
785-625-6942
Disability Served: all

Research and Training Center on Independent Living
University of Kansas
4089 Dole Building
Lawrence, KS 66045
913-864-4095
Disability Served: all

Resource Center for Independent Living
PO Box 257
Osage City, KS 66523
785-528-3105
Disability Served: all

Three Rivers Independent Living Center
408 Lincoln Avenue
Wamego, KS 66547
913-456-9915
Disability Served: all

Topeka Independent Living Program
VA Medical Center
2200 Gage Boulevard
Topeka, KS 66622
785-271-4350
Disability Served: all

Topeka Independent Living Resource Center
501 SW Jackson, Suite 100
Topeka, KS 66603
785-233-4572
Disability Served: all

KENTUCKY

Center for Accessible Living
1304-U Chestnut
Murray, KY 42071
270-753-7676, 888-261-6194
http://www.cfal.com
Disability Served: all

Center for Accessible Living
981 South Third Street
Louisville, KY 40203
502-589-6620
http://cfal.com
Disability Served: all

Community Alternatives Kentucky
1604 Louisville Road
Frankfort, KY 40601
502-875-5777
Disability Served: all

LOUISIANA

Independent Living Center, Inc.
320 North Carrollton Avenue, #2C
New Orleans, LA 70119
504-484-6400
Disability Served: all

New Horizons (Alexandria Satellite Office)
1756 Elliott Street
Alexandria, LA 71301
318-484-3596
Disability Served: all

New Horizons (Monroe Satellite Office)
2000A Tower Drive
Monroe, LA 71201
318-323-4374
Disability Served: all

New Horizons, Inc.
6670 Saint Vincent Avenue
Shreveport, LA 71106
318-865-1000
Disability Served: all

New Orleans Resources for Independent Living
1555 Poydras Street, Suite 1500
New Orleans, LA 70112
504-522-1955
Disability Served: all

New Orleans Resources for Independent Living
701 Main Street, Suite A
Baton Rouge, LA 70802
504-379-3840
Disability Served: all

Southwest Louisiana Independence Center
3505 5th Avenue, Suite A-2
Lake Charles, LA 70607
318-477-7194
Disability Served: all

Volunteers of America Independent Living Program
3900 North Causeway Boulevard, Suite 750
Metairie, LA 70002
504-834-7015
Disability Served: vision

MAINE

Maine Independent Living Services
424 Western Avenue
Augusta, ME 04330-6014
207-622-5434
http://www.mainetoday.koz.com/maine/mils
Disability Served: all

Maine Mental Health Connections
150 Union Street
Bangor, ME 04401
207-941-2907
Disability Served: mental health

Motivational Services, Inc.
114 State Street
Augusta, ME 04330
207-626-3465
Disability Served: all

Shalom House, Inc.
400 Congress Street
PO Box 560
Portland, ME 04112
207-874-1080
Disability Served: mentally disabled

MARYLAND

Independence Now, Inc.
818 Roeder Road, Suite 202
Silver Spring, MD 20910
301-587-4162
Disability Served: all

MCIL Resources for Independent Living
5807 Harford Road
Baltimore, MD 21214
410-444-1400
Disability Served: all

MASSACHUSETTS

AD-LIB, Inc.
215 North Street
Pittsfield, MA 01201
413-442-7047
Disability Served: all

Boston Center for Independent Living
95 Berkeley Street, Suite 206
Boston, MA 02116
617-338-6665
TTY: 617-338-6662
Disability Served: all

Cape Organization for the Rights of the Disabled
1019 Iyannough Road, #4
Hyannis, MA 02601
508-775-8300
http://www.capecod.net/cord
Disability Served: all

Center for Living & Working, Inc.
484 Main Street, Suite 345
Worcester, MA 01608
508-798-0350
Disability Served: all

Independence Associates, Inc.
10 Oak Street, Second Floor
Taunton, MA 02780
508-880-5325
Disability Served: all

Independent Living Center of the North Shore and Cape Ann
27 Congress Street, Suite 107
Salem, MA 01970
978-741-0077
Disability Served: all

Massachusetts Commission for the Blind—ILC
88 Kingston Street
Boston, MA 02111
617-727-5550
Disability Served: all

MetroWest Center for Independent Living
63 Fountain Street, Suite 401
Framingham, MA 01701
508-875-7853
Disability Served: all

Renaissance Program
21 Branch Street
Lowell, MA 01851
978-454-7944
Disability Served: all

Southeast Center for Independent Living
170 Pleasant Street, 3rd Floor East
Fall River, MA 02721
508-679-9210
Disability Served: all

Stavros Center for Independent Living
691 South East Street
Amherst, MA 01002
413-256-0473, 800-442-1185
Disability Served: all

Student Independent Living Experience
5 Randolph Street
Canton, MA 02021
617-828-2440
Disability Served: all

MICHIGAN

Ann Arbor Center for Independent Living
2568 Packard Road, Georgetown Mall
Ann Arbor, MI 48104-6831
734-971-0277
Disability Served: all

ARC Detroit
51 West Hancock
Detroit, MI 48201
313-831-0202
Disability Served: all

Association for Retarded Citizens of Muskegon County
1145 East Wesley Avenue
Muskegon, MI 49442
616-777-2006
Disability Served: all

Blue Water Center for Independent Living
310 Water Street
Port Huron, MI 48060
810-987-9337, 800-527-2167
Disability Served: all

Capital Area Center for Independent Living
3815 West St Joseph Street, #D
Lansing, MI 48917-3623
517-334-7830
Disability Served: all

CIL of Mid-Michigan
1206 James Savage Road
Midland, MI 48640
517-835-4041
Disability Served: all

Commission for the Blind
411-G East Genesee
Saginaw, MI 48603
517-758-1765
Disability Served: vision

Cristo Rey Hispanic Handicapper's Center
1717 North High Street
Lansing, MI 48906
517-372-4700
Disability Served: all

Family and Children Services
1608 Lake Street
Kalamazoo, MI 49001
616-344-0202
Disability Served: all

Grand Rapids Center for Independent Living
3600 Camelot Drive SE
Grand Rapids, MI 49546
616-949-1100
Disability Served: all

Grand Traverse Area Community Living Center
935 Barlow
Traverse City, MI 49684
616-941-7150
Disability Served: all

Great Lakes Center for Independent Living
4 East Alexandrine, Suite 104
Detroit, MI 48201
313-832-3371
Disability Served: all

Jewish Association for Residential Care for Persons with Developmental Disabilities
28366 Franklin Road
Southfield, MI 48034
248-352-5272
Disability Served: all

Lakeshore Center for Independent Living
426 Century Lane
Holland, MI 49423
616-396-5326
Disability Served: all

Oakland/Macomb Center for Independent Living
3765 East 15 Mile Road
Sterling Heights, MI 48310
810-268-4160
http://www.omcil.org
Disability Served: all

Southeastern Michigan Center for Independent Living
1200 6th Avenue, 15th Floor
Detroit, MI 48226
313-256-1524
Disability Served: all

MINNESOTA

Accessible Space, Inc.
2550 University Avenue West, Suite 330N
St Paul, MN 55114
651-645-7271, 800-466-7722
http://www.accessiblespace.org
Disability Served: all

Center for Independent Living of Northeastern Minnesota
205 West 2nd Street, #200
Duluth, MN 55802
218-722-8911
Disability Served: all

Center for Independent Living of Northeastern Minnesota, Inc.
Mesabi Mall, Suite 11
Hibbing, MN 55746
218-262-6675
Disability Served: all

Deaf Blind Services
2344 Nicollet Avenue, #420
Minneapolis, MN 55404
612-871-4788
Disability Served: all

Freedom Resource Center for Independent Living, Inc.
3505 8th Street South, Suite 7
Moorhead, MN 56560
218-236-0459
http://www.macil.org/freedom
Disability Served: all

Independence Crossroads, Inc.
8932 Old Cedar Avenue South
Bloomington, MN 55425
612-854-8004
Disability Served: all

Metropolitan Center for Independent Living, Inc.
1600 University Avenue West, Suite 16
St. Paul, MN 55104
612-646-8342
Disability Served: all

OPTIONS, Interstate Resource Center for Independent Living
1010 Central Avenue, NE
East Grand Forks, MN 56721
218-773-6100
Disability Served: all

Southeastern Minnesota Center for Independent Living
1306 Seventh Street NW
Rochester, MN 55901
507-285-1815, 888-460-1815
http://www.macil.orglsemcil#lsemcil
Disability Served: all

Southern Minnesota Independent Living Enterprises & Services
709 South Front Street
Mankato, MN 56001
507-345-7139
http://www.macil.org/smiles/
Disability Served: all

Southwestern Center for Independent Living
109 South Fifth Street, Suite 700
Marshall, MN 56258
507-532-2221
http://www.macil.org/swcil/swcil/
Disability Served: all

Vinland Center
PO Box 308, Lake Independence
Loretto, MN 55357
612-479-3555
http://www.vinlandcenter.org
Disability Served: all

MISSISSIPPI

Gulf Coast Independent Living Center
18 John M. Taturn Industrial Drive
Hattiesburg, MS 39401
601-544-4860
Disability Served: all

Jackson Independent Living Center
300 Capers Avenue
Jackson, MS 39203
601-961-4140
Disability Served: all

Living Independence for Everyone (MS)
754 North President Street, Suite 2
Jackson, MS 39202
601-969-0601
Disability Served: all

Signature Works, Inc.
PO Drawer 30
Hazelhurst, MS 39083
601-894-1771
Disability Served: all

MISSOURI

Access II Independent Living Center
1020 South Main Street
Gallatin, MO 64640
816-663-2423
Disability Served: all

Independence Center
4380 West Pine Boulevard
St Louis, MO 63108
314-533-6511
Disability Served: all

Life Skills Foundation
10176 Corporate Square Drive, Suite 100
St. Louis, MO 63132-2924
314-567-7705
Disability Served: all

Paraquad
311 North Lindbergh Boulevard
St Louis, MO 63141
314-567-1558
Disability Served: all

Places for People, Inc.
4120 Lindell Boulevard
St Louis, MO 63108
314-535-5600
http://placesforpeople.org
Disability Served: mental health

Rehabilitation Institute, Kansas City
3011 Baltimore
Kansas City, MO 64108
816-751-7700
Disability Served: all

Rural Advocates for Independent Living
715 South Baltimore
Kirksville, MO 63501
816-627-7245
Disability Served: all

SEMO Alliance for Disability Independence, Inc.
121 South Broadview, Suite 12
Cape Girardeau, MO 63703
573-651-6464
Disability Served: all

Services for Independent Living
1301 Vandiver Drive, Suite Q
Columbia, MO 65202
573-874-1646
Disability Served: all

Southwest Center for Independent Living
1856 East Cinderella
Springfield, MO 65804
417-886-1188
Disability Served: all

Whole Person, Inc.
3100 Main, Suite 206
Kansas City, MO 64111
816-561-0304
Disability Served: all

MONTANA

Living Independently for Today and Tomorrow, Inc.
929 Broadwater Square
Billings, MT 59101
406-259-5181, 800-669-6319
Disability Served: all

Montana Independent Living Project
PO Box 5415
Helena, MT 59604
406-442-5755
Disability Served: all

North Central Independent Living Services
104 Second Street South, Suite 101
Great Falls, MT 59405
406-452-9834
Disability Served: all

Summit Independent Living Center
700 Southwest Higgins, Suite 101
Missoula, MT 59803
406-728-1630
http://www.summitilc.com
Disability Served: all

NEBRASKA

Center for Independent Living of Central Nebraska, Inc.
1804 South Eddy Street
Grand Island, NE 68801
308-382-9255
Disability Served: all

League of Human Dignity Independent Living Center
400 Elm Street
Norfolk, NE 68701
402-371-4475
Disability Served: all

League of Human Dignity, Inc.
1701 P Street
Lincoln, NE 68508-1741
402-441-7871
Disability Served: all

League of Human Dignity, Omaha Center for Independent Living
5513 Center Street
Omaha, NE 68106
402-595-1256
Disability Served: all

NEVADA

Nevada Association for the Handicapped
6200 West Oakey
Las Vegas, NV 89102
702-870-7050
Disability Served: all

Northern Nevada Center for Independent Living
999 Pyramid Way
Sparks, NV 89431
702-353-3599
Disability Served: all

NEW HAMPSHIRE

Granite State Independent Living Foundation
PO Box 7268
Concord, NH 03301
603-228-9680
Disability Served: all

NEW JERSEY

Camden Independent Living Center
30 North Fifth Street, Suites 222-223
Camden, NJ 08102
856-966-0800
Disability Served: all

Center for Independent Living of South Jersey
1200 Delsea Drive
Westville, NJ 08093
609-853-6490
Disability Served: all

DAWN, Inc.
7 Boardwalk
Sparta, NJ 07871
973-729-7155
Disability Served: all

DIAL, Inc.
66 Mt Prospect Avenue, Building C-1
Clifton, NJ 07013-1918
973-470-8090
Disability Served: all

Heightened Independence & Progress
2815 Kennedy Boulevard, Suite 2G
Jersey City, NJ 07306
201-413-1200
Disability Served: all

MOCEANS Center for Independent Living, Inc.
279 Broadway, 1st Floor
Long Branch, NJ 07740
732-571-4884
Disability Served: all

Project Freedom, Inc.
PO Box 8898
Trenton, NJ 08650
609-448-2998
Disability Served: all

Resources for Independent Living
Masonville Square
115 Centerton Road, Suite 6
Mt Laurel, NJ 08054
609-273-7630
Disability Served: all

Total Living Center, Inc.
231 Philadelphia Avenue
PO Box 342
Egg Harbor City, NJ 08215
609-965-3734
Disability Served: all

NEW MEXICO

Independent Living Resource Center (NM)
4401 B Lomas, NE
Albuquerque, NM 87110
505-266-5022
Disability Served: all

New Vistas Adult Services
PO Box 2364
Santa Fe, NM 87504
505-471-1001
Disability Served: all

Southern New Mexico Center for Independent Living
424 North Downtown Mall, Suite 100
Las Cruces, NM 88001-1218
505-526-5016
Disability Served: all

NEW YORK

Access to Independence & Mobility
271 East First Street
Corning, NY 14830
607-962-8225
http://www.aim/auto.com
Disability Served: all

Action Toward Independence, Inc.
2927 Route 6
Slate Hill, NY 10973
914-355-2030
Disability Served: all

ARISE, Inc., Center for Independent Living
1065 James Street, Suite 110
Syracuse, NY 13203
315-472-3171
Disability Served: all

Barrier Free Living
270 East Second Street
New York, NY 10009
212-677-6668
http://barrierfreeliving.org
Disability Served: all

Batavia Center for Independent Living
61 Swan Street
Batavia, NY 14020
716-343-4524
Disability Served: all

Bronx Independent Living Services
3525 Decatur Avenue
Bronx, NY 10467
718-515-2800
Disability Served: all

Brooklyn Center for Independence
2044 Ocean Drive, Suite B3
Brooklyn, NY 11230
718-998-3000
Disability Served: all

Capital District Center for Independence
855 Central Avenue
Albany, NY 12206
518-459-6422
Disability Served: all

Center for Independence of the Disabled in New York
841 Broadway, Room 205
New York, NY 10003
212-674-2300
Disability Served: all

Directions in Independent Living
512 West State Street
Olean, NY 14760
716-373-4602
Disability Served: all

Finger Lakes Independence Center
609 West Clinton Street, Suite 112
Ithaca, NY 14850
607-272-2433
Disability Served: all

Glens Falls Independent Living Center
25 Sherman Avenue
PO Box 453
Glens Falls, NY 12801
518-792-3537
Disability Served: all

Harlem Independent Living Center
5-15 West 125th Street
New York, NY 10027
212-369-2371
Disability Served: all

Independent Living Center of Amsterdam, Inc.
12 Chestnut Street
Amsterdam, NY 12010
518-842-3561
Disability Served: all

Independent Living, Inc.
5 Washington Terrace
Newburgh, NY 12550-5338
914-565-1162
Disability Served: all

Long Island Center for Independent Living, Inc.
3601 Hempstead Turnpike, Suite 312
Levittown, NY 11756
516-796-0144
Disability Served: all

Massena Independent Living Center
156 Center Street
Massena, NY 13662
315-764-9442
Disability Served: all

Nassau County Office for the Physically Challenged
1550 Franklin Avenue
Mineola, NY 11501
516-535-3147
Disability Served: physically disabled

Native American Independent Living Services
3108 Main Street
Buffalo, NY 14214
716-836-0822
Disability Served: all

Niagara Frontier Center for Independent Living
1522 Main Street
Niagara Falls, NY 14305-2522
716-284-2452
Disability Served: all

North Country Center for Independent Living
159 Margaret Street, Suite 202
Plattsburgh, NY 12901-1837
518-563-9058
Disability Served: all

Northern Regional Center for Independent Living
165 Mechanic Street
Watertown, NY 13601-2711
315-785-8703
http://nrcil.org
Disability Served: all

Options for Independence
75 Genesee Street
Auburn, NY 13021
315-255-3447, 800-496-9148
Disability Served: all

Queens Independent Living Center
140-40 Queens Boulevard
Jamaica, NY 11435
718-658-2526
Disability Served: all

Resource Center for Accessible Living, Inc.
Center for Independent Living
602 Albany Avenue
Kingston, NY 12401
914-331-0541
Disability Served: all

Rochester Center for Independent Living
758 South Avenue
Rochester, NY 14620-2237
716-442-6470
http://rcil.org
Disability Served: all

Rockland Independent Living Center
238 North Main Street
Spring Valley, NY 10977-4001
914-426-0707
Disability Served: all

Southern Tier Independence Center
24 Prospect Avenue
Binghamton, NY 13901
607-724-2111
http://www.stic-cil.org
Disability Served: all

Southwestern Independent Living Center, Inc.
843 North Main Street
Jamestown, NY 14701
716-661-3010
Disability Served: all

Staten Island Center for Independent Living, Inc.
470 Castleton Avenue
Staten Island, NY 10301
718-720-9016
Disability Served: all

Taconic Resources for Independence
82 Washington Street, Suite 214
Poughkeepsie, NY 12601
914-452-3913
Disability Served: all

Troy Resource Center Independent Living
Troy Atrium, Broadway & 4th Street
Troy, NY 12180
518-274-0701
Disability Served: all

Visions/Services for the Blind and Visually Impaired
120 Wall Street, 16th Floor
New York, NY 10005
212-425-2255, 888-CIL-8333
http://www.cilpubs.com
Disability Served: vision

Westchester County Independent Living Center
297 Knollwood Road
White Plains, NY 10607
914-682-3926
Disability Served: all

Westchester Disabled on the Move
984 North Broadway, Suite L-1
Yonkers, NY 10701
914-968-4717
Disability Served: all

NORTH CAROLINA

Guilford Advocacy Project
PO Box 86
Greensboro, NC 27402
910-272-0501
Disability Served: all

Live Independently Networking Center
PO Box 1135
Newton, NC 28658
704-464-0331
Disability Served: all

Pathways for the Future
PO Box 2077
Sylva, NC 28779
704-631-1167
Disability Served: all

Programs for Accessible Living
5701 Executive Center, Suite 320
Charlotte, NC 28212
704-537-0550
Disability Served: all

NORTH DAKOTA

Dakota Center for Independent Living
3111 East Broadway Avenue
Bismark, ND 58501
701-222-3636
Disability Served: all

Fraser Hall, Inc.
2902 South University Drive
Fargo, ND 58103
701-223-3301
Disability Served: all

OHIO

Ability Center of Greater Toledo
5605 Monroe
Sylvania, OH 43560
419-885-5733
Disability Served: all

Access CIL, Inc.
35 South Jefferson
Dayton, OH 45402
937-341-5202
http://www.acils.com
Disability Served: all

Center for Independent Living Options
632 Vine Street, Suite 601
Cincinnati, OH 45202
513-241-2600
http://www.home.fuse.net/cilo/
Disability Served: all

HELP Foundation
3622 Prospect Avenue
Cleveland, OH 44115
216-361-3907
Disability Served: all

Independent Living Center of North Central Ohio
1 Marion Avenue, Suite 115C
Mansfield, OH 44903
419-526-6770
Disability Served: all

MOBILE, Inc. (Mid-Ohio Board for an Independent Living Environment, Inc.)
2040 Brice Road, Suite 100
Reynoldsburg, OH 43068
614-864-1199
TTY: 614-869-2038
http://mobileonline.org
Disability Served: all

Services for Independent Living
25100 Euclid Avenue, #105
Cleveland, OH 44117
216-731-1529
Disability Served: all

Tri-County Independent Living Center, Inc.
680 East Market Street, #205
Akron, OH 44304
330-762-0007
Disability Served: all

United Cerebral Palsy of Central Ohio
440 Industrial Mile Road
Columbus, OH 43228-2411
614-279-0109
Disability Served: all

OKLAHOMA

Ability Resources
110 South Hartford, Suite 115
Tulsa, OK 74120
918-592-1235
Disability Served: all

Green County Independent Living Resource Center
4100 SE Adams Road, Suite C-106
Bartlesville, OK 74006
918-335-1314, 800-559-0567
Disability Served: all

Oklahomans for Independent Living
321 South Third, Suite 2
McAlester, OK 74501
918-426-6220
Disability Served: all

Progressive Independence, Inc.
121 North Porter Avenue
Norman, OK 73071
405-321-3203
Disability Served: all

Sandra Beasley Independent Living Center
705 South Oakwood, Suite B-1
Enid, OK 73703
405-237-8508, 800-375-4358
Disability Served: all

OREGON

Central Oregon Resources for Independent Living
20436 Clay Pigeon Court
Bend, OR 97702
541-388-8103
Disability Served: all

Columbia Gorge Center
2940 Thomsen Road
Hood River, OR 97031
541-386-3520
Disability Served: all

Handicap Awareness & Support League II (Satellite)
222 West 6th Street
Medford, OR 97501
541-772-7820
Disability Served: all

Handicap Awareness & Support League—Independent Abilities Center
1252 Redwood Avenue
Grants Pass, OR 97527
541-479-4275
http://nonprof.edsnet.net/hasl
Disability Served: all

Independent Living Resources, Inc.
4506 SE Belmont Street, Suite 100
Portland, OR 97215
503-232-7411
Disability Served: all

Living Opportunities, Inc.
PO Box 1105
Medford, OR 97501
541-772-1503
Disability Served: all

SPOKES Unlimited
111 North 7th Street
Klamath Falls, OR 97601
541-883-7547
Disability Served: all

PENNSYLVANIA

Abilities in Motion
416 Blair Avenue
Reading, PA 19601
610-376-0010
Disability Served: all

Allied Services for the Handicapped
475 Morgan Highway
Scranton, PA 18501
717-348-2221
Disability Served: all

Anthracite Region Center for Independent Living
40 North Church Street, City Hall
Hazelton, PA 18201
717-455-9800, 800-777-9906
Disability Served: all

Brian's House, Inc.
1300 South Concord
West Chester, PA 19382
610-399-1175
Disability Served: all

Center for Independent Living of Central Pennsylvania
415 Fallowfield Road, Suite 101
Camp Hill, PA 17011-4906
717-731-1900, 800-323-6060
TTY: 717-737-1335
http://www.cilcp.org
Disability Served: all

Center for Independent Living of Southcentral Pennsylvania
3009 Walnut Avenue
Altoona, PA 16601
814-949-1905
Disability Served: all

Citizens for Independence and Access
3450 Industrial Drive
York, PA 17402-9050
717-840-9653
Disability Served: all

Community Resources for Independence
2222 Filmore Avenue
Erie, PA 16506
814-838-7222
http://www.crinet.org
Disability Served: all

Freedom Valley Disability Center
3607 Chapel Road
Newton Square, PA 19073
610-353-6640
Disability Served: all

Lehigh Valley Center for Independent Living
919 South Ninth Street
Allentown, PA 18103
610-770-9781
Disability Served: all

Liberty Resources, Inc.
1341 North Delaware Avenue, Suite 105
Philadelphia, PA 19125
215-634-2000
http://www.libertyresources.org
Disability Served: all

Life & Independence For Today
503 Arch Street Extension
St. Marys, PA 15857-1779
814-781-3050, 800-341-5438
http://users.penn.com/~lift
Disability Served: all

North Central Center for Independent Living
66 North Bull Run Crossing
Lewisburg, PA 17837
717-524-9695
Disability Served: all

Northeastern Pennsylvania Center for Independent Living
431 Wyoming Avenue, Lower Level
Scranton, PA 18503
717-344-7211
Disability Served: all

Three Rivers Center for Independent Living
7110 Penn Avenue
Pittsburgh, PA 15208-2434
412-371-7700
TTY: 412-371-9230
Disability Served: all

Tri-County Patriots for Independent Living
69 East Beau Street
Washington, PA 15301
412-223-5115
Disability Served: all

RHODE ISLAND

IN-SIGHT Independent Living
43 Jefferson Boulevard
Warwick, RI 02888
401-941-3322
Disability Served: vision

Ocean State Center for Independent Living
59 West Shore Road
Warwick, RI 02889
401-738-1013
http://www.oscil.org
Disability Served: all

PARI Independent Living Center
500 Prospect Street
Pawtucket, RI 02860
401-725-1966
Disability Served: all

SOUTH CAROLINA

SC Independent Living Council
810 Dutch Square Boulevard, Suite 214
Columbia, SC 29210
803-731-1607, 877-217-2331 (toll-free)
TTY: 803-731-1608
Disability Served: all

SOUTH DAKOTA

Adjustment Training Center, Inc.
607 North 4th Street
Aberdeen, SD 57401
605-229-0263
Disability Served: all

Opportunities for Independent Living
9 Fifth Avenue Southeast
Aberdeen, SD 57401
605-626-7037
Disability Served: all

Prairie Freedom Center for Independent Living
301 South Garfield Avenue, Suite 8
Sioux Falls, SD 57104
605-367-5630
Disability Served: all

Prairie Freedom Center for Independent Living of Yankton
413 West 15th, Suite 107
Yankton, SD 57078
605-668-2940
http://members.xoom.com/pfcily/index.htm
Disability Served: all

Western Resources for dis-ABLED Independence
36 East Chicago
Rapid City, SD 57701
605-394-1930, 800-226-3938 (SD)
Disability Served: all

TENNESSEE

Memphis Center for Independent Living
163 North Angelus
Memphis, TN 38104
901-726-6404
Disability Served: all

Tri-State Disability and Resource Center
5708 Uptain Road
Suite 350, Building 5800
Chattanooga, TN 37411
423-892-4774
Disability Served: all

TEXAS

ABLE Center for Independent Living
208 West 23rd Street
Odessa, TX 79761
915-580-3439
Disability Served: all

Austin Resource Center for Independent Living
400 West Hopkins, #101
San Marcos, TX 78666
512-396-5790
Disability Served: all

Crockett Resource Center for Independent Living
1020 Loop 304 East
Crockett, TX 75835
409-544-2811, 800-784-8710
Disability Served: all

Houston Center for Independent Living
7000 Regency Square Boulevard, #160
Houston, TX 77036-3209
713-974-4621
Disability Served: all

Independent Living Program
10118 Laurie Lane
Highlands, TX 77562
281-426-5765
Disability Served: all

Independent Living Research Utilization
2323 South Shepherd, Suite 1000
Houston, TX 77019
713-520-0232
Disability Served: all

LIFE/RUN Centers for Independent Living
3212 34th Street
Lubbock, TX 79410
806-795-5433
Disability Served: all

Panhandle Action Center for Independent Living Skills
3608 South Washington Street
Amarillo, TX 79110
806-352-1500
Disability Served: all

REACH of Dallas Resource Center on Independent Living
8625 King George, Suite 210
Dallas, TX 75235-2286
214-630-4796
http://web2.airmail.net/reachdal
Disability Served: all

REACH Resource Center on Independent Living of Denton
405 South Elm, Suite 202
Denton, TX 76201-6068
940-383-1062
Disability Served: all

REACH Resource Center on Independent Living of Ft. Worth
1205 Lake Street
Ft Worth, TX 76102-4501
817-870-9082
Disability Served: all

San Antonio Independent Living Services
1028 South Alamo
San Antonio, TX 78210
210-281-1878
Disability Served: all

Valley Association for Independent Living
105C East Expressway 83
Pharr, TX 78577
956-781-7733
Disability Served: all

UTAH

OPTIONS for Independence
1095 North Main
Logan, UT 84341
435-753-5353
http://www.optionsind.org
Disability Served: all

Redrock Center for Independence
515 West 300 North, #A
St George, UT 84770
801-673-7501
Disability Served: all

Utah Independent Living Center
3445 South Main Street
Salt Lake City, UT 84115-4453
801-466-5565
Disability Served: all

VERMONT

Vermont Center for Independent Living
11 East State Street
Montpelier, VT 05602
802-229-0501, 800-639-1522
Disability Served: all

Vermont Center for Independent Living—Bennington Office
532 Main Street
Bennington, VT 05201
802-447-0574
Disability Served: all

Vermont Center for Independent Living—Brattleboro Office
230 Main Street
Brattleboro, VT 05301
802-254-6851
Disability Served: all

VIRGINIA

Access Independence
312 West Cork Street
Winchester, VA 22601
540-662-4452
Disability Served: all

Appalachian Independence Center
230 Charwood Drive
Abingdon, VA 24210
540-628-2979
Disability Served: all

Blue Ridge Independent Living Center
1502-D Williamson Road, NE
Roanoke, VA 24012
540-342-1231
Disability Served: all

Central Virginia Independent Living Center
2900 West Broad Street
Richmond, VA 23230
804-353-6503
Disability Served: all

Endependence Center, Inc.
6320 North Center Drive
15 Koger Center, Suite 100
Norfolk, VA 23502
757-461-8007
Disability Served: all

Independence Resource Center
815 Cherry Avenue
Charlottesville, VA 22903
804-971-9629
Disability Served: all

Peninsula Center for Independent Living
2021-B Cunningham Drive, Suite 2
Hampton, VA 23666
757-827-0275
Disability Served: all

Virginia Department for the Visually Handicapped
210 Church Avenue SW, Suite 308
Roanoke, VA 24011
540-857-7122, 800-622-2155
http://www.cns.state.va.us/drh/
Disability Served: vision

Woodrow Wilson Center for Independent Living
Box 37, Route 250
Fishersville, VA 22939
540-332-7103
Disability Served: all

WASHINGTON

Center for Independence
PO Box 1247
Puyallup, WA 98372
253-845-5187
Disability Served: all

Community Services Center for the Deaf and Hard of Hearing
1609 19th Avenue
Seattle, WA 98122
206-322-4996
Disability Served: hearing

Designs for Independent Living
819 South Hatch
Spokane, WA 99202
509-535-9696
Disability Served: all

Epilepsy Association of Washington
3800 Aurora Avenue North, Suite 370
Seattle, WA 98103
206-547-4551
Disability Served: all

Greater Lakes Mental Health Care Access Center
9330 59th Avenue SW
Lakewood, WA 98499
253-581-6085
Disability Served: all

Independent Lifestyle Services
109 East 3rd, Suite 2
Ellensburg, WA 98926
509-962-9620
Disability Served: all

Independent Living Service Center
607 SE Everett Mall, Suite E
Everett, WA 98208
425-347-5768
Disability Served: all

Kitsap Community Action Program
1201 Park Avenue
Bremerton, WA 98337
360-377-0053
http://www.kcr.org
Disability Served: all

Lilac Blind Foundation
1212 North Howard
Spokane, WA 99201
509-328-9116, 800-422-7893
Disability Served: vision

Resource Center for the Handicapped
500 SW Seventh Street, Suite A
Renton, WA 98055
425-271-0587
http://www.rch.org
Disability Served: all

Tacoma Area Coalition of Individuals with Disabilities
6315 South 19th Street
Tacoma, WA 98466
253-565-9000
Disability Served: all

Washington Coalition of Citizens with Disabilitles
4649 Sunnyside North, Suite 100
Seattle, WA 98103
206-545-7055
Disability Served: all

WEST VIRGINIA

Appalachian Center for Independent Living
Elk Office Center
4710 Chimney Drive, Suite C
Charleston, WV 25302
304-965-0376, 800-642-3003
Disability Served: all

Mountain State Center for Independent Living
821 4th Avenue
Huntington, WV 25701
304-525-3324
Disability Served: all

Mountain State Center for Independent Living
329 Prince Street
Beckley, WV 25801
304-255-0122
Disability Served: all

Northern West Virginia Center for Independent Living
1130 Greenbag Road
Morgantown, WV 26505
304-296-6091, 800-834-4070
Disability Served: all

WISCONSIN

Access to Independence
2345 Atwod Avenue
Madison, WI 53704
608-242-8484, 800-362-9877
Disability Served: all

Center for Independent Living for Western Wisconsin, Inc.
University of Wisconsin
Stout Vocational Rehabilitation Building #106
Menomonie, WI 54751
715-232-2150
Disability Served: all

Great Rivers Independent Living Services, Inc.
4328 Mormon Coulee Road
La Crosse, WI 54601
888-474-5745
TTY: 888-378-2198
Disability Served: all

IndependenceFirst
600 West Virginia Street, Suite 301
Milwaukee, WI 53204
414-291-7520
http://www.independencefirst.org
Disability Served: all

Independent Living Program
1506 South Oneida Street
Appleton, WI 54915
920-738-2644
Disability Served: all

Inspiration Ministries
PO Box 948
Corner of Route 67 and County F
Walworth, WI 53184-0848
414-275-6131
http://inspirationministries.org
Disability Served: all

North Country Independent Living
2231 Catlin Avenue
Superior, WI 54880
715-392-9118, 800-924-1220
Disability Served: all

Options for Independent Living, Inc.
2900 Curry Lan
PO Box 9517
Green Bay, WI 54308-9517
920-465-1515, ext. 145, 888-465-1515, ext. 145
Disability Served: all

Wovenhearts
Wausau, WI 54401
715-675-4444
Disability Served: all

WYOMING

Rehabilitation Enterprises of Northeast Wyoming
245 Broadway
Sheridan, WY 82801
307-672-7481
http://www.renew-wyo.com
Disability Served: all

Western Wyoming Center for Independent Living
550 Main Street, #2
Lander, WY 82520
307-332-4889
Disability Served: all

Wyoming Independent Living Rehabilitation Center
305 West 1st Street
Casper, WY 82601
307-266-6956
Disability Served: all

CANADA

ALBERTA

Calgary Association for Independent Living
#7, 11th Street NE
Calgary, AB T2E 4Z2 Canada
403-263-6880
http://www.indie.ca/cailc/english/ilrcc/index.htm
Disability Served: all

BRITISH COLUMBIA

North Shore Disability Resource Centre
3158 Mountain Highway
North Vancouver, BC V7K 2H5 Canada
604-985-5371
http://nscweb.org/nsdrc
Disability Served: all

MANITOBA

Independent Living Resource Centre
201-294 Portage Avenue
Winnipeg, MB R3C 0B9 Canada
204-947-0194
http://www.pangea.ca/~ilrcwpg/
Disability Served: all

ONTARIO

Center for Independent Living in Toronto
205 Richmond Street West, #605
Toronto, ON M5V 1V3 Canada
416-599-2458
Disability Served: all

Daly Support Services Corporation
101-2410 Southvale Crescent
Ottawa, ON K1B 5K2 Canada
613-736-1182
Disability Served: all

Independent Living Center of Waterloo Region
3400 King Street East
Kitchener, ON N2A 4B2 Canada
519-894-8350
http://www.ilcwr.org/
Disability Served: all

Independent Living Resource Center (ONT)
1201 Jasper Drive, Suite B
Thunder Bay, ON P7B 6R2 Canada
807-345-6157, 800-461-3153
Disability Served: all

Niagara Center for Independent Living
211 Church Street
St. Catharines, ON L2R 3E8 Canada
905-684-7111, 800-668-1910
http://www.vaxxine.com/ncil/
Disability Served: all

Ottawa-Carleton Independent Living Center
369A Richmond Road
Ottawa, ON K2A 0E7 Canada
613-236-2558
Disability Served: all

Legal Assistance Organizations

These organizations provide legal assistance and advocacy services for persons with disabilities. Some of the agencies are governmental entities that provide protection and advocacy services.

ALABAMA

Alabama Disabilities Advocacy Program
PO Box 870395
Tuscaloosa, AL 35487-0395
205-348-4928, 800-826-1675
Disability Served: all

ALASKA

Alaska Protection & Advocacy for Persons with Developmental Disabilities
Advocacy Services of Alaska
615 East 82nd Avenue, Suite 101
Anchorage, AK 99518
907-344-1002
Disability Served: developmentally disabled

ARIZONA

Arizona Protection & Advocacy for Persons with Disabilities
Arizona Center for Law in the Public Interest
3724 North Third Street, Suite 300
Phoenix, AZ 85012
602-274-6287
Disability Served: all

DNA People's Legal Services, Inc.
PO Box 306
Window Rock, AZ 86515
520-871-4151
Disability Served: all

CALIFORNIA

Disability Rights Education and Defense Fund
2212 Sixth Street
Berkeley, CA 94710
510-644-2555, 800-466-4232
Disability Served: all

Legal Center for the Elderly and the Disabled
1722 J Street, Suite 19
Sacramento, CA 95814
916-446-4851
Disability Served: all

National Center for Youth Law
114 Sansome Street, Suite 900
San Francisco, CA 94104
415-543-3307
Disability Served: all

COLORADO

Estate Planning for Persons with Disabilities
3100 Arapahoe Avenue, #112
Boulder, CO 80303
Disability Served: all

The Legal Center for People with Disabilities and Older People
The Legal Center
455 Sherman Street, Suite 130
Denver, CO 80203
303-722-0300
Disability Served: all

CONNECTICUT

Office of Protection and Advocacy for Persons with Disabilities
60B Weston Street
Hartford, CT 06120
860-297-4300, 800-642-7303 (CT)
Disability Served: all

DELAWARE

Delaware Protection & Advocacy for Persons with Disabilities
144 East Market Street
Georgetown, DE 19947
302-856-0038
Disability Served: all

DISTRICT OF COLUMBIA

ABA Community on Legal Problems of the Elderly
1800 M Street, NW
Washington, DC 20036
202-331-2297
Disability Served: elderly

Commission on the Mentally Disabled
American Bar Assocation
1800 M Street, NW, 2nd Floor
Washington, DC 20036
202-331-2639
Disability Served: developmentally disabled

Information, Protection and Advocacy Center for Handicapped Individuals
4455 Connecticut Avenue, NW, #B100
Washington, DC 20008
202-966-8081
Disability Served: all

Legal Action Center
236 Massachusetts Avenue, NE, Suite 510
Washington, DC 20002
202-544-5478
Disability Served: all

National Senior Citizens Law Center
1101 14th Street, NW, Suite 400
Washington, DC 20005
202-289-6976
http://www.nsclc.org
Disability Served: elderly

United States Department of Labor
200 Constitution Avenue, NW
Washington, DC 20210
202-523-6666
Disability Served: all

FLORIDA

Florida Protection & Advocacy for Persons with Disabilities
2671 Executive Center Circle West
Tallahassee, FL 32301
850-488-9071
Disability Served: all

GEORGIA

Georgia Advocacy Office
1708 Peachtree Street, NW, Suite 505
Atlanta, GA 30309
404-885-1234, 800-537-2329
Disability Served: all

HAWAII

Hawaii Protection & Advocacy for Persons with Disabilities
1580 Makaloa Street, Suite 1060
Honolulu, HI 96814
808-949-2922
Disability Served: all

ILLINOIS

AIDS Legal Council of Chicago
220 South State Street
Chicago, IL 60604
312-427-8990
Disability Served: all

Attorney General's Office Disability Rights Advocacy Division
500 South Second Street
Springfield, IL 62706
217-524-6575
http://www.ag.state.il.us
Disability Served: all

Council for Disability Rights
176 West Adams, Suite 1830
Chicago, IL 60603
312-444-9484
http://www.disabilityrights.org
Disability Served: all

Disabled Americans Rally for Equality
4752 South Kilpatrick
Chicago, IL 60632
773-582-5930
Disability Served: all

Guardianship Services Associates
41 A South Boulevard
Oak Park, IL 60302
708-386-5398
Disability Served: all

Illinois Protection & Advocacy for Persons with Disabilities
11 East Adams, Suite 1200
Chicago, IL 60603
312-341-0022
Disability Served: all

Law Lab, Inc.
707 Skokie Boulevard
Northbrook, IL 60062
847-236-5920
Disability Served: all

Legal Clinic for the Disabled, Inc.
448 East Ontario Street, 6th Floor
Chicago, IL 60611
312-908-4463
Disability Served: all

United States Department of Health & Human Services Office for Civil Rights
105 West Adams Street, 16th Floor
Chicago, IL 60603
312-886-2359, 800-368-1019
Disability Served: all

United States Department of Labor/Office of Federal Contract Compliance Programs
Regional Office
230 South Dearborn, Suite 570
Chicago, IL 60604
312-353-1929
http://www.dol-esa.gov
Disability Served: all

INDIANA

Indiana Protection & Advocacy for Persons with Disabilities
850 North Meridian, Suite 2-C
Indianapolis, IN 46204
317-232-1150, 800-622-4845
Disability Served: all

IOWA

Iowa Protection & Advocacy Services, Inc.
3015 Merle Hay Road, Suite 6
Des Moines, IA 50310-1270
515-278-2502, 800-779-2502
Disability Served: mental health

KANSAS

Kansas Advocacy & Protective Services, Inc.
2601 Anderson Avenue, Suite 200
Manhattan, KS 66502
785-776-1541, 800-432-8276 (KS)
Disability Served: all

KENTUCKY

Kentucky Protection & Advocacy
100 Fair Oaks Lane, 3rd Floor
Frankfort, KY 40601
502-564-2967
Disability Served: physically disabled, mental health, developmentally disabled

LOUISIANA

Advocacy Center
225 Baronne Street, Suite 2112
New Orleans, LA 70112
504-522-2337
Disability Served: all

MARYLAND

Maryland Protection & Advocacy for Persons with Disabilities
2510 St Paul Street
Baltimore, MD 21218
410-235-4700
Disability Served: all

MASSACHUSETTS

Center for Public Representation
22 Green Street
Northampton, MA 01060
413-587-6265
Disability Served: mentally disabled

MICHIGAN

Michigan Protection & Advocacy for Persons with Disabilities
109 West Michigan, Suite 900
Lansing, MI 48933
517-487-1755
Disability Served: all

MINNESOTA

Minnesota Protection & Advocacy for Persons with Disabilities
430 First Avenue North, Suite 300
Minneapolis, MN 55401
612-332-1441, 800-292-4150
Disability Served: all

MISSOURI

Missouri Protection & Advocacy for Persons with Disabilities
925 South Country Club Drive
Jefferson City, MO 65109
573-893-3333
Disability Served: all

NEBRASKA

Nebraska Advocacy Services
215 Centennial Mall South, Suite 522
Lincoln, NE 68508
402-474-3183
Disability Served: mental health, physically disabled

NEVADA

Nevada Protection & Advocacy for Persons with Disabilities
2105 Capurro Way, Suite B
Sparks, NV 89431
702-789-0233
Disability Served: all

NEW HAMPSHIRE

New Hampshire Protection & Advocacy for Persons with Disabilities
PO Box 19
Concord, NH 03302
603-228-0432
Disability Served: all

NEW JERSEY

New Jersey Protection & Advocacy, Inc.
210 South Broad Street
Trenton, NJ 08625
609-292-1750
http://www.njpanda.org
Disability Served: all

NEW MEXICO

New Mexico Protection & Advocacy for Persons with Disabilities
1720 Louisiana Boulevard, NE
Albuquerque, NM 87110
505-256-3100, 800-432-4682 (NM)
Disability Served: all

NEW YORK

American Civil Liberties Union
132 West 43rd Street
New York, NY 10036
212-944-9800
Disability Served: all

NORTH DAKOTA

North Dakota Protection & Advocacy Project
400 East Broadway, Suite 616
Bismarck, ND 58501-4073
701-328-2950
http://www.ndcd.org/ndcpd/uapdis/pa.htmlndcp
Disability Served: all

OHIO

Ohio Protection & Advocacy for Persons with Disabilities
8 East Long Street, 5th Floor
Columbus, OH 43215
614-466-7264
Disability Served: all

OKLAHOMA

Oklahoma Protection & Advocacy for Persons with Disabilities
9726 East 42nd Street
Tulsa, OK 74146
918-664-5883
Disability Served: all

OREGON

Oregon Protection & Advocacy for Persons with Disabilities
310 SW 4th Avenue, Suite 625
Portland, OR 97204
503-243-2081
Disability Served: all

PENNSYLVANIA

David Ferleger, Esquire
37 South 20th Street, Suite 601
Philadelphia, PA 19103
215-567-2828
http://www.ferleger.com
Disability Served: all

Pennsylvania Protection & Advocacy for Persons with Disabilities
116 Pine Street
Harrisburg, PA 17101
717-236-8110, 800-692-7443
Disability Served: all

Public Interest Law Center of Philadelphia
125 South 9th Street, Suite 700
Philadelphia, PA 19107
215-627-7100
Disability Served: all

RHODE ISLAND

Rhode Island Protection & Advocacy for Persons with Disabilities
55 Bradford Street, 2nd Floor
Providence, RI 02903
401-831-3150
Disability Served: all

SOUTH CAROLINA

South Carolina Protection & Advocacy for Persons with Disabilities
3710 Landmark Drive, Suite 208
Columbia, SC 29204
803-782-0639
Disability Served: all

SOUTH DAKOTA

South Dakota Advocacy Services
221 South Central Avenue
Pierre, SD 57501-2453
605-224-8294, 800-658-4782
Disability Served: all

UTAH

Disability Law Center
455 East 400 South, Suite 201
Salt Lake City, UT 84111
801-363-1347
http://www.disabilitylawcenter.org
Disability Served: all

VERMONT

Vermont Protection & Advocacy for Persons with Disabilities
12 North Street
Burlington, VT 05402
802-863-2881
Disability Served: all

VIRGINIA

Department for Rights of Virginians with Disabilities
202 North Ninth Street, 9th Floor
Richmond, VA 23219
804-225-2042, 800-552-3962 (VA)
http://www.cns.state.va.us/drvd
Disability Served: all

National Center for State Courts
300 Newport Avenue
PO Box 8798
Williamsburg, VA 23187-8798
757-253-2000
http://www.ncsc.dni.us
Disability Served: all

WASHINGTON

Disabilities Law Project
Puget Sound Law School
4649 Sunnyside Avenue North, Suite 100
Seattle, WA 98103-6900
206-545-7055
Disability Served: all

Washington Protection & Advocacy for Persons with Disabilities
1401 East Jefferson, Suite 506
Seattle, WA 98122
206-324-1521
Disability Served: all

WEST VIRGINIA

West Virginia Protection & Advocacy for Persons with Disabilities
1524 Kanawha Boulevard East
Charleston, WV 25311
304-346-0847
Disability Served: all

WISCONSIN

Wisconsin Coalition for Advocacy
16 North Carroll Street, Suite 400
Madison, WI 53703
608-267-0214, 800-928-8778
Disability Served: all

WYOMING

Wyoming Protection & Advocacy for Persons with Disabilities
2424 Pioneer Avenue, Suite 101
Cheyenne, WY 82001
307-638-7668
Disability Served: all

Libraries & Research Centers

A Budget-Friendly Guide to Making Your Library More Accessible

Libraries have long played a vital role in connecting people with disabilities to information that can help them lead independent lives. Federal legislation has affirmed that role by mandating equal access for patrons with disabilities. Thanks to that legislation, most new library facilities are designed from the start to be user-friendly for all people. The San Francisco Public Library, for instance, was built in 1996 according to universal design principles, which ensure that an environment is usable by people with a broad range of abilities and disabilities. Throughout the library, patrons with vision impairments can browse the online card catalog on audio headsets; deaf patrons can view more than fifteen hundred videos in special viewing stations; and people with mobility impairments can access every nook and cranny of the building's seven floors. "We wanted the library to be accessible right from the time that a patron approaches the building," says Marti Goddard, Adaptive Technology Coordinator at the San Francisco Public Library. Community meetings and advisory groups representing various disabilities ensured that the goal of accessibility was met.

But what if your library is situated in an architecturally outdated, fifty-year-old building? What if recent budget cuts don't allow it to stay open evenings, let alone buy a slew of new computers? Believe it or not, making your library more accessible to people with disabilities doesn't have to drain the coffers.

This essay outlines how you can improve accessibility at your library through a combination of staff training, structural changes, technology, and outreach. To get your feet wet, contact a few similarly sized libraries near your own to ask if and how they have gone about improving accessibility. More often than not, they will be proud of the work they have done and enthusiastic about sharing their findings and plans. It is also crucial to include people with disabilities in the planning process.

Staff Training and Awareness

A library's staff is often the most overlooked resource when it comes to creating a great, usable environment for people with disabilities. Solicit ideas and opinions from the staff. They might have low-cost solutions, such as putting a nonskid surface on an entryway or creating large-print directional signs using the photocopier or computer printer.

It's also important to help staff members become comfortable communicating with people with disabilities. As part of regular meetings, set aside time when staffers can discuss their concerns. At this time, you can also explore ways for staff members to expand their training. Ask if anyone is interested in learning specialized skills such as using telecommunication devices for the deaf (TTD/TTY) or setting up and managing assistive technology on the computers. Is anyone interested in learning American Sign Language or taking a course in guiding people who are blind? These are also skills and interests to consider when interviewing and hiring new employees.

As new equipment or services for people with disabilities are incorporated, be sure to keep staff members up to date. For instance, has your staff stayed current on state and federal organizations such as talking book and Braille libraries that provide services to people with disabilities? Is every staff member trained on at least the very basics of using assistive technology that's installed on library computers? At one library in central Illinois, several part-time librarians didn't even realize that computer equipment for visually impaired users was available on site.

Accessing the Building and Its Services

"To get a book from the business section, just go to the information desk and ask if someone can escort you. A librarian will then take you up a steep ramp, through some closed stacks, then onto a freight elevator. You'll get off the freight elevator and go through some more closed stacks, then presto, you're in the business section." That's the odyssey that mobility-impaired patrons in wheelchairs used to face at one city's public library, prior to redesign. Imagine how many people thought twice before undergoing that trial.

With universal design, there is at least one route, preferably the main entrance, where people with disabilities can enter a library as freely and with as much dignity as everyone else. Equally important, once a person with a disability is inside the library, he or she needs to be able to access its services as easily as possible. To accomplish that, you'll need to determine what obstacles are currently standing in the way at your facility. The following checklist will get you started. To get a more extensive checklist, along with suggested solutions, contact your regional Disability and Business Technical Assistance Center (see "Sources" at the end of this essay).

- Can a person in a wheelchair navigate the parking areas, sidewalks, and doors to the building?
- Is there a way of entering that does not involve using stairs? Is the route of travel stable, firm, and slip-resistant?
- Are all doorways at least thirty-two inches wide, with a bottom lip no higher than half an inch?
- Are ramps or elevators provided as an alternative to stairs? Can someone in a wheelchair reach the elevator controls? Are the controls also written in Braille and large print?
- Are hallways kept clear for wheelchair users? Is carpeting low-pile, tightly woven, and securely attached along its edges? Can all protruding objects in the hallway be detected by a person with a visual disability who uses a cane?
- Does the emergency system have both visible and audible signals?
- At book return/checkout counters and information desks, is there a section of the counter that is no more than thirty-six inches high for wheelchair users?
- Are there Braille and large-print shelf identifiers? Are call numbers on the spines of books in large print for low-vision users?
- Are telecommunications devices (TTD/TTY) for the deaf available?
- Are wheelchair-accessible restrooms available and marked with large-print signs?

Computers and Assistive Technology

Computers have made it possible for libraries to serve a previously untapped segment of the population. For example, a person with a lifelong mobility impairment who has never handled a book can now have it scanned into a computer and read back aloud using a speech-output system. To create a facility that's more accessible to people with disabilities, your library should plan on purchasing and installing assistive hardware and software.

But how do you choose this technology? In an article outlining an eight-part library access strategy, Alan Cantor, a workplace accommodation consultant, tries to reassure librarians who feel they lack the expertise to select appropriate technology for disabled patrons. He writes, "The accessibility of your library will not be judged by the sophistication of the technologies you have, but the comprehensiveness of services you offer." That said, how much or how little equipment you have is ultimately dependent upon the needs of your patrons and your budget. Again, many of the best suggestions will come from people with disabilities. A designated staff member or committee can evaluate and respond to patrons' requests and keep abreast of technology developments.

It pays to scout around at various dealers for the best prices. Price differences of $100 to $400 per device are not unusual, and your library can save a bundle by shopping wisely. The list below offers a good—and affordable—selection of what's common at many libraries. (For greater detail about specific pieces of equipment, see "Understanding the Basics of Assistive Technology.")

Basic Computer Access

- Adjustable-height worktables that a wheelchair can easily fit beneath
- Adjustable chairs
- Large-print and Braille key labels for people with blindness or low vision
- Keyboard trays and alternate keyboards such as mini-keyboards or extended keyboards to help people with various mobility impairments
- Mouse alternatives such as trackballs or keyboard control of the mouse
- Wristrests for people who require extra wrist support while typing

Software and Hardware

- Screen-enlargement software that enlarges images to assist patrons with low vision and learning disabilities
- A speech-output system that converts text on the computer screen to speech can help patrons with low vision, blindness, and learning disabilities
- A scanner that allows books to be scanned into the computer, where they can be converted to speech for patrons with low vision or blindness
- Braille conversion software and a Braille printer for patrons who are blind
- Large-screen monitors for patrons with low vision
- Software that "speaks" text back as it is typed for those with blindness, low vision, or learning disabilities
- Software that modifies keyboard response (such as sticky keys or slow keys) for people with impaired mobility or dexterity
- Dictation software that allows people who are blind or mobility impaired to input text using their voice rather than a keyboard

Reaching Out

Sometimes, reaching out to patrons who are disabled can literally mean finding ways of transporting them to the library (minibus or taxi provisions) or delivering books to them (bookmobile). Reaching out also means offering text in alternative formats to patrons. Does your library have print materials available on cassette or CD-ROM? Captioned videocassettes? A CD-ROM dictionary in American Sign Language? A talking dictionary and calculator? Do your meeting rooms have assistive-listening devices for people with hearing impairments?

A number of accessibility solutions can sometimes be found in an office supply store. Whether you have a formal disability advisory council or not, be sure to talk to your patrons with disabilities to gather ideas. Chances are they've come up with low-cost solutions in their own homes that you can transfer to the library. For instance, a simple bookholder and a magnifying glass mounted on an adjustable arm can help people with low vision, as can a good desk lamp. A tape recorder will work nicely as a note-taking machine for people who can't use their hands, are blind, or have a learning disability. And having a basic walker with a hanging bin for books will greatly assist patrons who tire on their feet.

Lastly, once your library has achieved its goal of improved accessibility, don't forget to tell people about all you now have to offer. That means going beyond the mailing list of those who have already identified themselves as library patrons with disabilities. Put together a brochure in formats that everyone can access—such as Braille, large-print, and audio versions—and put the information on a web site. Send a press release to the local newspaper as well as radio and television stations. Get the word out! There are probably many people with disabilities in your community who would be happy to become patrons.

Sources

"The A-D-A-P-T-A-B-L-E Approach: Planning Accessible Libraries." Alan Cantor, *Information Technology and Disabilities,* December 1995. This article can be found at http://www.rit.edu/~easi/itd/itdv02n4/article2html.

Checklist for Readily Achievable Barrier Removal

This publication was created by Adaptive Environments, Inc. and Barrier Free Environments, Inc., which were authorized by the National Institute on Disability and Rehabilitation Research to develop information and materials on the Americans with Disabilities Act. For a copy of this extensive checklist, contact the regional Disability and Business Technical Assistance Center nearest you by calling 800-949-4ADA.

Disability Resources

http://www.disabilityresources.org

This site's Librarians' Connections section has a wealth of information on assistive technology for patrons with disabilities, connections to listservs and e-zines about library services for people with disabilities, and connections to libraries that have special collections for or about people with disabilities.

DO-IT

University of Washington
PO Box 354842
Seattle, WA 98195-4842
206-685 DOIT
doit@u.washington.edu
http://www.washington.edu/doit

DO-IT (Disabilities, Opportunities, Internetworking, and Technology) works to increase the participation of individuals with disabilities in academic programs and careers.

Library & Research Center Listings

Some of these library resources for persons with visual impairments and physical disabilities are private. Many are administered by the National Library Service for the Blind and Physically Handicapped, Library of Congress and provide free services.

ALABAMA

Alabama Institute for Deaf and Blind
Library & Resource Center for the Blind
705 South Street
PO Box 698
Talladega, AL 35160
205-761-3287, 800-848-4722
Disability Served: all

Alabama Radio Reading Service Network
1028 Seventh Avenue South
Birmingham, AL 35294
205-934-2606
Disability Served: all

Alabama Regional Library for the Blind and Physically Handicapped
6030 Monticello Drive
Montgomery, AL 36130-6000
334-213-3906, 800-392-5671
http://www.apls.state.al.us
Disability Served: vision, physically disabled, learning disabled

Birmingham Brailling Group
10 Monte Vallo Lane
Birmingham, AL 35213
205-879-3963
Disability Served: vision

Department for the Blind and Physically Handicapped
Houston-Love Memorial Library
PO Box 1369
Dothan, AL 36302
334-793-9767
Disability Served: all

Huntsville Subregional Library for the Blind & Physically Handicapped
PO Box 443
Huntsville, AL 35804
256-532-5980, 256-532-5981
Disability Served: all

Library for the Blind & Handicapped
Public Library of Anniston and Calhoun County
PO Box 308
Anniston, AL 36202
205-237-8501
Disability Served: all

Temple Emanu-El Sisterhood
2100 Highland Avenue
Birmingham, AL 35205
205-933-8037
Disability Served: vision

Tuscaloosa Subregional Library for the Blind and Physically Handicapped
1801 Jack Warner Parkway
Tuscaloosa, AL 35401
205-345-3994
http://www.tuscaloosa-library.org
Disability Served: vision, physically handicapped

ALASKA

Alaska State Library Talking Book Center
344 West Third Avenue, Suite 125
Anchorage, AK 99501
907-269-6575
http://www.ced.state.ak.us/lam/library/dev/tbc.html
Disability Served: all

ARIZONA

Arizona State Braille and Talking Book Library
1030 North 32nd Street
Phoenix, AZ 85008
602-255-5578, 800-255-5578
http://www.dlapr.lib.az.us
Disability Served: all

Books for the Blind of Arizona, Inc.
6120 East Fifth, A-107
Tucson, AZ 85719
Disability Served: vision

Desert Volunteer Braille Guild
The Foundation for Blind Children
1235 East Harmont Drive
Phoenix, AZ 85020
602-331-1470, 602-678-5810
Disability Served: vision

Flagstaff City—Coconino County Public Library
300 West Aspen Avenue
Flagstaff, AZ 86001
520-779-7670
Disability Served: all

FRB&D Recording Studio
Sun Cities Studio
9449 North 99th Avenue
Peoria, AZ 85345
602-977-6020
Disability Served: vision

Prescott Public Library/Talking Book Center
215 East Goodwin
Prescott, AZ 86303
520-445-8110
Disability Served: all

Recorded Recreational Reading for the Blind
9447 North 99th Avenue
Peoria, AZ 85345
623-933-0985
Disability Served: vision

RFB&D Recording Studio—Phoenix
3627 East Indian School Road, Suite 108
Phoenix, AZ 85018
602-468-9144
http://www.rfbd.org
Disability Served: vision

Special Needs Center/Phoenix Public Library
1221 North Central Avenue
Phoenix, AZ 85004
602-261-8690
http://www.ci.phoenix.az.us/library/spelneed.html
Disability Served: all

Trinity Braille Ministry
Trinity United Methodist Church
3104 West Glendale Avenue
Phoenix, AZ 85051
602-973-1415
Disability Served: vision

WAHEC Medical Library Consortium
Bullhead Community Hospital
2735 Silver Creek Road
Bullhead, AZ 86442
520-763-2273
Disability Served: all

ARKANSAS

Educational Services for the Visually Impaired
PO Box 668
Little Rock, AR 72203
Disability Served: vision

Fort Smith Public Library for the Blind and Handicapped
61 South Eighth Street
Ft Smith, AR 72901
501-783-0229
Disability Served: vision, physically disabled

Library for the Blind and Handicapped, Southwest
CLOC Regional Library
PO Box 668
Magnolia, AR 71753
501-234-1991
Disability Served: all

Library for the Blind and Physically Handicapped
One Capitol Mall
Little Rock, AR 72201
501-682-1155
Disability Served: all

Northwest Ozarks Regional Library for the Blind and Handicapped
217 East Dickson Street
Fayetteville, AR 72701
501-442-6253

http://www.uark.edu/ALADDIN/publib/lbph.html
Disability Served: all

CALIFORNIA

American Red Cross
Oakland Service Center
10771 San Pablo Avenue
El Cerrito, CA 94530
510-526-7206
Disability Served: vision

Beach Cities Braille Guild, Inc.
PO Box 712
Huntington Beach, CA 92648
714-536-9666
Disability Served: vision

Books Aloud, Inc.
180 West San Carlos Street
San Jose, CA 95150-5731
408-277-4839, 408-277-4878
Disability Served: all

Braille and Talking Book Library
900 North Street
Sacramento, CA 95814
916-654-0640, 800-952-5666
http://www.library.ca.gov
Disability Served: vision

Braille Institute Library Services
741 North Vermont Avenue
Los Angeles, CA 90029
323-660-3880, 800-808-2555
http://www.brailleinstitute.org
Disability Served: vision

Braille Transcribers Guild of San Diego, Inc.
1807 Upas Street
San Diego, CA 92103
619-298-4219
Disability Served: vision

Braille Transcribers of Humboldt
PO Box 6363
Seventh and A Streets
Eureka, CA 95501
707-442-4048
Disability Served: vision

Braille Transcribers of Santa Barbara
339 Loma Media Road
Santa Barbara, CA 93103
805-965-2212
Disability Served: vision

Braille Transcribers, Sacramento North Area
c/o Ralph Richardson Center, Braille Center
4848 Cottage Way
Carmichael, CA 95608
916-971-7912
Disability Served: vision

Braille Transcription Project of Santa Clara County, North Branch
PO Box 326
Los Altos, CA 94022
650-948-0139
Disability Served: vision

Contra Costa Braille Transcribers
514 Freya Way
Pleasant Hill, CA 94523
510-682-4734
Disability Served: vision

Golden Gate Braille Transcribers, Inc.
1466 44th Avenue
San Francisco, CA 94122
415-566-1641
Disability Served: vision

Herrick Health Sciences Library
Alta Bates Medical Center
2001 Dwight Way
Berkeley, CA 94704
510-204-4517
Disability Served: all

Laguna Hills Transcribers, Inc.
924-D Avenida Majorca
Laguna Hills, CA 92653-4444
714-830-2125
Disability Served: vision

Monterey County Braille Transcribers, Inc.
PO Box DF
Pacific Grove, CA 93950
Disability Served: vision

National Association for Visually Handicapped—West
3201 Balboa Street
San Francisco, CA 94121
415-221-3201
http://www.navh.org
Disability Served: vision

Pomona Valley Transcribers Guild
Ontario Public Library
215 East C Street
Ontario, CA 91764
714-986-5060
Disability Served: vision

RFB&D Recording Studio—Los Angeles
5022 Hollywood Boulevard
Los Angeles, CA 90027
213-664-5520
http://www.rfbd.org
Disability Served: vision, learning disabled, physically disabled

RFB&D Recording Studio—Manhattan Beach
1230 Rosecrane Avenue
Manhattan Beach, CA 90265-2416
310-536-5301
Disability Served: vision

RFB&D Recording Studio—Palo Alto
488 West Charleston Road
Palo Alto, CA 94306
650-493-3717
Disability Served: vision

RFB&D Recording Studio—Santa Barbara
3970 La Colina Road
Santa Barbara, CA 93110
805-687-6393
Disability Served: vision

RFB&D Recording Studio—Upland
1844-C West 11th Street
Upland, CA 91786
909-949-4316
Disability Served: vision

Sacramento Braille Transcribers, Inc.
2791 24th Street, Room 7
Sacramento, CA 95818
916-455-9121
Disability Served: vision

San Fernando Valley Braille Transcribers Guild
4784 Park Encino Lane, #303
Encino, CA 91436
818-905-1256
Disability Served: vision

San Francisco Public Library
Talking Books Program
Civic Center, 100 Larkin Street
San Francisco, CA 94102
415-557-5253
Disability Served: vision

San Gabriel Valley Braille Guild
PO Box 255
Covina, CA 91723
818-331-2071
Disability Served: vision

Santa Cruz County Transcribers Guild
809 Bay Avenue
Capitola, CA 95010
408-476-7140, ext. 319
Disability Served: vision

Sequoia Braille Transcribers
PO Box 3435
Visalia, CA 93278
559-732-1912
Disability Served: vision

Sisterhood Temple Beth Israel
12326 Riverside Drive
North Hollywood, CA 91607
818-763-9148, 213-877-3431
Disability Served: vision

Sixth District California State BTA
Braille Transcription Project
101 North Bascom Avenue
San Jose, CA 95128
408-298-4468
Disability Served: vision

Sonoma County Braille Transcribers Guild
908 Stevenson Street
Santa Rosa, CA 95404
707-546-6930
Disability Served: vision

Talking Book Library for the Blind
Fresno County Public Library
770 North San Pablo
Fresno, CA 93728
209-488-3217, 800-742-1011
Disability Served: vision

Transcribers of Orange County
10982 Paddock Lane
Santa Ana, CA 92705
714-731-5899
Disability Served: vision

Transcribing Mariners
PO Box 4232
San Rafael, CA 94913
415-721-7150
Disability Served: vision

Volunteer Transcribing Services
205 East Third Avenue
San Mateo, CA 94401-4077
650-344-8664
Disability Served: vision

Volunteers of Soledad
Project for the Visually and Physically Handicapped
PO Box 686
Soledad, CA 93960-0686
408-675-2411, ext. 2186
Disability Served: vision

Volunteers of Vacaville—Blind Project
1600 California Drive
PO Box 670
Vacaville, CA 95696-0670
707-448-6841, ext. 2044
Disability Served: vision

COLORADO

Boulder Public Library
1000 Canyon Boulevard
Boulder, CO 80302
303-441-3098
Disability Served: all

Colorado Talking Book Library
180 Sheridan Boulevard
Denver, CO 80226
303-727-9277, 800-685-2136
http://cde.state.co.us/ctbl.htm
Disability Served: all

RFB&D Recording Studio—Denver
2696 South Colorado Boulevard, Suite 330
Denver, CO 80222
303-767-0787
Disability Served: vision

Volunteer Transcribers for the Visually Impaired
833-3 East Platte Avenue
Colorado Springs, CO 80903
719-632-2299
Disability Served: vision

CONNECTICUT

Connecticut Braille Association, Inc.
Woman's Club Building
44 Imperial Avenue
Westport, CT 06880
203-227-5243
Disability Served: vision

Connecticut Braille Association, Inc.
Large Type Division
664 Oakwood Avenue
West Hartford, CT 06110
860-953-9692
Disability Served: vision